The Liver in Systemic Diseases

Hiromasa Ohira
Editor

The Liver in Systemic Diseases

Springer

Editor
Hiromasa Ohira
Department of Gastroenterology and Rheumatology
Fukushima Medical University School of Medicine
Fukushima, Japan

ISBN 978-4-431-56693-9 ISBN 978-4-431-55790-6 (eBook)
DOI 10.1007/978-4-431-55790-6

Softcover reprint of the hardcover 1st edition 2016

Printed on acid-free paper

This Springer imprint is published by Springer Nature
The registered company is Springer Japan KK

Preface

The liver plays a central role in maintaining life and functions in association with various organs. The liver is anatomically formed from a common development source that forms the biliary tract, gallbladder, and pancreas, and there is an inflow of many materials through the portal vein from the intestinal tract and spleen. Also, the liver is affected by circulatory dynamics from the heart and lungs through the hepatic vein. Based on results of studies on autoimmunity, the endocrine system, nutrients, metal metabolism, and intestinal bacterial flora, attention has been given to the functional correlations of the liver with the spleen, visceral fat, intestinal tract, and central nervous system. Associations with dysbiosis and nonalcoholic steatohepatitis and with hepatocellular carcinoma are hot topics. Diseases of the liver itself have effects on other organs, and it is known that hepatic lesions are often complicated with diabetes, endocrine diseases, and rheumatic diseases. Therefore, it is important to determine the associations of the liver with systemic organs and with clinical conditions of diseases.

For *The Liver in Systemic Diseases*, I invited leading Japanese scientists in this field to write about associations of organs with the liver from basic and clinical points of view. I hope that this book will enhance the specialties of clinicians and provide an opportunity to consider clinical conditions of diseases from a wider standpoint.

I also hope that the book will be helpful in facilitating clinical and research activities on liver diseases. It would be an honor if this book earned a place in your library and perhaps on your reading list. Finally, I would like to thank all of the authors for their contributions as well as Springer for their efforts in publishing this book.

Fukushima, Japan Hiromasa Ohira

Contents

Part I
Basics

Chapter 1
Innate Immunity and the Liver

Kouichi Miura and Hirohide Ohnishi

Abstract The liver contains a wide array of immune cells such as macrophages, dendritic cells, and lymphocytes. In addition, nonimmune liver cells participate in the immune system by producing soluble pattern recognition receptors (PRRs) and complement proteins. This liver-mediated immune system maintains the local defense against microbial infection as well as systemic homeostasis. In fact, patients with advanced liver diseases have a high risk for infection due to impaired biosynthesis of secreted PRRs. Thus, the liver is to be considered as an immune organ.

The innate immune system can promptly eliminate nonspecific pathogens using several types of PRRs, including Toll-like receptors, NOD-like receptors, RIG-I-like receptors, and complement proteins. Representative products that act through PRR signaling are cytokines, which have antibacterial and antiviral effects. These mediators are used to kill pathogens with the assistance of other immune cells. Indeed, mice deficient in PRRs are susceptible to infection. However, an excessive immune response may lead to a sustained elevation of harmful cytokines. As a result, mice deficient in PRRs also show rather mild liver injuries, indicating that the lack of PRR signaling can provide beneficial effects. Thus, the innate immune system has dual functions in the prevention of infection as well as the development of liver diseases.

Keywords Innate immunity • Pattern recognition receptor • Toll-like receptor • Liver disease

K. Miura (✉)
Liver Disease Consultation Center, Akita University Hospital, 1-1-1 Hondo, Akita-shi, Akita 010-8543, Japan
e-mail: miura116@doc.med.akita-u.ac.jp

H. Ohnishi
Department of Gastroenterology and Hepato-Biliary-Pancreatology, Akita University Graduate School of Medicine, 1-1-1 Hondo, Akita-shi, Akita 010-8543, Japan
e-mail: hohnishi@doc.med.akita-u.ac.jp

H. Ohira (ed.), *The Liver in Systemic Diseases*, DOI 10.1007/978-4-431-55790-6_1

1.1 Components of the Innate Immune System in the Liver

The innate immune system promptly eliminates nonspecific pathogens using membrane-bound pattern recognition receptors (PRRs), intracellular PRRs, phagocytic PRRs, and secreted PRRs. These PRRs include Toll-like receptors (TLRs), NOD-like receptors, RIG-I-like receptors, and complement proteins. TLRs are located on the cell surface or in endosomes. NOD-like receptors and RIG-I-like receptors are located in the cytosol and participate in intracellular immune surveillance. PRR signaling leads to the production of a wide variety of cytokines. In addition, complement proteins are secreted from liver cells such as hepatocytes. This hepatic innate immune system contributes to the prevention of microbial infection as well as the development of liver diseases (Fig. 1.1). We herein describe TLRs, NOD-like receptors, RIG-I, and their downstream molecules, and complement proteins in the liver, followed by a discussion of the association between the hepatic innate immune system and hepatic manifestations observed in liver diseases.

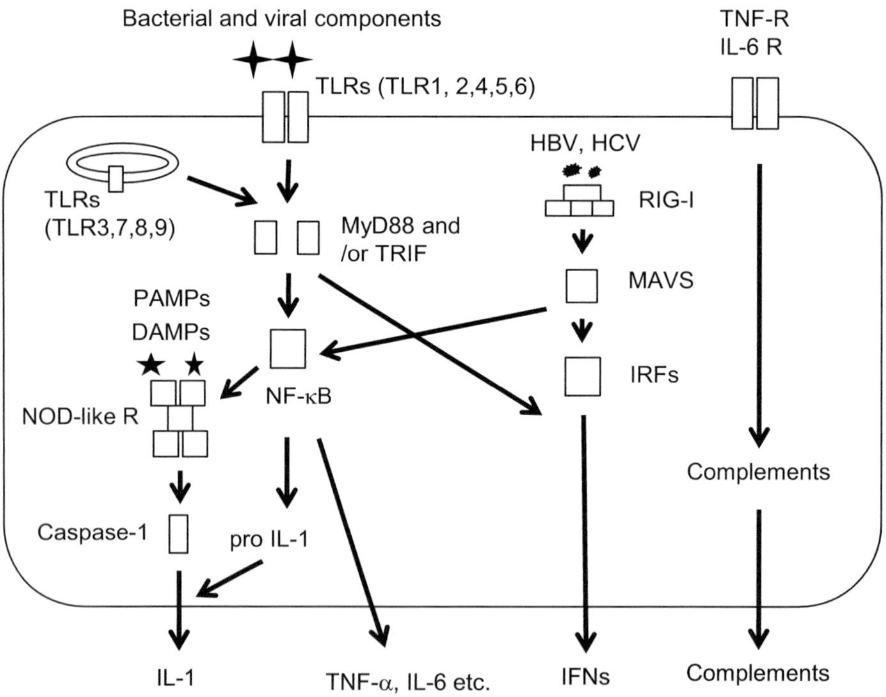

Fig. 1.1 Signaling of pattern recognition receptors and mediators in the liver cells. *TLR* Toll-like receptor, *PAMP* pathogen-associated molecular pattern, *DAMP* danger-associated molecular pattern, *MAVS* mitochondrial antiviral signaling adaptor, *IRF* interferon regulatory factor, *IFN* interferon

1.2 TLRs

1.2.1 TLRs, Adaptor Proteins, and TLR Ligands

TLRs are representative PRRs that recognize bacterial and viral components. In addition to pathogen-associated molecular patterns, TLRs recognize the extracellular matrix (ECM) and abnormal nucleic acids derived from the host cells. Currently, 10 and 13 TLRs have been identified in human and rodent, respectively (Table 1.1); the genes for TLR11, TLR12, and TLR13 do not exist in human [1]. TLRs are located on the cell surface (TLR1, TLR2, TLR4, TLR5, TLR6) or in intracellular vesicles (TLR3, TLR7, TLR8, TLR9). Although more than 10 TLRs have been identified, TLR signaling is divided into two pathways, namely, MyD88- and TRIF-dependent pathways. TLR3 uses only the TRIF-dependent pathway, while TLR4 uses both MyD88- and TRIF-dependent pathways. The other TLRs use the MyD88-dependent pathway only. The majority of proinflammatory cytokines and chemokines depend on the MyD88 pathway, while TRIF-dependent pathways are associated with the production of type I interferons (IFNs). However, cross talk between these pathways exists at downstream molecules. Thus, the MyD88-dependent pathway can also induce type I IFNs, and TRIF signaling can induce proinflammatory cytokines. MyD88-deficient mice and TRIF-deficient mice exhibit different phenotypes regarding liver injuries. Mice deficient in TLR4, which use both adaptor proteins, are protected from the development of nonalcoholic steatohepatitis (NASH) and alcoholic liver disease (ALD), which share several features. Interestingly, TRIF- but not MyD88-deficient mice exhibit decreased inflammation in an ALD model [2, 3], whereas MyD88-deficient mice show decreased inflammation in a NASH model [4]. TNF-α is a key cytokine in the

Table 1.1 TLRs, adaptor proteins, ligands, and expressing cells

	Location	Adaptor proteins	Exogenous ligands	Endogenous ligands	Cells
TLR2-TLR1	Cell surface	MyD88	Lipoprotein, LTA, PGN	Fatty acids	Macrophage, HSC, DC
TLR2-TLR6	Cell surface	MyD88	Lipoprotein, LTA, PGN	Fatty acids	Macrophage, HSC, DC
TLR3	Intracellular	TRIF	Double strand RNA		Macrophage, DC
TLR4	Cell surface	MyD88, TRIF	LPS	Fatty acids, ECM	Macrophage, HSC, DC
TLR5	Cell surface	MyD88	Flagellin		DC
TLR7	Intracellular	MyD88	Single strand RNA	miRNA	DC, macrophage
TLR8	Intracellular	MyD88	Single strand RNA		Monocytes
TLR9	Intracellular	MyD88	CpG DNA	Host DNA	pDC, HSC, macrophage

progression of NASH and ALD according to the results of gene-modified mice. Although TNF-α production depends largely on the MyD88 pathway [5], the TRIF/IRF3 pathway may also transactivate the TNF-α gene in hepatic macrophages.

The liver has a unique blood supply system; 70–80 % is supplied from the gut via the portal vein with the remaining from the hepatic artery. Hence, the liver is constantly exposed to gut-derived factors including bacterial products, environmental toxins, and food antigens [6]. The hepatic immune system is strictly regulated as a barrier between the gastrointestinal tract and whole body. Although the gut microbiota is a source of TLR ligands, the hepatic cells can remove these gut-derived TLR ligands without harmful effects under normal physiological conditions, referred as liver tolerance. However, this tolerance is broken in liver diseases, leading to the susceptibility to TLR ligands. In addition, plasma levels of gut-derived TLR ligands are elevated during liver injury [7], which is caused by increased gut permeability and compositional changes in the gut microbiota. As a result, a larger amount of TLR ligands translocate into the portal circulation and stimulate liver cells to produce many cytokines. For instance, ethanol feeding disrupts the tight junctions of intestinal epithelial cells and increases gut permeability. TLR ligands migrate into the portal vein and then stimulate macrophages to produce TNF-α in the liver. TNF-α further promotes gut permeability by disrupting the tight junctions of the intestinal epithelium. In addition, ethanol feeding induces compositional changes in the gut microbiota. In a murine ALD model, the relative abundance of *Bacteroidetes*, a group of Gram-negative bacteria, is increased, whereas commensal probiotics, including *Lactobacillus*, are decreased [8]. Indeed, TLR4-deficient mice are protected from alcoholic liver injury [9]. Alcohol feeding further induces the overgrowth of intestinal bacteria, which can alter the metabolism with intestinal inflammation. Antibiotic treatment to sterilize the gut can reduce the severity of liver injury in ALD [10]. These data indicate that the gut microbiota contributes to the pathogenesis of liver diseases as a source of TLR ligands.

1.2.2 TLR2

TLR2 senses many components from pathogens, including Gram-positive bacteria, fungi, parasites, and viruses. TLR2 forms a heterodimer with either TLR1 or TLR6. The TLR2-TLR6 dimer recognizes diacylated lipopeptides, while the TLR2-TLR1 dimer recognizes triacylated lipopeptides in Gram-positive bacteria. Although TLR2 ligands induce proinflammatory cytokines and fibrogenic factors in in vitro experiments, the phenotype of TLR2-deficient mice varies depending on the model used. For instance, lesser degrees of hepatic steatosis and inflammation are observed in TLR2-deficient mice on a choline-deficient amino acid-defined (CDAA) diet [11], a NASH model. On the other hand, severe inflammation is induced by feeding methionine- and choline-deficient (MCD) diet [12]. Although both diets are well known as NASH models, the metabolic parameters largely differ between TLR2-deficient mice on a CDAA versus an MCD diet; the CDAA diet induces insulin resistance with obesity, while the MCD diet promotes insulin signaling with body weight loss. Enhanced sensitivity to lipopolysaccharide (LPS) likely accounts for the deterioration in TLR2-deficient mice on the MCD diet [12]. However, this phenomenon does not appear to occur in other obesity-inducible diets including the CDAA diet and a high-fat (HF) diet. Indeed, TLR2-deficient mice are protected from obesity and insulin resistance induced by the CDAA or HF diet. Currently, different gut microbiota compositions have been reported between obese and lean individuals; *Firmicutes*, Gram-positive bacteria, are increased in obese individuals, while *Bacteroidetes*, Gram-negative bacteria, are increased in lean individuals, as well as mice. These data suggest that compositional changes in the gut microbiota may provide different results.

Conflicting results have also been reported in experimental hepatocellular carcinoma (HCC) models. TLR2-deficient mice show an increased incidence of HCC induced by diethylnitrosamine (DEN) [13], suggesting that Gram-positive bacteria may protect from the development of HCC. The lack of TLR2 signaling decreases the infiltration of inflammatory cells and expression of proinflammatory cytokines, leading to the suppression of senescence and autophagy, which possess barrier function against HCC. However, inflammation is observed in most livers which develop HCC. On the other hand, Gram-positive bacteria contribute to the increased incidence of HCC in a model using a chemical carcinogen combined with HF diet [14]. In this model, Gram-positive bacteria *Clostridium* generate cytotoxic bile acids such as deoxycholic acid, which induce senescence of activated HSCs.

In contrast to the conflicting findings in NASH and HCC models, TLR2-deficient mice are not protected from ALD. TLR2 signaling is attenuated in monocytes isolated from patients with ALD [15]. In addition, Gram-negative bacteria are prominent in the gut of mice with ALD. These data suggest that TLR2 signaling has minor effects on the development of ALD. Furthermore, higher concentrations of TLR2 ligands are required for TLR2 activation compared with the TLR4 ligand LPS in in vitro experiments [16]. In this case, it is believed that LPS activates TLR4 signaling before TLR2 ligands are at sufficient concentrations to activate TLR2 in this case.

1.2.3 TLR3 and TLR7

TLR3 and TLR7 recognize double-strand and single-strand RNA, respectively. TLR3 and TLR7 ligands are derived from viruses, endogenous dying cells, and microRNAs. Although TLR3 and TLR7 signaling use different adaptor proteins, these TLRs are mostly responsible for IFN-mediated immune responses in liver diseases.

TLR3 recognizes hepatitis C virus (HCV) and subsequently induces type I IFNs. However, HCV can reduce the production of type I IFNs by inhibiting TLR3 signaling, which allows the replication of HCV. In in vitro experiments, HCV and its related proteins degrade TRIF, an adaptor protein for TLR3 [17]. TLR7 in DCs is believed to recognize HCV and its signaling is crucial for IFN production through IRF7. TLR7 agonists have been developed as agents for HCV treatment through IFN-mediated HCV elimination [18]. However, oral directly acting antiviral therapies for chronic HCV infection are currently widely used because these agents are highly effective and have a lower incidence of adverse effects. On the other hand, IFN-based therapies induce many adverse effects in patients. Thus, the use of IFN-based therapies is limited at present. HBV can also inhibit TLR signaling. The expression of TLR3 and IFN-β was significantly decreased in monocyte-derived DCs in patients with chronic HBV infection compared with normal subjects [19]. As expected, the expression of TLR3 was inversely correlated with the severity of hepatitis. Currently, nucleoside analogues (NAs) are widely used to treat patients with chronic HBV infection. The issues associated with NA administration include a long treatment period and the emergence of NA-resistant HBV. Because type I IFNs have anti-HBV effects and promote the seroconversion of HBe antigen [20], there are advantages utilizing IFN-mediated therapy in chronic HBV infection. Thus, TLR7 agonists have gained as an adjuvant therapy in combination with NAs.

Although TLRs have been originally identified as sensors for nonself-components, recent data demonstrate that TLRs recognize self-components, such as modified nucleic acids released from injured cells. In autoimmune diseases, including primary biliary cholangitis (PBC), TLR3-expressing immune cells recognize self-derived nucleic acids as nonself substances. The hepatic expression of TLR3 and IFN-α in PBC is higher than other liver diseases including autoimmune hepatitis and chronic HCV infection. Furthermore, there is a positive correlation between TLR3 and IFN-α/β expression in PBC [21]. TLR3 expression and its downstream molecule IFN-α are enhanced in the portal areas, where liver injury is most prominent in PBC. Indeed, macrophages and plasma cells express both TLR3 and IFN-α in the portal tract of PBC. These data suggest that the TLR3-TRIF pathway contributes to the development of PBC, and this signaling is a potential target for treatment of PBC. Although TLR3 recognizes double-strand RNA, the TLR3 ligands in PBC have not yet been identified. On the other hand, TLR7 expression was not increased in PBC.

In experimental models, TLR7-deficient mice show increased fibrosis in liver injuries induced by bile duct ligation or CCl_4 [22]. Moreover, the antifibrotic effects of IFNs are suppressed in TLR7-deficient mice.

1.2.4 TLR4

TLR4 recognizes LPS, a cell wall component of Gram-negative bacteria. LPS binds to TLR4 after forming a complex between LPS and TLR4 coreceptors including MD2 and CD14, which do not have intracellular domains. TLR4 is a unique TLR that transduces its signal using two major adaptor proteins, MyD88 and TRIF. Upon

TLR4 activation, the MyD88-dependent pathway is promptly initiated and subsequently activates its downstream molecules, IRAK1/IRAK4 and TRAF6, to induce NF-κB-related genes. Behind the initiation of MyD88 signaling, the TRIF-dependent pathway is activated through IKK/TAK1 and IRF3, resulting in the induction of IFN-inducible genes and NF-κB.

It is well known that LPS contributes to inflammation and liver fibrosis by stimulating liver cells to produce various cytokines. As expected, many reports have demonstrated that TLR4 signaling is associated with the progression of liver injuries. TLR4-deficient mice are protected from NAFLD/NASH, even mice on MCD diet, CDAA diet, and HF diet [23]. Apart from TLR2-deficient mice, other TLR signaling is not likely enhanced in TLR4-deficient mice.

1.2.5 TLR5

TLR5 is a receptor for flagellin, a component of bacterial flagella. TLR5-deficient mice spontaneously develop colitis and metabolic syndrome even in specific pathogen-free conditions [24], indicating that TLR5 signaling maintains gut homeostasis. Anti-flagellin antibody levels are low in TLR5-deficient mice and MyD88-deficient mice [25], suggesting that TLR5 signaling controls the production of anti-flagellin antibodies [26]. Many types of cells express TLR5 in the gut. Chassaing et al. have reported that mice lacking TLR5 specifically on intestinal epithelial cells exhibit colitis and metabolic syndrome similar to systemic TLR5-deficient mice [27], indicating that TLR5 on intestinal epithelial cells plays a key role in the development of manifestations observed in TLR5-deficient mice. Although initial studies have reported that compositional changes in the gut microbiota are a potential cause of manifestations observed in TLR5-deficient mice, recent findings demonstrate that the gut microbiota of TLR5-deficient mice is vastly diverse, that is, TLR5-deficient mice do not always exhibit colitis and steatohepatitis under different environmental conditions in other facilities [28]. Prolonged separated bleeding results in a different composition of gut microbiota in TLR-deficient mice [29]. Interestingly, there are minimal changes between TLR5-deficient mice and WT littermates regarding the composition of gut microbiota when they are housed at the same place. A time-series analysis of the gut microbiota provides further information particular to TLR5-deficient mice. TLR5-deficient mice show a greater diversity of gut microbiota depending on the conditions in which they are housed. The ability to stimulate TLR5 is not always equivalent in potency in flagellin-producing bacteria. For instance, flagellin from *Salmonella typhimurium* has a 1,000-fold greater ability to stimulate TLR5 compared with *Helicobacter pylori* [30]. Thus, minor changes in the gut microbiota may amplify the differences in gene expression in TLR5-deficient mice [31]. As a result, TLR5-deficient mice show a wide variety of manifestations due to the volatility of the gut microbiota and gene expression over time. TLR5 loss allows the expansion of specific gut microbiota that can cause injury to the intestinal epithelium.

Carvalho et al. have reported that TLR5-deficient mice show sporadic increases of Proteobacteria including *E. coli* [32], which is associated with intestinal inflammation [33] and human Crohn's disease [34]. Thus, TLR5 may be associated with the development of inflammatory bowel diseases [35].

1.2.6 TLR9

TLR9 recognizes bacteria- and virus-derived DNA and modified self-DNA from injured cells. TLR9 signaling induces proinflammatory cytokines and type I IFNs through the MyD88-dependent manner. These mediators contribute to the hepatic inflammation, liver fibrosis, and replication of hepatitis virus. TLR-mediated IFN production can prevent the replication of hepatitis virus including HBV. However, TLR9 expression and the subsequent production of IFN-α are reduced in mononuclear cells and DCs in patients with chronic HBV infection [36], suggesting that HBV inhibits TLR9 signaling.

The TLR9 ligand bacterial DNA is elevated in alcoholic liver injury [37] and NASH [4], in which gut permeability is increased. A TLR9 ligand stimulates macrophages to induce proinflammatory cytokines including IL-1β, which can also induce profibrogenic factors such as tissue inhibitor of metalloproteinase-1 (TIMP-1). Indeed, TLR9-deficient mice are protected from inflammation and fibrosis in a CDAA diet-induced NASH model [4]. Thus, the stimulation of TLR9-mediated macrophages leads to inflammation and fibrosis.

In contrast to the NASH model, the role of TLR9 is complex in CCl_4-induced inflammation and liver fibrosis [38]. Although the administration of a TLR9 ligand attenuates CCl_4-induced liver fibrosis, TLR9-deficient mice show decreased fibrosis in the same model. A TLR9 ligand increases the number of NK cells in WT mice, in which TLR9 ligand-stimulated natural killer (NK) cells inhibit the proliferation of hepatic stellate cells (HSCs). However, HSCs undergo senescence in TLR9-deficient mice, resulting in decreased fibrosis. In the CCl_4 model, different types of liver cells participate in TLR9-mediated liver injury. For instance, DCs are one of the cell types that abundantly express TLR9. In response to TLR9 ligands, DCs produce TNF-α that promotes inflammation-mediated fibrosis, whereas they also produce IFNs that suppress liver fibrosis. On the other hand, DCs can produce IL-10 that suppresses inflammation, while they can also produce proinflammatory IFNs. These data indicate that the role of TLR9 signaling depends on the disease models used and the function of the liver cells and cytokines.

1.2.7 TLR Polymorphisms

Experimental data have demonstrated that TLRs are associated with many liver disease models. Thus, single nucleotide polymorphisms (SNPs) in TLRs have been gained much attention in the development of human liver diseases. In chronic HCV infection and HCV-based HCC, patients with the TLR2 -196 to -174 del/ins polymorphism are at increased risk for HCC in HCV genotype 1 infection. Interestingly, these patients are characterized by higher viral load with similar clinical presentations, including serum alanine transaminase (ALT) levels and the stages of liver fibrosis. Monocytes isolated from patients with the TLR2 -196 to -174 del/ins polymorphism have low expression levels of TLR2 and IL-8 in response to TLR2 ligands [39], suggesting that a low immune response is a feature of patients with the TLR2 -196 to -174 del/ins polymorphism. On the other hand, patients with TLR2 rs3804099 C/T and rs3804100 C/T genotypes have a low risk of HCC [40]. Several studies have shown the association of TLR4 SNPs in HCV-related liver diseases. TLR4 D229G and T399I SNPs are reported to protect against hepatic inflammation and liver fibrosis [41]. These TLR4 SNPs are linked to liver cirrhosis in patients with chronic HCV infection [42] and the outcomes of liver transplantation [43]. TLR3 SNPs rs5743305 (T/A) and rs3775291 (C/T) were reported in patients with chronic HCV infection. However, no association was found between these SNPs and the clinical parameters [44]. The TLR3 L412F SNP may protect against acute graft rejection in the recipients of liver transplantation with HCV-related cirrhosis [45]. Most of the currently reported TLR SNPs have been associated with HCV-related liver diseases, although TLR SNPs may be found in association with nonviral hepatitis in the near future.

1.3 NOD-Like Receptors

NOD-like receptors (NLRs) and its related proteins form a large molecular platform referred to as the inflammasome, in which procaspase-1 is processed to active caspase-1, and the subsequent maturation of IL-1 and IL-18. There are 22 members of NLRs in human and 34 in mouse [46]. Although NLRs were initially identified as sensors for pathogens, emerging data demonstrate that NLRs also recognize danger-associated molecular patterns (DAMPs), such as ATP and uric acids. Of the NLRs, NACHT, LRR and PYD domains-containing protein 3 (NLRP3) has been well investigated in the development of liver injuries including acetaminophen-induced liver injury, ischemic reperfusion liver injury, alcoholic liver injury, and NASH. The NLRP3-mediated inflammasome requires two steps for activation: an increase in NLRP3 expression and the aggregation of inflammasome components. First, TLR ligands such as LPS increase the NLRP3 expression through NF-κB. Then, various DAMPs induce the aggregation of inflammasome components and process caspase-1 activation.

Of the human liver diseases, NASH is characterized by increased inflammasome activation compared with chronic HCV infection [47]. Many substances that can stimulate inflammasome components are increased in NASH. For instance, saturated fatty acid and cholesterol crystal are substances that can form a complex of inflammasome components in NASH [48, 49]. These lipids activate the inflammasome when its components are sufficiently expressed. In addition, host-derived modified DNA has been shown to function as a DAMP. TLR9-deficient mice on a CDAA diet show an interesting cytokine profile. These mice exhibit lesser degrees of steatosis and inflammation compared with WT mice. Although WT macrophages produce several proinflammatory cytokines in response to a TLR9 ligand, only IL-1β expression is suppressed in TLR9-deficient mice on a CDAA diet [4]. The CDAA diet increases several components of the inflammasome including NLRP3, NLRP1, ASC, AIM-2, and caspase-1 [11]. This diet also increases the number of apoptotic cells and bacterial DNA levels, which can aggregate inflammasome components. Thus, the inflammasome is activated in an experimental NASH model.

One of the final products of inflammasome activation is IL-1β, which is increased at the mRNA and protein levels in experimental NASH models. Mice deficient in either IL-1R or IL-1β are protected from steatosis, cell death, and liver fibrosis, indicating that IL-1β promotes the progression of NASH. IL-1β has multiple functions in the development of steatohepatitis. IL-1β increases steatosis by activating PPAR-α and DGAT2, a converter of diglyceride to triglyceride. In addition, IL-1β may induce cell death in lipid-laden hepatocytes or support TNF-α-mediated cell injury [50].

1.4 RIG-I

RIG-I-like receptors (RLRs) include RIG-I, melanoma differentiation-associated gene 5 (MDA5), and laboratory of genetics and physiology 2 (LGP2). These PRRs sense RNA viruses such as HCV and subsequently produce type I IFNs. RIG-I is expressed by most cells at a low level with resting state in the cytosol. Once RIG-I senses RNA pathogens, RIG-I moves to the mitochondrial-associated membrane and engages MAVS (Cardif), which initiates the signaling cascade. Finally, IFNs and proinflammatory cytokines are produced through IRF3 and NF-κB activation. Type I IFNs are used for the treatment of chronic HBV/HCV infections because they have potent antiviral effects. Because IFNs can increase the expression of RIG-I, the activation of RIG-I signaling is a target for the treatment of viral hepatitis. However, HCV protein NS3/4A inhibits IFN production by degrading MAVS [51] as well as the TLR3 adaptor protein TRIF. HCV NS5A also suppresses RIG-I signaling [52] as well as TLR4-mediated antiviral effects. Although hepatocytes contribute to the production of type I IFNs by recognizing HCV through RIG-I, HCV can evade this signaling. Hence, IFN treatment alone is not sufficient for eradicating HCV. At present, directly acting antivirus agents are available as anti-HCV agents, including asunaprevir and daclatasvir, which are inhibitors of HCV proteins N3/4A and NS5A, respectively. These agents are highly effective against HCV without mutations at Y93 and L31 in the NS5 region. Although HBV is a DNA virus, RIG-I senses HBV [53, 54], which inhibits the RIG-I pathway by downregulating MAVS. As a result, the production of type I and III IFNs is suppressed in hepatocytes, which allows for the replication of HBV.

1.5 Complements

The liver is responsible for the production of 80–90 % of complement proteins [6]. The complement system comprises more than 35 proteins. There are three pathways for activating the complement system: the classical, lectin, and alternative pathways. All three pathways use C3 to activate the complement cascade. After C3 is cleaved into C3a and C3b, C3b cleaves C5 into C5a and C5b, and the C5b-9 complex is formed to attack infected cells (Fig. 1.2).

Although the primary role of the complement system is to defend against microbial infection, its activation is closely associated with the development of

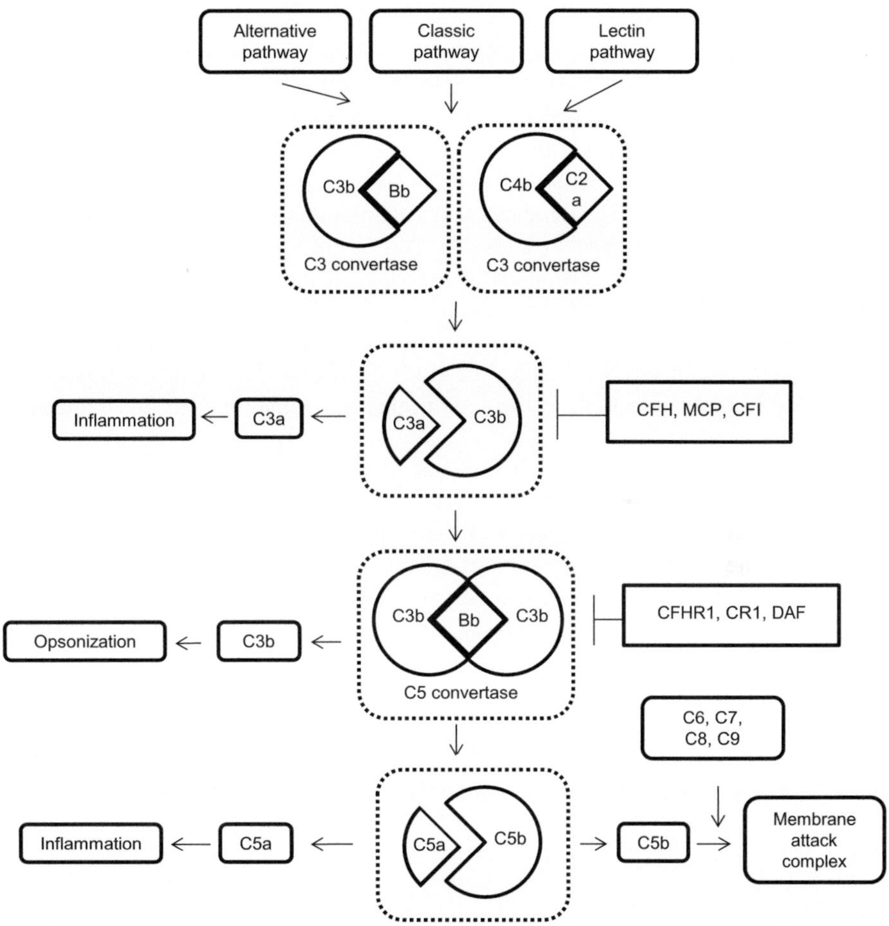

Fig. 1.2 Cascade of complement proteins. CHF (factor F), MCP (membrane cofactor protein), CFI (factor I), CFHR1 (complement factor H-related protein), CR1 (complement receptor 1), and DAF (decay-accelerating factor) are inhibitors against complement activation

liver diseases. For instance, patients with nonalcoholic fatty liver disease (NAFLD) had increased plasma concentrations of complement proteins and complement activation [55] because IL-6 and TNF-α levels, which enhance the hepatic production of complement proteins, are increased in these patients. In addition, gut-derived products and apoptotic cells that activate the complement cascade are increased in NASH [56]. As a result, the hepatic deposition of complement proteins is correlated with the severity of NASH, an advanced stage of NAFLD. NAFLD is a predictor for type 2 diabetes, and the major cause of death in NAFLD patients is cardiovascular diseases. Thus, complements produced by the liver may be associated with systemic diseases, including diabetes and cardiovascular diseases.

In experimental ALD models, the deposition of C3, C8, and C9 is increased in the liver [57, 58]. C5 is also associated with the development of ALD. C5-deficient mice show low expression levels of proinflammatory cytokines and attenuated histological inflammation in ALD [59]. In a liver fibrosis model by bile duct ligation, mice deficient in C5 (Hc^0/Hc^0 mice) showed an attenuation of liver fibrosis at an early time point [60]. Decreased leukocyte infiltration and TNF-α expression accounted for the decreased fibrosis. Because hepatic macrophages and HSCs produce proinflammatory cytokines and profibrogenic factors through C5 activation, the blockade of C5R1 attenuates hepatic inflammation and fibrosis in mice.

Although the plasma concentration of complement is elevated in early stages of liver diseases, the activity is suppressed at advanced stages of liver diseases due to impaired biosynthesis and increased consumption [61]. This condition results in infectious diseases in patients with liver diseases, such as spontaneous bacterial peritonitis, a common complication of liver cirrhosis. C3 and C5 activation is reported to recruit neutrophils to the site of infection, which prevent the expansion of microbial infection by promoting phagocytic activity and opsonization. However, these defense mechanisms weaken due to low levels of complement. In liver transplantation, the recipients have a higher risk of infection when the donor liver has a genetically decreased capacity of complement production [62]. In an experimental murine model, mice deficient in decay-accelerating factor (CD55/DAF), an inhibitor of complement, demonstrated severe steatosis and elevated ALT levels following ethanol feeding. Collectively, these studies show that appropriate concentrations of complement proteins provide a healthy condition.

1.6 Innate Immune System and Hepatic Manifestations

1.6.1 Inflammation

Many liver cells are engaged in the development of inflammation, in which macrophages contribute to both the progression and suppression of inflammation (Fig. 1.3). Several classifications have been proposed to divide inflammatory and anti-inflammatory macrophages. One of the representatives is the M1/M2

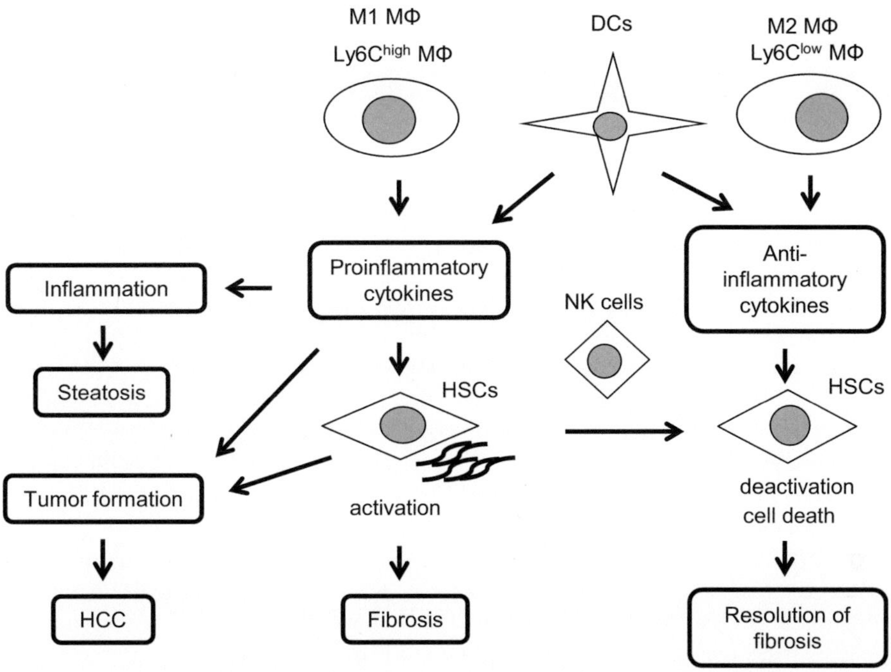

Fig. 1.3 Liver cells and mediators that induce inflammation, steatosis, fibrosis, and tumor formation. A wide array of liver cells participates in the innate immune system and contributes to the development of liver diseases

classification [63], which depends on the catabolism of L-arginine. M1 macrophages express inducible nitric oxide synthase (iNOS), which converts L-arginine to L-citrulline and nitric oxide. M1 macrophages are classical macrophages that produce proinflammatory cytokines. On the other hand, M2 macrophages express arginase I, which converts L-arginine to L-ornithine. M2 macrophages are referred to as alternatively activated macrophages and demonstrate anti-inflammatory responses. The abundance of M1 macrophages and M2 macrophages is altered in systemic diseases including liver diseases. For instance, the switch from M2 anti-inflammatory macrophages to M1 inflammatory macrophages occurs in the liver of mice with NASH [64]. The number of macrophages expressing the M2 markers is increased during mild liver injury caused by ALD and obesity compared with those during severe injury [65], suggesting that M2 macrophages have protective roles. These are debating on the M1/M2 polarization in Kupffer cells, hepatic tissue macrophages. Wan et al. have reported that Kupffer cells include both M1 and M2 phenotypes [66]. Of Kupffer cells, the M2 type is 20 % and 40 % in Th1-biased C57/BL6 mice and Th2-biased Balb/c mice, respectively. T helper cell-derived Th1 and Th2 cytokines can activate M1 and M2 macrophages, respectively. In Th2-biased Balb/c mice, ethanol feeding increases expression of the M2 markers but not M1 markers in macrophages. In this model, M2-type Kupffer cells induce the apoptosis of M1 Kupffer cells by an IL-10-mediated arginase-dependent mechanism [66]. As a result, Th2-biased Balb/c mice are resistant against alcohol-induced liver injury and high-fat-induced steatosis.

Ly6C, a glycoprotein on the cell surface, has emerged as a marker for bone marrow-derived inflammatory macrophages. We have previously reported that Ly6C-positive macrophages are recruited in experimental NASH along with the progression of inflammation [67]. Interestingly, CCR2-deficient mice show a decreased number of Ly6C macrophages in the liver, suggesting that CCR2 contributes to the recruitment of Ly6C macrophages. In other injury models, the recruitment of Ly6C macrophages depends on CCR2 expression [68]. In acetaminophen-induced liver injury, $Ly6C^{high}$ macrophages are predominantly recruited in the inflammatory phase, while $Ly6C^{low}$ macrophages are recruited in the recovery phase [69]. In CCl_4-induced liver injury, $Ly6C^{high}$ macrophages are recruited in both the inflammatory and recovery phases. On the other hand, $Ly6C^{low}$ macrophages are predominantly recruited in the recovery phase and contribute to tissue repair by producing angiogenetic factors and inhibiting of neutrophils [68]. Thus, the expression of Ly6C on macrophages is a potential marker to know hepatic inflammation. Although the phenotype of M1 macrophages is similar to that of $Ly6C^{high}$ macrophages, these macrophages are not always identical.

Several investigators have described the phenotype of inflammatory macrophages using classical markers including CD11b and CD68, which are receptors for C3b and oxidized low-density lipoprotein (LDL), respectively. Kinoshita et al. have reported that F4/80 and CD11b double-positive macrophages are recruited from the circulation, spleen, and BM. These recruited macrophages possess an increased ability to produce proinflammatory cytokines [70]. On the other hand, F4/80 and CD68 double-positive macrophages are classical hepatic macrophages Kupffer cells and have potent phagocytic ability and ROS production.

DCs, a small population in the liver, are comprised from heterogeneous populations and exhibit vastly different functions depending on the expressing surface markers. Monocyte-derived DCs (moDCs) contribute to inflammation by producing TNF-α in the bile duct ligation model [71]. moDCs expressing CD11b differentiate into inflammatory DCs, which are recruited to inflammatory sites in a CCR2-dependent manner. The phenotype of these moDCs is similar to M1 macrophages that produce proinflammatory cytokines in response to TLR ligands. On the other hand, CD1c+ DCs secrete anti-inflammatory cytokine IL-10 in response to LPS [72]. CD1c+ DCs represent a major population in the liver among the three major classes of DCs [73]. DCs are mainly located in the portal area of the liver, where the cells have the advantage to detect foreign bodies from the gut. However, hepatic DCs represent an immature phenotype and have decreased antigen-presenting ability compared with DCs in the skin and spleen. Thus, hepatic DCs are associated with hepatic tolerance as well as the suppression of inflammation in the liver.

1.6.2 Steatosis

Hepatic steatosis is observed in NAFLD/NASH and ALD as a result of imbalance between the lipid input and output. Interestingly, the innate immune system is associated with the development of hepatic steatosis (Fig. 1.3). For example, the polarization of hepatic macrophages is linked to the development of steatosis, in which the polarization of M1 macrophages contributes to steatosis. TNF-α is a potential mediator of inducing steatosis by several mechanisms [23]. TNF-α induces insulin resistance by inhibiting insulin receptors, insulin receptors substrate-1, and GLUT4 expression. Insulin resistance promotes subsequent release of free fatty acids (FFAs) from adipocytes. Increased serum FFA levels further promote insulin resistance. On the other hand, TNF-α increases the uptake of FFAs and cholesterol accumulation in hepatocytes by inducing LDL receptor and by inhibiting the efflux of cholesterol [74], resulting in aberrant steatosis. A representative chemokine CCL2 contributes to the development of steatosis by recruiting TNF-α-producing macrophages, resulting in an increased lipid accumulation in the liver. CCL2 also promotes steatosis by increasing lipid synthesis through PEPCK activity. In addition, CCL2 inhibits lipid efflux through Apo B suppression in hepatocytes. Hepatocytes have been reported not to express CCR2, a receptor for CCL2, suggesting that hepatocytes use other pathways. Indeed, mice deficient in these proinflammatory cytokines or chemokine exhibit decreased hepatic steatosis.

In contrast to M1 macrophages, steatosis is mild when macrophages are polarized to the M2 phenotype in human ALD and obese individuals [75]. In addition, M2 Kupffer cells inhibit steatosis in ALD and NASH through the production of IL-6 [65]. These data indicate that M2 macrophages reduce the accumulation of lipids in the liver. On the other hand, TGF-β promotes lipid accumulation in hepatocytes through SMAD signaling [76], although certain M2 macrophages produce TGF-β. Because M2 macrophages can be divided into at least three subpopulations, further investigation is required to elucidate the mechanism by which M2 macrophages contribute to the development of steatosis.

1.6.3 Liver Fibrosis

Liver fibrosis is a common consequence of any chronic liver diseases. The innate immune system also contributes to the development of liver fibrosis (Fig. 1.3). HSCs are well known as the primary cells that promote liver fibrosis by producing ECM proteins, such as type I collagen. Recently, the immunologic functions of HSCs have gained much attention in liver fibrosis because HSCs express PRRs, including TLR2, TLR4, TLR9, and complement receptor C5R1. TLR ligands further increase the expression of chemokines and PRRs in HSCs. Although TLR ligands do not always directly drive HSCs to produce collagen, some TLR ligands render HSCs to sense TGF-β, a potent fibrogenic factor. Bambi, a pseudoreceptor for TGF-β, is a molecular target of TLR ligands, which can downregulate the expression of Bambi in HSCs [77]. As a result, HSCs stimulated with the TLR4 ligand LPS show enhanced TGF-β signaling, which accelerates the transformation from HSCs to collagen-producing myofibroblast-like cells. Thus, TLR4 signaling in HSCs promotes liver fibrosis through the downregulation of Bambi. Although TLR2 ligands can decrease the expression of Bambi in HSCs, the role of TLR2 on liver fibrosis is dependent on the models. For example, TLR2-deficient mice are not predispose to liver fibrosis induced by bile duct ligation [77], whereas TLR2-deficient mice showed decreased fibrosis in a NASH model induced by a CDAA diet [11]. A higher concentration of ligands is required to stimulate TLR2 in HSCs [16], suggesting that limited conditions allow the predominant activation of TLR2 signaling in the liver. In mice, a CDAA diet induces obesity, in which Gram-positive bacteria are abundant in the gut. Thus, an increase in Gram-positive bacteria is a potential cause of TLR2 activation in mice on a CDAA diet.

Macrophages play a role in the progression, as well as regression, of liver fibrosis. $Ly6C^{high}$ macrophages have been reported to promote liver fibrosis by producing higher levels of TGF-β and proinflammatory cytokines. These $Ly6C^{high}$ macrophages are recruited from circulating monocytes. On the other hand, resident Kupffer cells contribute to liver fibrosis regardless of Ly6C expression [78]. Macrophages are one of the sources of TGF-β, a potent activator of HSCs. In addition, hepatic macrophages produce IL-1 and TNF in response to TLR ligands. IL-1 and TNF subsequently prolong the survival period of HSCs [78]. These proinflammatory cytokines induce TIMP-1 expression, which can inhibit apoptosis of HSCs. In contrast to $Ly6C^{high}$ macrophages and Kupffer cells, $Ly6C^{low}$ macrophages contribute to resolution of liver fibrosis [79]. $Ly6C^{low}$ macrophages are derived from $Ly6C^{high}$ macrophages and are distinct from typical M2 macrophages [79], which contribute to tissue remodeling by producing TGF-β.

The contribution of DCs to liver fibrosis is exceptionally complex. DCs regulate NK cells to kill activated HSCs, resulting in the resolution of liver fibrosis. In addition, DCs secrete large concentration of matrix metalloproteinases (MMPs), including MMP-9 [80]. MMPs play a role in the resolution of ECM, resulting in the improvement of liver fibrosis. These data show that DCs are able to attenuate liver fibrosis. On the other hand, a subset of DCs significantly can increase in number during bile duct ligation-induced liver fibrosis [81], suggesting that DCs promote liver fibrosis. A recently published paper has demonstrated that hepatic DCs play a lesser role in liver fibrosis [78]. Further investigation is required to address the role of DCs during liver fibrosis.

NK cells are considered to suppress liver fibrosis by killing activated HSCs. The ability of NK cells to kill activated HSCs is reduced in chronic exposure to ethanol via several molecules including NKG2D, TRAIL, FAS ligands, and IFN-γ [82]. In addition, increased TGF-β, a potential inhibitor of NK cells, suppresses the function of NK cells.

1.6.4 Hepatic Malignancies

HCC is the primary cancer caused by the chronic HBV/HCV infection, NASH, and exposure to alcohol/aflatoxin. The innate immune system has dual functions in the development of HCC. Although TLR4-deficient mice are protected from precancerous liver injuries, conflicting data exist regarding the role of TLR4 in experimental HCC models using chemical carcinogens. TLR4-deficient mice exhibit a decreased incidence of HCC induced by DEN [83] or DEN combined with CCl_4 [84]. TLR4 deficiency suppresses the production of proinflammatory cytokines and ECM proteins, suggesting that TLR4-mediated inflammation and fibrosis contribute to the development of HCC. In these settings, TLR4 expression on non-parenchymal cells plays an important role in tumor growth by producing growth factors, ECM, and angiogenetic factors. HCC generally develops during chronic inflammation and liver fibrosis, in which tumor-associated macrophages and cancer-associated fibroblasts are components of the tissue microenvironment of the tumors. Indeed, the depletion of macrophages or fibroblasts inhibits tumor growth in mice [85, 86]. In addition to macrophages and fibroblasts, emerging data demonstrate that human HCC cells express TLRs, and the expression is correlated with the prognosis and tumor size [87]. TLR ligands can activate TLR signaling in human HCC cell lines. The TLR4 ligand LPS induces the expression of IL-6, a tumor-promoting factor, and the proliferation of HCC cell lines [88]. In addition, LPS induces the epithelial-mesenchymal transition of HCC cells. Thus, TLR4 signaling in tumor cells is also activated during the development of tumors.

Conversely, Wang et al. have demonstrated that the lack of TLR4 signaling promotes the development of DEN-induced HCC. A deficiency in TLR4 signaling inhibits the function of DNA repair protein Ku70 and senescence [89], which are potential factors for cancer promotion. Although the discrepancy of these studies remains unknown, TLR4 signaling in different cell types may lead to conflicting data.

The liver is rich in lymphocytes including NK cells and NKT cells. For instance, approximately 30–50 % of human hepatic lymphocytes are NK cells. NK cells have antitumor effects by killing tumor cells. However, the function and the number of NK cells are decreased in hepatic malignancies, resulting in a poor prognosis. NK cells express a wide variety of immune recognition receptors that recognize tumor cells. The expression of several receptors is decreased in HCC, allowing tumor cells to evade the anticancer immune system [90]. Thus, new immune therapies to restore the function of NK cells are under development.

1.7 Concluding Remarks

The innate immune system in the liver contributes to the prevention against microbial infection. Recent work has demonstrated that the innate immune system is also closely associated with the development of liver diseases. The involvement of the innate immune system in liver diseases is a complex process, in which many liver cells and mediators participate in the modulation of disease activity. Thus, innate immunity contributes to the amelioration, as well as deterioration, of liver diseases. Therefore, further investigations are required to determine how to control the innate immune system in order to prevent microbial infection as well as liver diseases.

References

1. Kawai T, Akira S. The role of pattern-recognition receptors in innate immunity: update on Toll-like receptors. Nat Immunol. 2010;11:373–84.
2. Hritz I, Mandrekar P, Velayudham A, Catalano D, Dolganiuc A, Kodys K, et al. The critical role of toll-like receptor (TLR) 4 in alcoholic liver disease is independent of the common TLR adapter MyD88. Hepatology. 2008;48:1224–31.
3. Zhao X-J, Dong Q, Bindas J, Piganelli JD, Magill A, Reiser J, et al. TRIF and IRF-3 binding to the TNF promoter results in macrophage TNF dysregulation and steatosis induced by chronic ethanol. J Immunol. 2008;181:3049–56.
4. Miura K, Kodama Y, Inokuchi S, Schnabl B, Aoyama T, Ohnishi H, et al. Toll-like receptor 9 promotes steatohepatitis by induction of interleukin-1beta in mice. Gastroenterology. 2010;139:323–34.e7.
5. Hirotani T, Yamamoto M, Kumagai Y, Uematsu S, Kawase I, Takeuchi O, et al. Regulation of lipopolysaccharide-inducible genes by MyD88 and Toll/IL-1 domain containing adaptor inducing IFN-β. Biochem Biophys Res Commun. 2005;328:383–92.
6. Gao B, Jeong WI, Tian Z. Liver: an organ with predominant innate immunity. Hepatology. 2008;47:729–36.
7. Rivera CA, Bradford BU, Seabra V, Thurman RG. Role of endotoxin in the hypermetabolic state after acute ethanol exposure. Am J Physiol. 1998;275:G1252–8.
8. Yan AW, Fouts DE, Brandl J, Stärkel P, Torralba M, Schott E, et al. Enteric dysbiosis associated with a mouse model of alcoholic liver disease. Hepatology. 2011;53:96–105.
9. Uesugi T, Froh M, Arteel GE, Bradford BU, Thurman RG. Toll-like receptor 4 is involved in the mechanism of early alcohol-induced liver injury in mice. Hepatology. 2001;34:101–8.
10. Adachi Y, Moore LE, Bradford BU, Gao W, Thurman RG. Antibiotics prevent liver injury in rats following long-term exposure to ethanol. Gastroenterology. 1995;108:218–24.
11. Miura K, Yang L, van Rooijen N, Brenner DA, Ohnishi H, Seki E. Toll-like receptor 2 and palmitic acid cooperatively contribute to the development of nonalcoholic steatohepatitis through inflammasome activation in mice. Hepatology. 2013;57:577–89.
12. Rivera CA, Gaskin L, Allman M, Pang J, Brady K, Adegboyega P, et al. Toll-like receptor-2 deficiency enhances non-alcoholic steatohepatitis. BMC Gastroenterol. 2010;10:52.
13. Lin H, Yan J, Wang Z, Hua F, Yu J, Sun W, et al. Loss of immunity-supported senescence enhances susceptibility to hepatocellular carcinogenesis and progression in Toll-like receptor 2-deficient mice. Hepatology. 2013;57:171–82.
14. Yoshimoto S, Loo TM, Atarashi K, Kanda H, Sato S, Oyadomari S, et al. Obesity-induced gut microbial metabolite promotes liver cancer through senescence secretome. Nature. 2013;499:97–101.
15. Pimentel-Nunes P, Roncon-Albuquerque R, Gonçalves N, Fernandes-Cerqueira C, Cardoso H, Bastos RP, et al. Attenuation of toll-like receptor 2-mediated innate immune response in patients with alcoholic chronic liver disease. Liver Int. 2010;30:1003–11.

16. Paik Y-H, Lee KS, Lee HJ, Yang KM, Lee SJ, Lee DK, et al. Hepatic stellate cells primed with cytokines upregulate inflammation in response to peptidoglycan or lipoteichoic acid. Lab Invest. 2006;86:676–86.
17. Wang N, Liang Y, Devaraj S, Wang J, Lemon SM, Li K. Toll-like receptor 3 mediates establishment of an antiviral state against hepatitis C virus in hepatoma cells. J Virol. 2009;83:9824–34.
18. Funk E, Kottilil S, Gilliam B, Talwani R. Tickling the TLR7 to cure viral hepatitis. J Transl Med. 2014;12:129.
19. Li N, Li Q, Qian Z, Zhang Y, Chen M, Shi G. Biochemical and biophysical research communications impaired TLR3 / IFN- b signaling in monocyte-derived dendritic cells from patients with acute-on-chronic hepatitis B liver failure: relevance to the severity of liver damage. Biochem Biophys Res Commun. 2009;390:630–5.
20. Yeh M-L, Peng C-Y, Dai C-Y, Lai H-C, Huang C-F, Hsieh M-Y, et al. Pegylated-interferon alpha therapy for treatment-experienced chronic hepatitis B patients. PLoS One. 2015;10: e0122259.
21. Takii Y, Nakamura M, Ito M, Yokoyama T, Komori A, Shimizu-yoshida Y, et al. Enhanced expression of type I interferon and toll-like receptor-3 in primary biliary cirrhosis. Lab Investig. 2005;85:908–20.
22. Roh YS, Park S, Kim JW, Lim CW, Seki E, Kim B. Toll-like receptor 7-mediated type I interferon signaling prevents cholestasis- and hepatotoxin-induced liver fibrosis. Hepatology. 2014;60:237–49.
23. Miura K, Seki E, Ohnishi H, Brenner DA. Role of toll-like receptors and their downstream molecules in the development of nonalcoholic Fatty liver disease. Gastroenterol Res Pract. 2010;2010:362847.
24. Vijay-Kumar M, Aitken JD, Carvalho FA, Cullender TC, Mwangi S, Srinivasan S, et al. Metabolic syndrome and altered gut microbiota in mice lacking Toll-like receptor 5. Science. 2010;328:228–31.
25. Cullender TC, Chassaing B, Janzon A, Kumar K, Muller CE, Werner JJ, et al. Innate and adaptive immunity interact to quench microbiome flagellar motility in the gut. Cell Host Microbe. 2013;14:571–81.
26. Letran SE, Lee SJ, Atif SM, Uematsu S, Akira S, McSorley SJ. TLR5 functions as an endocytic receptor to enhance flagellin-specific adaptive immunity. Eur J Immunol. 2011;41:29–38.
27. Chassaing B, Ley RE, Gewirtz AT. Intestinal epithelial cell toll-like receptor 5 regulates the intestinal microbiota to prevent low-grade inflammation and metabolic syndrome in mice. Gastroenterology. 2014;147:1363–77.e17.
28. Flores-Langarica A, Marshall JL, Hitchcock J, Cook C, Jobanputra J, Bobat S, et al. Systemic flagellin immunization stimulates mucosal CD103+ dendritic cells and drives Foxp3+ regulatory T CELL and IgA responses in the mesenteric lymph node. J Immunol. 2012;189:5745–54.
29. Ubeda C, Lipuma L, Gobourne A, Viale A, Leiner I, Equinda M, et al. Familial transmission rather than defective innate immunity shapes the distinct intestinal microbiota of TLR-deficient mice. J Exp Med. 2012;209:1445–56.
30. Gewirtz AT, Yu Y, Krishna US, Israel DA, Lyons SL, Peek RM. Helicobacter pylori flagellin evades toll-like receptor 5-mediated innate immunity. J Infect Dis. 2004;189:1914–20.
31. Leifer CA, Mcconkey C, Li S, Chassaing B, Gewirtz AT, Ley RE. Linking genetic variation in human Toll-like receptor 5 genes to the gut microbiome' s potential to cause inflammation. Immunol Lett. 2014;162:3–9.
32. Carvalho FA, Koren O, Goodrich JK, Johansson ME V, Nalbantoglu I, Aitken JD, et al. Transient inability to manage proteobacteria promotes chronic gut inflammation in TLR5-deficient mice. Cell Host Microbe. 2012;12:139–52.
33. Frank DN, St Amand AL, Feldman RA, Boedeker EC, Harpaz N, Pace NR. Molecular-phylogenetic characterization of microbial community imbalances in human inflammatory bowel diseases. Proc Natl Acad Sci U S A. 2007;104:13780–5.

34. Darfeuille-Michaud A, Boudeau J, Bulois P, Neut C, Glasser AL, Barnich N, et al. High prevalence of adherent-invasive Escherichia coli associated with ileal mucosa in Crohn's disease. Gastroenterology. 2004;127:412–21.
35. Sheridan J, Mack DR, Amre DK, Israel DM, Cherkasov A, Li H, et al. A Non-synonymous coding variant (L616F) in the TLR5 gene is potentially associated with Crohn's disease and influences responses to bacterial flagellin. PLoS One. 2013;8:1–6.
36. Xu N, Yao HP, Lv GC, Chen Z. Downregulation of TLR7/9 leads to deficient production of IFN-?? from plasmacytoid dendritic cells in chronic hepatitis B. Inflamm Res. 2012;61:997–1004.
37. Romics L, Dolganiuc A, Kodys K, Drechsler Y, Oak S, Velayudham A, et al. Selective priming to Toll-like receptor 4 (TLR4), not TLR2, ligands by P. acnes involves up-regulation of MD-2 in mice. Hepatology. 2004;40:555–64.
38. Abu-Tair L, Axelrod JH, Doron S, Ovadya Y, Krizhanovsky V, Galun E, et al. Natural killer cell-dependent anti-fibrotic pathway in liver injury via toll-like receptor-9. PLoS One. 2013;8:1–11.
39. Nischalke HD, Coenen M, Berger C, Aldenhoff K, Müller T, Berg T, et al. The toll-like receptor 2 (TLR2) -196 to -174 del/ins polymorphism affects viral loads and susceptibility to hepatocellular carcinoma in chronic hepatitis C. Int J Cancer. 2012;130:1470–5.
40. Junjie X, Songyao J, Minmin S, Yanyan S, Baiyong S, Xiaxing D, et al. The association between Toll-like receptor 2 single-nucleotide polymorphisms and hepatocellular carcinoma susceptibility. BMC Cancer. 2012;12:57.
41. Guo J, Loke J, Zheng F, Hong F, Yea S, Fukata M, et al. Functional linkage of cirrhosis-predictive single nucleotide polymorphisms of toll-like receptor 4 to hepatic stellate cell responses. Hepatology. 2009;49:960–8.
42. Huang H, Shiffman ML, Friedman S, Venkatesh R, Bzowej N, Abar OT, et al. A 7 gene signature identifies the risk of developing cirrhosis in patients with chronic hepatitis C. Hepatology. 2007;46:297–306.
43. Dhillon N, Walsh L, Krüger B, Ward SC, Godbold JH, Radwan M, et al. A single nucleotide polymorphism of Toll-like receptor 4 identifies the risk of developing graft failure after liver transplantation. J Hepatol. 2010;53:67–72.
44. Yin S, Gao B. Toll-like receptor 3 in liver diseases. Gastroenterol Res Pract. 2010;1–7.
45. Citores MJ, Baños I, Noblejas A, Rosado S, Castejon R, Cuervas-Mons V. Toll-like receptor 3 L412F polymorphism may protect against acute graft rejection in adult patients undergoing liver transplantation for hepatitis C-related cirrhosis. Transplant Proc. 2011;43:2224–6.
46. Motta V, Soares F, Sun T, Philpott DJ. NOD-like receptors: versatile cytosolic sentinels. Physiol Rev. 2015;95:149–78.
47. Csak T, Ganz M, Pespisa J, Kodys K, Dolganiuc A, Szabo G. Fatty acid and endotoxin activate inflammasomes in mouse hepatocytes that release danger signals to stimulate immune cells. Hepatology. 2011;54:133–44.
48. Wen H, Gris D, Lei Y, Jha S, Zhang L, Huang MT-H, et al. Fatty acid-induced NLRP3-ASC inflammasome activation interferes with insulin signaling. Nat Immunol. 2011;12:408–15.
49. Rajamäki K, Lappalainen J, Öörni K, Välimäki E, Matikainen S, Kovanen PT, et al. Cholesterol crystals activate the NLRP3 inflammasome in human macrophages: a novel link between cholesterol metabolism and inflammation. PLoS One. 2010;5:1–9.
50. Petrasek J, Dolganiuc A, Csak T, Kurtjones EA, Szabo G. Type i interferons protect from toll-like receptor 9associated liver injury and regulate IL-1 receptor antagonist in mice. Gastroenterology. 2011;140:697–708.
51. Meylan E, Curran J, Hofmann K, Moradpour D, Binder M, Bartenschlager R, et al. Cardif is an adaptor protein in the RIG-I antiviral pathway and is targeted by hepatitis C virus. Nature. 2005;437:1167–72.
52. Hiet M-S, Bauhofer O, Zayas M, Roth H, Tanaka Y, Schirmacher P, et al. Control of temporal activation of hepatitis C virus-induced interferon response by domain 2 of nonstructural protein 5A. J Hepatol. 2015;63(4):829–37.

53. Wei C, Ni C, Song T, Liu Y, Yang X, Zheng Z, et al. The hepatitis B virus X protein disrupts innate immunity by downregulating mitochondrial antiviral signaling protein. J Immunol. 2010;185:1158–68.
54. Sato S, Li K, Kameyama T, Hayashi T, Ishida Y, Murakami S, et al. Article the RNA sensor RIG-I dually functions as an innate sensor and direct antiviral factor for hepatitis B virus. Immunity. 2015;42:123–32.
55. Rensen SS, Slaats Y, Driessen A, Peutz-Kootstra CJ, Nijhuis J, Steffensen R, et al. Activation of the complement system in human nonalcoholic fatty liver disease. Hepatology. 2009;50:1809–17.
56. Ogden CA, DeCathelineau A, Hoffmann PR, Bratton D, Ghebrehiwet B, Fadok VA, et al. C1q and mannose binding lectin engagement of cell surface calreticulin and CD91 initiates macropinocytosis and uptake of apoptotic cells. J Exp Med. 2001;194:781–95.
57. Järveläinen HA, Väkevä A, Lindros KO, Meri S. Activation of complement components and reduced regulator expression in alcohol-induced liver injury in the rat. Clin Immunol. 2002;105:57–63.
58. Bykov IL, Väkevä A, Järveläinen HA, Meri S, Lindros KO. Protective function of complement against alcohol-induced rat liver damage. Int Immunopharmacol. 2004;4:1445–54.
59. Pritchard MT, McMullen MR, Stavitsky AB, Cohen JI, Lin F, Medof ME, et al. {A figure is presented}differential contributions of C3, C5, and decay-accelerating factor to ethanol-induced fatty liver in mice. Gastroenterology. 2007;132:1117–26.
60. Schmitt J, Roderfeld M, Sabrane K, Zhang P, Tian Y, Mertens JC, et al. Complement factor C5 deficiency significantly delays the progression of biliary fibrosis in bile duct-ligated mice. Biochem Biophys Res Commun. 2012;418:445–50.
61. Bird G, Senaldi G, Panos M, Rolando N, Alexander G, Vergani D, et al. Activation of the classical complement pathway in spontaneous bacterial peritonitis. Gut. 1992;33:307–11.
62. Verspaget HW, Berger SP, Daha MR, Frölich M. Mannose binding lectin gene polymorphisms confer a major. Gastroenterology. 2005;129:408–14.
63. Sica A, Mantovani A. Science in medicine macrophage plasticity and polarization : in vivo veritas. J Clin Invest. 2012;122:787–95.
64. Seth RK, Das S, Pourhoseini S, Dattaroy D, Igwe S, Ray JB, et al. M1 polarization bias and subsequent nonalcoholic steatohepatitis progression is attenuated by nitric oxide donor DETA NONOate via inhibition of CYP2E1-induced oxidative stress in obese mice s. J Pharmacol Exp Ther. 2015;352:77–89.
65. Wan J, Benkdane M, Alons E, Lotersztajn S, Pavoine C. M2 kupffer cells promote hepatocyte senescence: an IL-6-dependent protective mechanism against alcoholic liver disease. Am J Pathol. 2014;184:1763–72.
66. Wan J, Benkdane M, Teixeira-Clerc F, Bonnafous S, Louvet A, Lafdil F, et al. M2 Kupffer cells promote M1 Kupffer cell apoptosis: a protective mechanism against alcoholic and nonalcoholic fatty liver disease. Hepatology. 2013;130–42.
67. Miura K, Yang L, van Rooijen N, Ohnishi H, Seki E. Hepatic recruitment of macrophages promotes nonalcoholic steatohepatitis through CCR2. Am J Physiol Gastrointest Liver Physiol. 2012;302:G1310–21.
68. Karlmark KR, Weiskirchen R, Zimmermann HW, Gassler N, Ginhoux F, Weber C, et al. Hepatic recruitment of the inflammatory $Gr1^+$ monocyte subset upon liver injury promotes hepatic fibrosis. Hepatology. 2009;50:261–74.
69. Zigmond E, Samia-Grinberg S, Pasmanik-Chor M, Brazowski E, Shibolet O, Halpern Z, et al. Infiltrating monocyte-derived macrophages and resident kupffer cells display different ontogeny and functions in acute liver injury. J Immunol. 2014;193:344–53.
70. Kinoshita M, Uchida T, Sato A, Nakashima M, Nakashima H, Shono S, et al. Characterization of two F4/80-positive Kupffer cell subsets by their function and phenotype in mice. J Hepatol. 2010;53:903–10.
71. Domínguez PM, Ardavín C. Differentiation and function of mouse monocyte-derived dendritic cells in steady state and inflammation. Immunol Rev. 2010;234:90–104.

72. Kassianos AJ, Hardy MY, Ju X, Vijayan D, Ding Y, Vulink AJE, et al. Human CD1c (BDCA-1) + myeloid dendritic cells secrete IL-10 and display an immuno-regulatory phenotype and function in response to Escherichia coli. Eur J Immunol. 2012;42:1512–22.
73. Bamboat ZM, Stableford JA, Plitas G, Burt BM, Nguyen HM, Welles AP, et al. Human liver dendritic cells promote T cell hyporesponsiveness. J Immunol. 2009;182:1901–11.
74. Ma KL, Ruan XZ, Powis SH, Chen Y, Moorhead JF, Varghese Z. Inflammatory stress exacerbates lipid accumulation in hepatic cells and fatty livers of apolipoprotein E knockout mice. Hepatology. 2008;48:770–81.
75. Louvet A, Teixeira-Clerc F, Chobert MN, Deveaux V, Pavoine C, Zimmer A, et al. Cannabinoid CB2 receptors protect against alcoholic liver disease by regulating Kupffer cell polarization in mice. Hepatology. 2011;54:1217–26.
76. Yang L, Roh YS, Song J, Zhang B, Liu C, Loomba R, et al. Transforming growth factor beta signaling in hepatocytes participates in steatohepatitis through regulation of cell death and lipid metabolism in mice. Hepatology. 2014;59:483–95.
77. Seki E, De Minicis S, Osterreicher CH, Kluwe J, Osawa Y, Brenner DA, et al. TLR4 enhances TGF-beta signaling and hepatic fibrosis. Nat Med. 2007;13:1324–32.
78. Pradere J-P, Kluwe J, De Minicis S, Jiao J-J, Gwak G-Y, Dapito DH, et al. Hepatic macrophages but not dendritic cells contribute to liver fibrosis by promoting the survival of activated hepatic stellate cells in mice. Hepatology. 2013;58:1461–73.
79. Ramachandran P, Pellicoro A, Vernon MA, Boulter L, Aucott RL, Ali A. Differential Ly-6C expression identifies the recruited macrophage phenotype, which orchestrates the regression of murine liver fibrosis. Proc Natl Acad Sci U S A. 2012;109:E3186–95.
80. Yen JH, Kocieda VP, Jing H, Ganea D. Prostaglandin E2 induces matrix metalloproteinase 9 expression in dendritic cells through two independent signaling pathways leading to activator protein 1 (AP-1) activation. J Biol Chem. 2011;286:38913–23.
81. Bleier JI, Katz SC, Chaudhry UI, Pillarisetty VG, Kingham TP, Shah AB, et al. Biliary obstruction selectively expands and activates liver myeloid dendritic cells. J Immunol. 2006;176:7189–95.
82. Jeong WI, Park O, Gao B. Abrogation of the antifibrotic effects of natural killer cells/ interferon-gamma contributes to alcohol acceleration of liver fibrosis. Gastroenterology. 2008;134:248–58.
83. Yu L-X, Yan H-X, Liu Q, Yang W, Wu H-P, Dong W, et al. Endotoxin accumulation prevents carcinogen-induced apoptosis and promotes liver tumorigenesis in rodents. Hepatology. 2010;52:1322–33.
84. Dapito DH, Mencin A, Gwak G-Y, Pradere J-P, Jang M-K, Mederacke I, et al. Promotion of hepatocellular carcinoma by the intestinal microbiota and TLR4. Cancer Cell. 2012;21:504–16.
85. Fan Q, Jing Y, Yu G, Kou X, Ye F, Gao L, et al. Tumor-associated macrophages promote cancer stem cell-like properties via transforming growth factor-beta1-induced epithelial – mesenchymal transition in hepatocellular carcinoma. Cancer Lett. 2014;352:160–8.
86. Mertens JC, Fingas CD, Christensen JD, Smoot RL, Bronk SF, Werneburg NW, et al. Therapeutic effects of deleting cancer-associated fibroblasts in cholangiocarcinoma. Cancer Res. 2013;73:897–907.
87. Eiró N, Altadill A, Juárez LM, Rodríguez M, González LO, Atienza S, et al. Toll-like receptors 3, 4 and 9 in hepatocellular carcinoma: relationship with clinicopathological characteristics and prognosis. Hepatol Res. 2014;44:769–78.
88. Wang L, Zhu R, Huang Z, Li H, Zhu H. Lipopolysaccharide-induced toll-like receptor 4 signaling in cancer cells promotes cell survival and proliferation in hepatocellular carcinoma. Dig Dis Sci. 2013;58:2223–36.
89. Wang Z, Yan J, Lin H, Hua F, Wang X, Liu H, et al. Toll-like receptor 4 activity protects against hepatocellular tumorigenesis and progression by regulating expression of DNA repair protein Ku70 in mice. Hepatology. 2013;57:1869–81.
90. Sun C, Sun H, Zhang C, Tian Z. NK cell receptor imbalance and NK cell dysfunction in HBV infection and hepatocellular carcinoma. Cell Mol Immunol. 2015;12:292–302.

Chapter 2
Microbiota and Liver

Kazumichi Abe, Atsushi Takahashi, and Hiromasa Ohira

Abstract The gut microbiota plays a key role in the development of chronic inflammatory liver disease. The gut-liver axis involves inflammatory cells, cytokines, and other molecules that cause liver deterioration. Dysbiosis is important in understanding several liver diseases, especially in relation to the development of nonalcoholic fatty liver disease, cirrhosis, and hepatocellular carcinoma. The aim of this report is to provide a current overview of alterations in the gut microbiota associated with liver diseases.

Keywords Microbiota • NAFLD/NASH • Cirrhosis • Hepatocellular carcinoma • LPS • SASP

2.1 Microbiota and Liver

2.1.1 Gut-Liver Axis

The gut and liver are closely related. The liver is significantly affected by the gut and its contents, as 70 % of the blood supplied to the liver is collected from the intestinal region through the portal venous system. Both the gut and liver play a pivotal role in absorption and metabolism of various nutrients and drugs. Abnormal bile acid homeostasis may lead to diarrhea and bacterial overgrowth [1]. Bacterial overgrowth, increased intestinal permeability, failure to inactivate endotoxin, and activated innate immunity all contribute to the pathological states of bacterial translocation.

K. Abe (✉) • A. Takahashi • H. Ohira
Department of Gastroenterology and Rheumatology, Fukushima Medical University School of Medicine, 1 Hikarigaoka, Fukushima City, Fukushima 960-1295, Japan
e-mail: k-abe@fmu.ac.jp

H. Ohira (ed.), *The Liver in Systemic Diseases*, DOI 10.1007/978-4-431-55790-6_2

2.1.2 Gut Microbiota

The gut microbiota collectively refers to 100 trillion bacteria, with an estimated mass of 1–2 kg, that inhabit the human gastrointestinal tract. This very diverse ecosystem comprises over 2000 distinct species and has a collective genome containing 150-fold more genes than the human genome [2]. The metabolic activity of gut microbiota provides benefits to human health by supplying essential nutrients and maximizing the efficiency of energy harvest from ingested food. However, the microbiota also contains numerous potential opportunistic pathogens. Moreover, gut microbial products activate Toll-like receptors (TLR) and induce inflammation that defines disease. Maintaining the homeostasis of the gut microbiota has thus necessitated the development of a specialized mucosal immune system [3]. The characterization of microbiota composition has been performed by culture and biochemical typing, i.e., the gold standards for identification of bacterial species. Recently, however, advances in culture-independent techniques have revolutionized our knowledge about the gut microbiota. These techniques, based on the sequence divergences of the small subunit ribosomal ribonucleic acid (16S rRNA), allow for demonstration of the diversity of the gut microbiota, providing qualitative and quantitative information on bacterial species, as well as alterations in the gut microbiota in healthy and diseased states [4].

2.1.3 NAFLD/NASH

Nonalcoholic fatty liver disease (NAFLD) is associated with obesity, insulin resistance (IR), and type 2 diabetes. NAFLD is a hepatic manifestation of metabolic syndrome and is thought to progress to nonalcoholic steatohepatitis (NASH) in about 10 % of patients, with a potential to develop into cirrhosis and even hepatocellular carcinoma (HCC) [5]. Although the pathogenesis of NAFLD has not been fully elucidated, the "two-hit" theory has been proposed to explain its development. The "first hit" involves hepatic lipid accumulation due to IR [6], which is followed by the "second hit" characterized by oxidative stress, leading to lipid peroxidation, secretion of pro-inflammatory cytokines such as tumor necrosis factor α and adipokines, and mitochondrial dysfunction. Subsequently, simple steatosis progresses to NASH [6, 7]. Currently, NAFLD is considered by some a pathogenetically "multiple-hit" disease [8].

The gut-liver axis has attracted much interest in the context of NAFLD pathogenesis [9]. The gut microbiota consists of about 10^{14} microorganisms that live in a symbiotic relationship with the host and is influenced by several factors such as diet, age, antibiotic therapy, hygienic habit, and infection. These intestinal bacteria produce endotoxin, which reaches the liver and is phagocyted by Kupffer cells. As such, the liver is constantly exposed to gut-derived TLR ligands including lipopolysaccharide (LPS) that may evoke an intense inflammatory reaction and thereby contribute to steatosis progression to NASH [10]. Assessments of the fecal microbiota of NAFLD and NASH patients using culture-independent techniques, such as quantitative polymerase chain reaction (PCR) and deep sequencing of a conserved region of the bacterial 16S rRNA gene [11–13], have shown that microbiota samples from these patients contain a lower proportion of the members of the *Ruminococcaceae* family compared to healthy subjects [11, 13]. At the genus level, *Escherichia coli* is the only abundant species in the intestinal microbiota that shows a significantly disproportionate distribution between obese children and pediatric NASH patients [13]. Moreover, extensive analyses of the gut microbiota in adult patients with NAFLD revealed that, at the phylum level, NAFLD patients have a lower percentage of *Bacteroidetes* and a higher percentage of *Firmicutes* compared to healthy controls [11]. At the genus level, adult patients with NASH have a significantly higher percentage of *Clostridium* compared to those with steatosis or healthy controls [12] (Table 2.1).

Small intestinal bacterial overgrowth (SIBO) is a disorder characterized by the growth of abnormally large numbers of bacteria in the small intestine. Patients with obesity or NAFLD have a higher prevalence of SIBO [14, 15]. Patients with NASH have also been reported to develop SIBO at a significantly higher rate (50 %) than that reported for healthy controls [16]. However, the results of studies comparing the bacterial taxonomic composition between patients with NAFLD and those with NASH have been variable or even contradictory. Since this discrepancy could be partially attributed to the small sample sizes in those studies, studies with larger and better-characterized cohorts are warranted in order to determine whether patients with NAFLD and NASH have distinct intestinal microbiome compositions [17, 18].

2.1.4 Cirrhosis

Cirrhosis is a common liver histological alteration observed in several end-stage hepatic diseases, characterized by the presence of regenerative nodules that cause portal hypertension. Major clinical complications include infection, ascites, renal failure, variceal hemorrhage, and hepatic encephalopathy (HE). Patients with these complications have poor prognoses, and liver transplantation is often indicated [19]. Dysbiosis, or altered gut microbiota, resulting from decreased autochthonous or commensal taxa has been observed in stool and colonic mucosa of patients with cirrhosis, which is, in turn, linked with disease severity and systemic inflammation [20, 21].

In previous studies, culture-based techniques were used to characterize the gut microbiota in patients with cirrhosis, including studies that assessed the taxonomic composition of the intestinal microbiota [22–26] (Table 2.1). Chen et al. were the first to use pyro-sequencing of the 16S rRNA V3 region and real-time quantitative PCR to characterize the fecal microbiota of patients with cirrhosis [22]. They demonstrated that, when compared with controls at the phylum level, the proportion of *Bacteroidetes* was significantly reduced in patients with cirrhosis, whereas

Table 2.1 Alterations in the gut microbiota associated with human liver diseases

Disease	Comparison	Implicated microbiota			Ref.
		Phylum	Family	Genus	
NAFLD ($n = 30$)	Healthy vs. NAFLD	*Firmicutes*	*Lactobacillaceae*↑	*Lactobacillus*↑	[11]
			Lachnospiraceae↑	*Roseburia*↑	
			Ruminococcaceae↓		
NASH ($n = 22$)	Healthy vs. NASH	*Bacteroidetes*↑	*Prevotellaceae*↑	*Prevotella*↑	[13]
			Rikenellaceae↓		
		Firmicutes↓	*Lachnospiraceae*↓		
			Eubacteriaceae	*Eubacterium*↓	
			Ruminococcaceae↓	*Oscillospira*↓	
		Actinobacteria↓	*Bifidobacteriaceae*↓	*Bifidobacterium*↓	
		Proteobacteria↑	*Enterobacteriaceae*↑	*Escherichia*↑	
	Obese vs. NASH	*Proteobacteria*↑	*Enterobacteriaceae*↑	*Escherichia*↑	
NASH ($n = 22$)	Healthy vs. NASH	*Bacteroidetes*↓			[12]
	Steatosis vs. NASH	*Bacteroidetes*↓			
		Firmicutes		*Clostridium*↑	
Cirrhosis ($n = 31$)	Healthy vs. cirrhosis	*Bacteroidetes*		*Prevotella*↓	[24]
		Firmicutes		*Enterococcus*↓	
				Faecalibacterium↓	
				Lactobacillus↓	
		Actinobacteria		*Bifidobacterium*↓	
		Proteobacteria	*Enterobacteriaceae*↑		
Cirrhosis ($n = 16$)	Healthy vs cirrhosis	*Actinobacteria*		*Bifidobacterium*↓	[25]
Cirrhosis ($n = 61$)	Healthy vs. cirrhosis	*Firmicutes*		*Lactobacillus*↓	[26]
Cirrhosis ($n = 24$)	Healthy vs. cirrhosis	Bacteroidetes↓			[22]
		Firmicutes		*Enterococcus*↑	
			Streptococcaceae↑		

			Lachnospiraceae↓		
			Veillonellaceae↑		
				Clostridium↑	
		Proteobacteria↑	*Enterobacteriaceae*↑		
			Pasteurellaceae↑		
		Fusobacteria↑	*Fusobacteriaceae*↑		
Alcoholic cirrhosis ($n = 12$)	Healthy vs. alcoholic cirrhosis	*Bacteroidetes*	*Prevotellaceae*↑		
Cirrhosis ($n = 25$)	Healthy vs. cirrhosis	*Firmicutes*	*Lachnospiraceae*↓		[23]
			Ruminococcaceae↓		
			Lactobacillaceae↑		
		Proteobacteria	*Enterobacteriaceae*↑		
			Alcaligenaceae↑		
		Fusobacteria	*Fusobacteriaceae*↑		
Cirrhosis with HE ($n = 17$)	Healthy vs. cirrhosis with HE	*Bacteroidetes*	*Porphyromonadaceae*↑		
		Proteobacteria	*Alcaligenaceae*↑		
Cirrhosis ($n = 98$)	Healthy vs. cirrhosis	*Bacteroidetes*↓		*Bacteroides*↓	[27]
		Firmicutes		*Prevotella*↑	
				Veillonella↑	
				Streptococcus↑	
				Clostridium↑	
		Proteobacteria↑			
		Fusobacteria↑			

NAFLD nonalcoholic fatty liver disease, *NASH* nonalcoholic steatohepatitis

Proteobacteria and *Fusobacteria* were abundant. At the family level, *Enterobacteriaceae*, *Veillonellaceae*, and *Streptococcaceae* were increased, whereas *Lachnospiraceae* was less prevalent. Interestingly, Child-Turcotte-Pugh (CTP) scores were positively correlated with *Streptococcaceae* and negatively correlated with *Lachnospiraceae*, suggesting the contribution of gut microbiota to the prognosis of patients with cirrhosis [22]. In a recent study, Qin et al. analyzed the gut microbiota of patients with cirrhosis by quantitative metagenomics and found that, at the phylum level, the gut microbiota of these patients contained fewer *Bacteroidetes*, with higher proportions of *Proteobacteria* and *Fusobacteria* compared to controls. At the genus level, the proportions of *Veillonella*, *Streptococcus*, *Clostridium*, and *Prevotella* were higher, whereas the proportion of *Bacteroides* was lower [27]. Another study by Bajaj et al. reported that the fecal microbiota of cirrhotic patients showed significantly higher levels of *Enterobacteriaceae*, *Alcaligenaceae*, and *Fusobacteriaceae* families and lower levels of *Ruminococcaceae* and *Lachnospiraceae* families, compared to controls. Moreover, in cirrhotic patients with HE, a correlation between *Porphyromonadaceae* and *Alcaligenaceae* was observed in poor performance on cognitive tests [23]. There was also evidence of pervasive immune-microbiota interface change in the saliva of patients with cirrhosis, similar to that found in stool [28]. These findings could help develop a new therapeutic strategy against cirrhosis by focusing on the gut microbiota.

2.1.5 Hepatocellular Carcinoma (HCC)

Chronic liver inflammation is a well-recognized risk factor for carcinogenesis. Indeed, 80 % of all HCC cases are associated with cirrhosis or fibrosis, diseases characterized by the persistent cycle of liver injury, inflammation, and compensatory hepatocyte proliferation. The major risk factor for HCC is chronic hepatitis, mostly related to hepatitis B and hepatitis C virus infection [29]. As obesity has become more prevalent in most developed countries, NAFLD/NASH is also on the rise. While NASH has been proposed as one of the most common causes of HCC, it is still unclear whether NASH leads to HCC in the absence of cirrhosis.

A previous report indicated the association between intestinal microbiota alteration and obesity [30]. Furthermore, the activation of TLR4 by LPS from intestinal Gram-negative bacteria has been shown to promote HCC development in an HCC model using DEN plus carbon tetrachloride treatment [31]. The progression of HCC depends on the balance between TRL4-induced proliferative, prosurvival, and apoptotic signals in chronically injured hepatocytes. Chronically inflamed liver is associated with intestinal dysbiosis, gut permeability changes, and LPS translocation to the liver. The TLR4 signaling is activated by LPS in hepatic stellate cells (HSCs), resulting in extracellular matrix remodeling, fibrogenesis, and secretion of the epiregulin growth factor, which triggers tumor hepatocyte proliferation (Fig. 2.1).

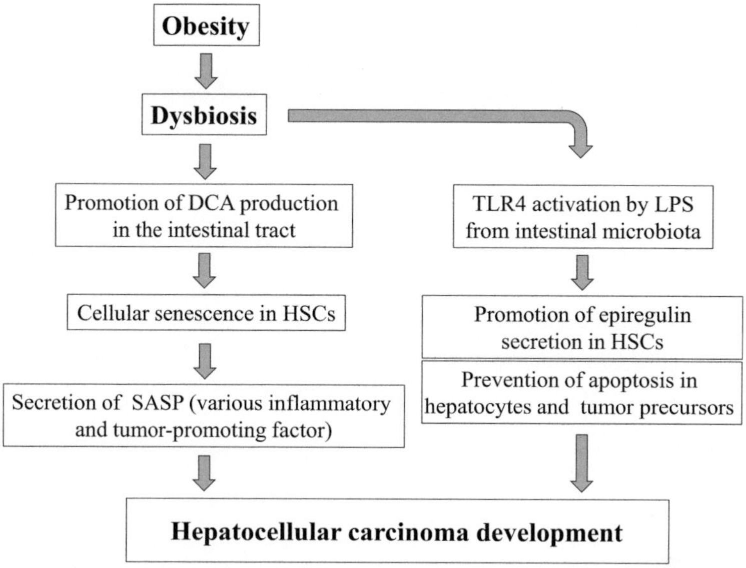

Fig. 2.1 Obesity-induced hepatocellular carcinoma development via senescence secretome or LPS. *DCA* deoxycholic acid, *HSCs* hepatic stellate cells, *SASP* senescence-associated secretory phenotype, *TLR* Toll-like receptor, *LPS* lipopolysaccharide

Cellular senescence is the state of irreversible cell-cycle arrest. It is primarily induced by persistent DNA damage responses triggered by a variety of potentially oncogenic stimuli, such as telomere erosion, oxidative stress, or activation of certain oncogenes [32–34]. Thus, cellular senescence has been considered an important tumor suppression mechanism [35, 36]. Yoshimoto et al. found that senescence-associated secretory phenotype (SASP) plays crucial roles in promoting obesity-associated HCC development in mice [37, 38]. Obesity induces an alteration of the gut microbiota (dysbiosis), thereby promoting deoxycholic acid (DCA) production in the intestinal tract. Elevated DCA levels provoke SASP in HSCs presumably through enterohepatic circulation, which, in turn, secrete various inflammatory and tumor-promoting factors in the liver (Fig. 2.1). Moreover, it was also demonstrated that obese mice, but not lean mice, developed HCC with the upregulated expression of $p21^{Waf1/Cip1}$ gene (a critical inducer of cellular senescence) in HSCs, adjacent to HCC nodules detected by bioluminescence signals. These findings indicate the possible benefits of treatments with prebiotics or probiotics in the prevention of DCA-producing gut bacterial growth.

2.1.6 Conclusion

There appears to be an association between intestinal dysbiosis and liver diseases. Future studies should assess microbial gene expression, proteins, and metabolites, with a particular focus on patients. It might be more effective to directly target the gut microbiota, as restoring it to a healthier state would presumably reduce pro-inflammatory gene expression in the host. Manipulation of the microbiota could be achieved with prebiotics, probiotics, antibiotics, or microbiota transplant. Our understanding of the homeostasis between the gut and its microbes could lead to new insights into the pathogenesis of liver diseases and therapeutic strategies.

References

1. Rai R, Saraswat VA, Dhiman RK. Gut microbiota: its role in hepatic encephalopathy. J Clin Exp Hepatol. 2015;5:29–36.
2. Qin J, Li R, Raes J, Arumugam M, Burgdorf KS, Manichanh C, et al. A human gut microbial gene catalogue established by metagenomic sequencing. Nature. 2010;464:59–65.
3. Hooper LV, Macpherson AJ. Immune adaptations that maintain homeostasis with the intestinal microbiota. Nat Rev Immunol. 2010;10:159–69.
4. Fraher MH, O'Toole PW, Quigley EM. Techniques used to characterize the gut microbiota: a guide for the clinician. Nat Rev Gastroenterol Hepatol. 2012;9:312–22.
5. Rozman D. From nonalcoholic fatty liver disease to hepatocellular carcinoma: a systems understanding. Dig Dis Sci. 2014;59:238–41.
6. Day CP. Pathogenesis of steatohepatitis. Best Pract Res Clin Gastroenterol. 2002;16:663–78.
7. Kojima H, Sakurai S, Uemura M, Fukui H, Morimoto H, Tamagawa Y. Mitochondrial abnormality and oxidative stress in nonalcoholic steatohepatitis. Alcohol Clin Exp Res. 2007;31:S61–6.
8. Polyzos SA, Kountouras J, Zavos C, Deretzi G. Nonalcoholic fatty liver disease: multimodal treatment options for a pathogenetically multiple-hit disease. J Clin Gastroenterol. 2012;46:272–84.
9. Loguercio C, De Simone T, Federico A, Terracciano F, Tuccillo C, Di Chicco M, Cartenì M. Gut-liver axis: a new point of attack to treat chronic liver damage? Am J Gastroenterol. 2002;97:2144–6.
10. Iacono A, Raso GM, Canani RB, Calignano A, Meli R. Probiotics as an emerging therapeutic strategy to treat NAFLD: focus on molecular and biochemical mechanisms. J Nutr Biochem. 2011;22:699–711.
11. Raman M, Ahmed I, Gillevet PM, Probert CS, Ratcliffe NM, Smith S, Greenwood R, Sikaroodi M, Lam V, Crotty P, Bailey J, Myers RP, Rioux KP. Fecal microbiome and volatile organic compound metabolome in obese humans with nonalcoholic fatty liver disease. Clin Gastroenterol Hepatol. 2013;11:868–75.
12. Mouzaki M, Comelli EM, Arendt BM, Bonengel J, Fung SK, Fischer SE, McGilvray ID, Allard JP. Intestinal microbiota in patients with nonalcoholic fatty liver disease. Hepatology. 2013;58:120–7.
13. Zhu L, Baker SS, Gill C, Liu W, Alkhouri R, Baker RD, Gill SR. Characterization of gut microbiomes in nonalcoholic steatohepatitis (NASH) patients: a connection between endogenous alcohol and NASH. Hepatology. 2013;57:601–9.
14. Miele L, Valenza V, La Torre G, Montalto M, Cammarota G, Ricci R, Mascianà R, Forgione A, Gabrieli ML, Perotti G, Vecchio FM, Rapaccini G, Gasbarrini G, Day CP,

Grieco A. Increased intestinal permeability and tight junction alterations in nonalcoholic fatty liver disease. Hepatology. 2009;49:1877–87.
15. Sabaté JM, Jouët P, Harnois F, Mechler C, Msika S, Grossin M, Coffin B. High prevalence of small intestinal bacterial overgrowth in patients with morbid obesity: a contributor to severe hepatic steatosis. Obes Surg. 2008;18:371–7.
16. Wigg AJ, Roberts-Thomson IC, Dymock RB, McCarthy PJ, Grose RH, Cummins AG. The role of small intestinal bacterial overgrowth, intestinal permeability, endotoxaemia, and tumour necrosis factor alpha in the pathogenesis of non-alcoholic steatohepatitis. Gut. 2001;48:206–11.
17. Schnabl B, Brenner DA. Interactions between the intestinal microbiome and liver diseases. Gastroenterology. 2014;146:1513–24.
18. Minemura M, Shimizu Y. Gut microbiota and liver diseases. World J Gastroenterol. 2015;21:1691–702.
19. Ginès P, Cárdenas A, Arroyo V, Rodés J. Management of cirrhosis and ascites. N Engl J Med. 2004;350:1646–54.
20. Bajaj JS, Heuman DM, Hylemon PB, Sanyal AJ, White MB, Monteith P, Noble NA, Unser AB, Daita K, Fisher AR, Sikaroodi M, Gillevet PM. Altered profile of human gut microbiome is associated with cirrhosis and its complications. J Hepatol. 2014;60:940–7.
21. Bajaj JS, Hylemon PB, Ridlon JM, Heuman DM, Daita K, White MB, Monteith P, Noble NA, Sikaroodi M, Gillevet PM. Colonic mucosal microbiome differs from stool microbiome in cirrhosis and hepatic encephalopathy and is linked to cognition and inflammation. Am J Physiol Gastrointest Liver Physiol. 2012;303:75–85.
22. Chen Y, Yang F, Lu H, Wang B, Chen Y, Lei D, Wang Y, Zhu B, Li L. Characterization of fecal microbial communities in patients with liver cirrhosis. Hepatology. 2011;54:562–72.
23. Bajaj JS, Ridlon JM, Hylemon PB, Thacker LR, Heuman DM, Smith S, Sikaroodi M, Gillevet PM. Linkage of gut microbiome with cognition in hepatic encephalopathy. Am J Physiol Gastrointest Liver Physiol. 2012;302:68–75.
24. Lu H, Wu Z, Xu W, Yang J, Chen Y, Li L. Intestinal microbiota was assessed in cirrhotic patients with hepatitis B virus infection. Intestinal microbiota of HBV cirrhotic patients. Microb Ecol. 2011;61:693–703.
25. Xu M, Wang B, Fu Y, Chen Y, Yang F, Lu H, Chen Y, Xu J, Li L. Changes of fecal Bifidobacterium species in adult patients with hepatitis B virus-induced chronic liver disease. Microb Ecol. 2012;63:304–13.
26. Wu ZW, Lu HF, Wu J, Zuo J, Chen P, Sheng JF, Zheng SS, Li LJ. Assessment of the fecal lactobacilli population in patients with hepatitis B virus-related decompensated cirrhosis and hepatitis B cirrhosis treated with liver transplant. Microb Ecol. 2012;63:929–37.
27. Qin N, Yang F, Li A, Prifti E, Chen Y, Shao L, Guo J, Le Chatelier E, Yao J, Wu L, Zhou J, Ni S, Liu L, Pons N, Batto JM, Kennedy SP, Leonard P, Yuan C, Ding W, Chen Y, Hu X, Zheng B, Qian G, Xu W, Ehrlich SD, Zheng S, Li L. Alterations of the human gut microbiome in liver cirrhosis. Nature. 2014;513:59–64.
28. Bajaj JS, Betrapally NS, Hylemon PB, Heuman DM, Daita K, White MB, Unser A, Thacker LR, Sanyal AJ, Kang DJ, Sikaroodi M, Gillevet PM. Salivary microbiota reflects changes in gut microbiota in cirrhosis with hepatic encephalopathy. Hepatology. 2015;62(4):1260–71.
29. Parkin DM, Bray F, Ferlay J, Pisani P. Global cancer statistics, 2002. CA Cancer J Clin. 2005;55:74–108.
30. Ley RE, Turnbaugh PJ, Klein S, Gordon JI. Microbial ecology: human gut microbes associated with obesity. Nature. 2006;444:1022–3.
31. Dapito DH, Mencin A, Gwak GY, Pradere JP, Jang MK, Mederacke I, Caviglia JM, Khiabanian H, Adeyemi A, Bataller R, Lefkowitch JH, Bower M, Friedman R, Sartor RB, Rabadan R, Schwabe RF. Promotion of hepatocellular carcinoma by the intestinal microbiota and TLR4. Cancer Cell. 2012;21:504–16.
32. d'Adda di Fagagna F. Living on a break: cellular senescence as a DNA damage response. Nat Rev Cancer. 2008;8:512–22.

33. Kuilman T, Michaloglou C, Mooi WJ, Peeper DS. The essence of senescence. Genes Dev. 2010;24:2463–79.
34. Ohtani N, Hara E. Cellular senescence: roles and mechanisms of cellular senescence in regulation of tissue homeostasis. Cancer Sci. 2013;104:525–30.
35. Campisi J. Senescent cells, tumor suppression, and organismal aging: good citizens, bad neighbors. Cell. 2005;120:513–22.
36. Collado M, Serrano M. Senescence in tumours: evidence from mice and humans. Nat Rev Cancer. 2010;10:51–7.
37. Yoshimoto S, Loo TM, Atarashi K, Kanda H, Sato S, Oyadomari S, Iwakura Y, Oshima K, Morita H, Hattori M, Honda K, Ishikawa Y, Hara E, Ohtani N. Obesity-induced gut microbial metabolite promotes liver cancer through senescence secretome. Nature. 2013;499:97–101.
38. Ohtani N, Yoshimoto S, Hara E. Obesity and cancer: a gut microbial connection. Cancer Res. 2014;74:1885–9.

Chapter 3
Spleen and Liver

Takuji Torimura

Abstract In liver cirrhosis, the spleen is a source of nitric oxide which affects a hyperdynamic state typical of portal hypertension. It is generally accepted that pancytopenia results predominantly from the increased phagocytosis and destruction of hemocytes in splenic macrophages. In addition, liver fibrosis is amplified by migrated Th2 lymphocytes and transforming growth factor beta from the spleen. There is a possibility that increase of the spleen stiffness is the primary factor of idiopathic portal hypertension. Spleen stiffness is caused by bleeding, fibrosis, and calcareous deposits after increase in red pulp pressure due to venous congestion. In nonalcoholic steatohepatitis, macrophage activity in the spleen is upregulated. In addition, high levels of inflammatory cytokines are produced and T cell shows increased proliferation in the spleen. In autoimmune hepatitis model, $CD4^+$ T cells are differentiated into follicular helper T cells (T_{FH}) in the spleen. T_{FH} cells promoted hypergammaglobulinemia and antinuclear antibodies production. T_{FH} cells migrate from the spleen to the liver, triggering induction of autoimmune hepatitis in this model. IgM-positive B cells localize in the CD21-positive lymph follicle in the spleen of primary biliary cholangitis. These findings prove that the spleen influences on the pathogenesis and severity of several kinds of liver disease.

Keywords Hyperdynamic state • Immune cell • Hypersplenism • TGF beta-1 • Follicular helper T cells

3.1 Introduction

The spleen, in healthy adult humans, is approximately 12 cm in length and usually 100–200 g in weight. It consists of red pulp and white pulp. The spleen is the largest lymphoid organ in the human body. However, it was considered a neglected organ. Since 1952, when King and Schumacker reported overwhelming post-splenectomy infection [1], there has been a growing recognition of the importance of the spleen

T. Torimura (✉)
Division of Gastroenterology, Department of Medicine, Kurume University School of Medicine, 830-0011, 67 Asahi-machi, Kurume City, Japan
e-mail: tori@med.kurume-u.ac.jp

H. Ohira (ed.), *The Liver in Systemic Diseases*, DOI 10.1007/978-4-431-55790-6_3

in the human body. Especially, in recent years, studies of spleen organization and structure, cell function, secretion, and innervations, a better understanding of the function has been gained. It has a fundamental role as the destruction of red blood cells, as the modulation of the immune system, and as the maintenance of peripheral tolerance via clearance of circulating apoptotic cells, the differentiation and activation of T and B cells, and production of antibodies in the white pulp [2, 3].

In the spleen, splenic macrophages and endothelial cells of the marginal sinus compose the blood-spleen barrier. The cells of the blood-spleen barrier can trap circulating infectious organisms and monocytes clear them from the blood stream and providing a selective environment for monocyte differentiation into macrophages and subsequent phagocytosis of the microorganisms. The interactions between the circulating lymphocytes and macrophages may regulate the entry of lymphocytes into the white pulp. The functions of the blood-spleen barrier in the spleen are to filter antigens, to keep the microenvironment of the white pulp stable, and to present antigen information to white pulp through the effects of the mechanical barrier which depends on the connection between cells and the phagocytosis of macrophages. The blood-spleen barrier in the spleen is relatively loose without the tight junction between cells. However, the blood-spleen barrier has more ability to stop and phagocytize more xenobiotic materials than other barriers, such as the blood-brain barrier and the blood-thymus barrier [4, 5].

Table 3.1 summarizes the functions of the spleen. As the spleen is strictly linked to liver, it influences on several kinds of liver disease, such as liver cirrhosis,

Table 3.1 Function of the spleen

Red pulp
Extramedullary hematopoiesis
Facilitating an environment wherein erythrocytes rid themselves of solid waste material
Blood filter for foreign material and damaged and senescent blood cells
Storage site for iron, erythrocytes, platelets, plasmablasts, and plasma cells
Rapid release of antigen-specific antibodies into the circulation produced by red pulp plasma cells
Defense against bacteria using iron metabolism by its macrophages
White pulp
T-cell zone (peripheral lymphatic sheath) and B cell zone (follicles)
Storage site for B and T lymphocytes
Development of B and T lymphocytes upon antigenic challenge
Release of immunoglobulins upon antigenic challenge by B lymphocytes
Production of immune mediators involved in clearance of bacteria
Marginal zone
Phagocytosis of circulating microorganisms and immune complexes by marginal zone macrophages
Development of marginal zone B lymphocytes upon T1-2 antigenic challenge
Blood trafficking of B and T lymphocytes
Release of immunoglobulins upon antigenic challenge by splenic B lymphocytes

idiopathic portal hypertension, nonalcoholic steatohepatitis, autoimmune hepatitis, and primary biliary cholangitis. In this chapter, I would like to review the participants of the spleen in liver diseases.

3.2 Liver Cirrhosis

Portal hypertension, pancytopenia, liver fibrosis, and regeneration and insulin resistance are common symptoms of liver cirrhosis. I will describe the participation of the spleen to such symptom [6, 7].

In patients with liver cirrhosis, increase of splenic blood flow is a common finding. There is a good correlation between the spleen volume and portal flow volume [8]. Kayacetin et al. [9] reported that splenic vein congestion was significantly increased in the Child-Pugh class C compared with the Child-Pugh class A. In addition, liver cirrhosis patients with esophageal varices bleeding as well as ascites have greater splenic blood flow volume, high splenic vein congestion, and high portal vein congestion.

In liver cirrhosis, a number of vasoactive substances have been implicated as potential mediators of portal hypertension. Especially, nitric oxide (NO), angiotensin II (Ang II), and endothelins (ETs) have received the greatest attention [10]. NO is a potent vasodilator, and there are 3 isoforms of NO synthase (NOS): inducible NO (iNOS), endothelial NOS (eNOS), and neuronal NOS [11, 12]. ETs are a family of 3 related peptides, ETs1, 2, 3. ETs act as potent vasoconstrictors [13]. The respective roles of NOS and ET-1 have been well studied in cirrhotic liver [14, 15]. The mechanical obstruction is assumed to be caused by distortion and compression of the hepatic vasculature by increased fibrosis and nodule formation [16]. In addition, intrahepatic vascular bed is typified by an increase in resistance to blood flow in cirrhotic liver. Liver injury causes a reduction in the production of vasodilators by sinusoidal endothelial cells such as NO; concomitantly, there is an increase in the synthesis of vasoconstrictors such as ET1 and Ang II by other cells in the sinusoids. In mesenteric vasculature, increased portal blood flow from the splanchnic circulation augments portal pressure and thereby contributes to the maintenance and exacerbation of portal hypertension. In cirrhotic condition, the expression of ET-1 and Ang II is reduced in splanchnic circulation. On the contrary, eNOS phosphorylation and NO production are increased. Arterial vasodilatation in the splanchnic circulation plays a critical role in increasing the blood flow to the portal vein. Increased eNOS-derived NO plays a principal role in arterial vasodilatation [17] (Fig. 3.1). In liver cirrhosis, the spleen is also a source of NO and secreted into portal blood flow affects a hyperdynamic state typical of patients with liver cirrhosis. A recent study indicates the possibility of the involvement of renin-angiotensin (Ang) system [18]. Ang II is a vasoconstrictor generated by Ang-converting enzyme (ACE) and is further cleaved by ACE2 to Ang-(1-7). Ang-(1-7) is a vasodilator, which binds to the G-protein coupled receptor Mas (MasR) and leads to eNOS activation and NO production in endothelial cells

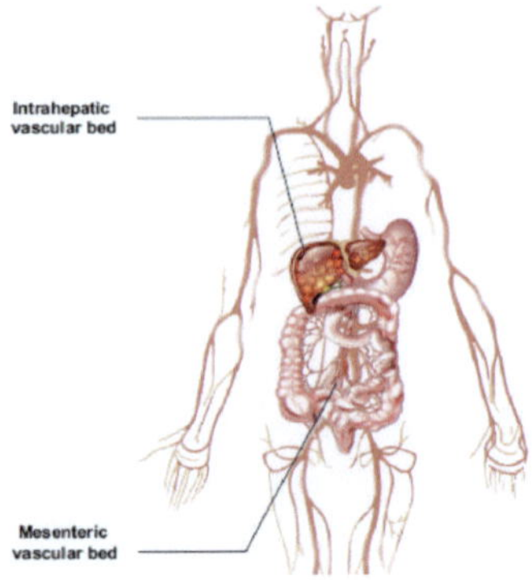

Molecular biology	Physiology
Intrahepatic vascular bed	
Increased expression of vasoconstrictors(ET-1, Ang II)	Increased resistance Increased pressure
Reduced eNOS phosphorylation, activity and NO production	Reduced portal blood flow
Splanchnic vascular bed	
Reduced expression of vasoconstrictors(ET-1, Ang II)	Arterial vasodilatation
Increased eNOS phosphorylation, activity and NO production	Increased portal blood flow

Fig. 3.1 Prominent vascular beds and their pathophysiology. *ET-1* endothelin-1, *Ang II* angiotensin II, *NO* nitric oxide, *eNOS* endothelial nitric oxide synthase, *VEGF* vascular endothelial growth factor, *PDGF* platelet-derived growth factor, *PlGF* placental growth factor (Image from Published Paper Iwakiri et al. 2014)

[19, 20]. Besides NO, other vasodilators, such as CO, prostacyclin, adrenomedullin, endocannabinoids, and endothelium-derived hyperpolarizing factor, also mediate arterial vasodilatation. These multiple factors seem to be involved in the excessive vasodilatation, observed in the splanchnic circulation.

3.2.1 Pancytopenia

Abnormalities in hematological parameters are common in patients with liver cirrhosis. The pathogenesis of abnormal hematological indices in liver cirrhosis is multifactorial such as portal hypertension, alterations of bone marrow stimulating factors, viral- and toxin-induced bone marrow suppression, and consumption loss (Table 3.2).

Splenic sequestration and destruction of platelets, white blood cells, and red blood cells in the portal hypertension-induced enlarged spleen is defined as hypersplenism. Liangpunsakul et al. [21] reported that 33 % patients with chronic liver disease were associated with severe hypersplenism. Although a number of factors contribute to hematological indices in patients with liver cirrhosis, portal hypertension and alterations in bone marrow hormones appear to be the strongest

Table 3.2 Causes of pancytopenia in liver cirrhosis

Portal hypertension-induced splenic sequestration
Alteration in thrombopoietin
Bone marrow suppression mediated by hepatitis B virus, hepatitis C virus, and alcohol
Consumptive coagulopathy (low-grade DIC, acquired intravascular coagulation, and fibrinolysis)
Increased blood loss
Alterations in granulocyte-colony stimulating factor and granulocyte macrophage-colony stimulating factor
Alterations in erythropoietin

contributions. It is generally accepted that pancytopenia results predominantly from the increased phagocytosis and destruction of hemocytes in splenic macrophages [22]. The rate of phagocytosis and the index of phagocytosis of splenic macrophages are notably in negative correlation with the count of leukocyte and platelet in peripheral blood. Regarding thrombocytopenia, the mechanisms include decreased production, splenic sequestration, endothelial dysfunction, and autoimmune destruction. Tana et al. [23] reported that the peripheral platelet count in patients with chronic hepatitis C was associated with liver fibrosis, thrombopoietin level, immature platelet fraction, and spleen size. Other factors that may influence the platelet count include platelet-associated antibodies and antiplatelet immunoglobulins. However, previous reports described that the presence of antiplatelet antibodies did not affect the platelet count [24].

Regarding the relationship between thrombocytopenia and liver fibrosis, Kondo et al. [25] clarified that patients with liver cirrhosis had a more extensive platelet area in the liver compared with those with normal liver. In cirrhotic liver, most platelets were present in the sinusoidal space of the periportal area with inflammation, where hepatic stellate cells expressing platelet-derived growth factor (PDGF) receptor-beta were frequently observed. Hepatic stellate cell is a key mediator of liver fibrosis. PDGF is the basic mediator involved in platelet granules. PDGF stimulates the proliferation of hepatic stellate cells [26]. So, they speculate that the accumulation of platelets in the liver may be involved in thrombocytopenia and liver fibrosis through the activation of hepatic stellate cells.

Recently, Li et al. [27] investigated the expression of microRNA of splenic macrophages in hypersplenism due to portal hypertension in hepatitis B virus-related liver cirrhosis. In this study, they identified 99 microRNA differences in expression between splenic macrophages associated with hypersplenism and those from the normal spleen. In those microRNAs, has-miR-615-3p was significantly upregulated in hypersplenism. As dysregulation of microRNA levels would affect the translation of multiple protein-coding genes, they speculated that has-miR-615-3p might regulate the activation of splenic macrophages and involved in the pathogenesis of hypersplenism due to portal hypertension.

3.2.2 Liver Fibrosis and Regeneration

Clinical observations have revealed that splenectomy not only increases the platelet count but also improves liver function [28, 29]. Some basic studies have shown that splenectomy suppresses the progression of liver fibrosis. For instance, platelets are able to inhibit the development of liver fibrosis, and splenectomy exerts an antifibrotic effect via thrombocytosis [30, 31]. The loss of spleen-derived transforming growth factor beta (TGF beta)-1 mediates the inhibitory effect of splenectomy on liver fibrosis. TGF beta-1 induces the phenotypic transition of hepatic stellate cells to proliferating myofibroblast-like cells that increase the production of extracellular matrix components and reduce the degradation of extracellular matrix proteins. Decreases in portal flow and portal pressure are other possible mechanisms of the antifibrotic effect of splenectomy.

The spleen also plays important roles in the immune system. The immune system can affect the progression of liver fibrosis because strain-specific differences in murine hepatic fibrosis are mediated by divergent T helper cytokine response [32]. In addition, immunosuppressants differently modulate hepatic fibrosis in mice and humans [33, 34]. These findings suggest that the spleen modulates hepatic fibrosis through its immunological functions. Previous studies have revealed that Th1 cytokines have a suppressive effect on liver fibrosis. In particular, interferon-r is a potent inhibitor of the activation of hepatic stellate cells [35, 36]. In contrast, Th2 cytokines such as IL-4 and IL-13 promote activation of hepatic stellate cells and progression of liver fibrosis [37, 38]. In mouse liver fibrosis model, $CD4^+$ cells in the spleen migrated to the liver in response to liver injury. As Th2 lymphocytes are the main constituent of the immune environment in the spleen, most of the spleen-derived $CD4^+$ cells in the fibrotic liver were Th2 cells. These findings as well as previous reports indicate that Th2-predominant splenic T lymphocytes migrate to the injured liver and promote liver fibrosis by modifying the Th1/Th2 balance in the liver toward Th2 dominance. Splenectomy decreases the absolute number of Th2 lymphocytes in the liver and reverses this Th1/Th2 imbalance, resulting in inhibition of liver fibrosis [39]. In human samples, Nomura et al. [40] reported that splenectomy significantly decreased liver fibrosis and the $CD4^+/CD8^+$, suggesting that splenectomy modified Th1/Th2 balanced to Th2 dominant and improved liver fibrosis in human.

Experimental studies have reported that splenomegaly inhibits liver regeneration in liver cirrhosis [41, 42] and splenectomy improves liver regeneration [43]. After a partial splenectomy in cirrhotic patients with splenomegaly, the remnant liver tends to regenerate to a small volume than in patients without splenomegaly [44]. However, the exact underlying mechanism for this effect has been elusive thus far. Two general mechanisms have been put forward. First, it has been proposed that the cytokines or growth factors released from the spleen influence liver regeneration by way of the portal circulation. The spleen promotes liver regeneration via preferential upregulation of heme oxygenase 1 and downregulation of tumor necrosis factor alpha [45]. In addition, spleen-derived TGF beta-1 has been reported to play a critical role in inhibiting the growth of hepatocytes [46]. TGF beta-1 induces liver fibrosis. However, it also acts directly on hepatocytes by inhibiting cell proliferation and inducing apoptosis [47]. TGF beta-1 plays an essential role in the normal quiescent liver by inducing a tonic effect to hepatocytes to keep them in the G0 phase [48]. Although TGF beta-1 is produced principally in the hepatic stellate cells in the liver, it is also produced by the macrophages in the spleen and secreted into the portal vein in a liver injury model (Fig. 3.2). Morinaga et al. reported that splenectomy significantly improved liver regeneration with reduction of plasma TGF beta-1 in cirrhotic model. Second, the hemodynamic alterations induced by a splenectomy are proposed to provide a favorable environment for liver regeneration. The splenectomy-induced increase in hepatic arterial flow with increased oxygen supply is also suggested to induce liver regeneration [49]. It is noteworthy that other spleen-derived factors such as hepatocyte growth factor (HGF) activator-inhibitor (HAI) and ET-1 also impair liver regeneration in cirrhotic liver. Furthermore, Lee et al. [21] reported that splenectomy-induced upregulation of hepatocyte growth factor (HGF) and downregulation of TGF beta-1 in the injured liver. TGF beta-receptor II was more highly expressed in the injured liver, and c-Met, a HGF receptor, was more highly expressed in the injured liver with splenectomy. TGF beta-1 binds to its receptor, TGF beta-receptor II, at the end of the regeneration phase, and it induces the production of extracellular matrix in the liver. Newly synthesized extracellular matrix, especially glycosaminoglycans, would be capable of inhibiting urokinase-induced HGF activation by binding to HGF itself. This set of events would bring hepatocytes back into a stage of quiescence, surrounded by HGF and TGF beta-1. Splenectomy increased HGF level in the portal vein and also upregulated the expression of HGF in the liver. HGF in the liver is mainly produced in the hepatic stellate cells [50] and is known to be essential to initiate the process of liver regeneration. Activated HGF binds to c-Met and stimulates hepatocytes DNA synthesis via endocrine or paracrine mechanism.

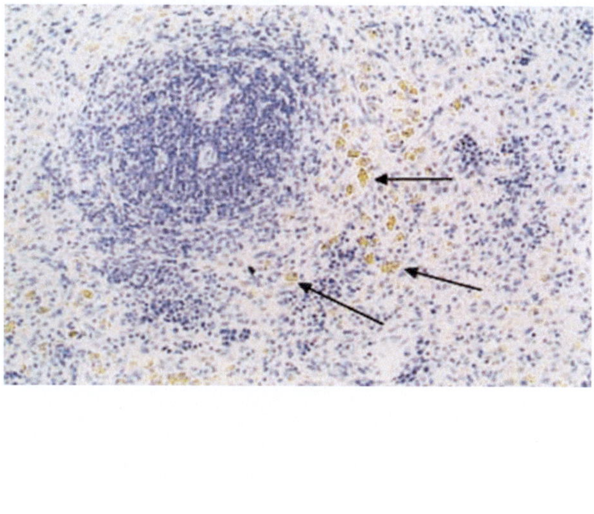

Fig. 3.2 Localization of TGF beta1-positive cells in the spleen. TGF beta1 was produced by macrophages in the red pulp (*arrows*). TGF beta1, transforming growth factor-beta1 (Image from Published Paper Akahoshi et al. 2002)

3.2.3 Insulin Resistance

Shimizu et al. [51] clarified that partial splenectomy reversed insulin resistance in patients with liver cirrhosis. The mechanism by which partial splenectomy reverses insulin resistance primarily involves hemodynamic improvements in the intestinal venous flow into the liver. In case of portal hypertension, the intestinal venous flow to the liver is disturbed due to the overflow of splenic venous return. The decrease in the splenic venous flow achieved with partial splenectomy may contribute to the increase in the intestinal venous flow relative to the total portal venous flow.

3.3 Idiopathic Portal Hypertension

Idiopathic portal hypertension is a disease that is characterized by splenomegaly and portal hypertension without liver cirrhosis. Occlusion of peripheral portal veins in the liver and increased splenic blood flow as a result of splenomegaly have been reported to be the causes that give rise to portal hypertension. The presence of fibrotic portal tracts and thin fibrous septa in the absence of cirrhosis are pathological criteria for making a diagnosis of idiopathic portal hypertension. Clinically, the median value of liver stiffness in patients with idiopathic portal hypertension is lower than that in patients with liver cirrhosis. To the contrary, spleen stiffness is higher in patients with idiopathic portal hypertension [52]. Histologically, splenomegaly in idiopathic portal hypertension was attributed to an increase in venous sinuses in the red pulp [53]. In addition, the lymph follicles and the reticular fibers and collagen fibers around the splenic cords grow thicker in a diffuse manner, and narrowing of cord width and narrowing of the sinus lumens is seen. Moreover, the rod-shaped cells became deformed, fall into disarray, and diversify, and the slits between the rod-shaped cells enlarge [54, 55]. The basal lamina of the sinuses also thickens. Therefore, the splenic tissue hyperplasia characterized by fibrogenesis enlargement and passive spleen congestion are likely to cause the increase of spleen tissue stiffness. The spleen is also known to undergo fibrosis in liver cirrhosis, primarily, in the red pulp. The appearance of venous sinus hyperplasia in patients with liver cirrhosis is not so marked as in patients with idiopathic portal hypertension, and the rod-shaped cells in the venous sinuses do not diversify as much. The degree of splenic congestion and fibrosis in patients with liver cirrhosis might be smaller than that in patients with idiopathic portal hypertension. Regarding the pathological difference of the spleen between idiopathic portal hypertension and liver cirrhosis, Sato et al. [44] reported that there is increase of Gamna-Gandy nodules, which developed in the lymphocyte sheaths around arteries and the splenic trabeculae, in idiopathic portal hypertension. Gamna-Gandy nodules are formed as a result of bleeding, fibrosis, and calcareous deposits after an increase in red pulp pressure due to venous congestion [56]. Gamna-Gandy nodules seem to be involved in increase of splenic stiffness. There is a strong possibility that portal hypertension due to narrowing of portal vein branches in the liver is not the only cause of idiopathic portal hypertension, and specific increase of spleen stiffness is the material primary factor.

3.4 Non-alcoholic Steatohepatitis

Non-alcoholic fatty liver disease (NAFLD), the most common cause of steatosis, is associated with obesity, mainly visceral, and insulin resistance. In the presence of more severe risk factors, simple hepatic steatosis may be complicated by liver inflammation named non-alcoholic steatohepatitis (NASH). NASH can lead to perisinusoidal fibrosis. Fat-laden hepatocytes are swollen, and in steatohepatitis, further swelling occurs due to ballooning of hepatocytes to cause sinusoidal distortion. It reduces intrasinusoidal volume and microvascular blood flow. Involvement of other cell types, such as sinusoidal endothelial cells, Kupffer cells, and hepatic stellate cells, and recruitment of inflammatory cells as well as platelets lead to dysregulation of microvascular blood flow. In animal models, the net effect of such changes is a marked reduction of sinusoidal space by approximately 50 % and a decrease in the number of normally perfused sinusoids. Such microvascular damage could accentuate further liver injury and disease progression in NASH.

NASH is a progressive liver disease characterized by Kupffer cell dysfunction which contributes to its pathogenesis. It is noteworthy that the reticular-endothelial system also plays a key role in the spleen. Colloid scintigraphy is a good method of reflecting Kupffer cell activity. Duman et al. [57] Reported that Colloid shift to the spleen was observed in patients with NASH comparing with simple steatosis. In a nutritional model of NASH in rats fed a methionine-and choline-deficient diet, the liver/spleen uptake ratio was significantly decreased in rats after 8 weeks of a methionine-and choline-deficient diet in comparison with control diet-fed rats [58]. In addition, the patients with NASH demonstrated higher IL-6 blood levels, spleen longitudinal diameter values, and VEGF concentrations than those of healthy subjects [59].

The relationship between NAFLD and immune functions is still under investigation. The spleen may have an important role. In the splenic lymphocytes of obese rats, the expression of glucose transporter 1 (GLUT-1) was lower compared to lean rats. The decreased expression of GLUT-1 in obese rats was associated with a decreased uptake of glucose into immune cells [60]. Miyake et al. [61] reported that in NAFLD mice immunized with hepatitis B vaccine containing hepatitis B surface antigen (HBsAg) and hepatitis B core antigen (HBcAg), levels of anti-HBs and proliferation activity of HBsAg and HBcAg-specific lymphocytes were significantly lower compared to controls. In addition, higher levels of inflammatory cytokines were produced and T cells showed increased proliferation rate in splenic cells of NAFLD than control. Splenic dendritic cells processing and presenting antigen activities were significantly decreased in NAFLD mice.

3.5 Autoimmune Hepatitis

Autoimmune hepatitis is characterized by mononuclear cell infiltration in the liver and elevated levels of gamma globulins as well as by the production of a variety of characteristic autoantibodies, including antinuclear antibodies. Liver-infiltrating T cells are considered the primary disease mediators of inflammatory liver damage, and circulating autoantibodies are diagnostic hallmarks. However, clinical manifestations are varied in patients with autoimmune hepatitis, ranging from non-symptomatic mild chronic hepatitis to fulminant hepatic failure.

Aoki et al. [62] reported that in programmed cell death-1 (PD-1)-deficient mice underwent thymectomy 3 days after birth, immune dysregulation by a concurrent loss of Foxp3$^+$ regulatory T cells and PD-1-mediated signaling induced fatal autoimmune hepatitis resembling acute-onset autoimmune hepatitis. In this model, CD4$^+$ and CD8$^+$ T-cell infiltration from the spleen with massive lobular necrosis in the liver, hypergammaglobulinemia, and production of antinuclear antibodies were observed. The spleen is an induction site for autoimmune hepatitis in this model, and splenic CD4$^+$ T cells were differentiated into follicular helper T cells (T_{FH}) in the spleen. T_{FH} cells expressing inducible costimulatory (ICOS) and C-X-C chemokine receptor (CXCR) five comprise a newly defined effector T-cell subset that powerfully assists B cells in forming germinal centers [63]. Dysregulated T_{FH} cells promoted hypergammaglobulinemia and antinuclear antibody production in this model. T_{FH} cells migrated from the spleen to the liver through the C-C chemokine receptor 6/C-C chemokine ligand 20 axis, triggering induction of autoimmune hepatitis. Regarding the fetal progression of autoimmune hepatitis in the model, they also reported that dendritic cells (DC)-derived IL-18 induced the differentiation of Th1 and CD8$^+$ effector cells in the spleen and hepatic macrophages/Kupffer cells producing CXC ligand 9 (CXCL9) induced the migration of these cells to the liver. TNF-alpha directly induces maturation of DCs, TNF-alpha and IL-18 may directly induce inflammasome upregulation and skew toward IL-18 production. TNF-alpha induces cell death of hepatocytes and free DNA released from apoptotic hepatocytes activates Toll-like receptor 9, triggering a signal cascade to induce pro-IL-18 [64]. Therefore, TNF-alpha may induce apoptosis of hepatocytes, triggering canonical IL-18 production. However, IL-18 may act as an autocrine for skewing prolonged IL-18 secretion in DCs. They concluded that IL-18 induced differentiation of CD4$^+$ T into Th1 cells and CD8$^+$ cells into effector T cells, following CXCR3-CXCL9 axis-dependent migration of these cells to the liver which induce fatal progression of autoimmune hepatitis [65] (Fig. 3.3). In addition, they showed that although corticosteroid therapy was effective for autoimmune hepatitis in mice, it allows residual splenic dysregulated T_{FH} cells to remain after treatment, which appear to be responsible for relapse. Splenectomy overcomes this insufficiency, including prolonged remission of autoimmune hepatitis in mice [66]. Furthermore, they reported that in another mouse model which developed chronic autoimmune hepatitis with fibrosis, hypergammaglobulinemia, and antinuclear antibody production, neonatal splenectomy suppressed the onset of

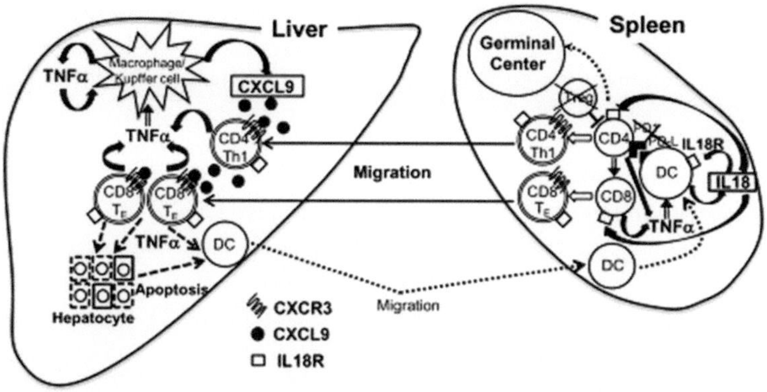

Fig. 3.3 Mechanistic links of cytokines and chemokines in the spleen and the liver in the progression of autoimmune hepatitis. *TN alpha* tumor necrosis factor alpha, *CXCL9* C-X-C motif ligand9, T_E effector T cell, *Th1* helper T cell, *DC* dendritic cell, *PD-1* programed cell death-1, *IL-18R* interleukin 18 receptor (Image from Published Paper Ikeda et al. 2014)

chronic autoimmune hepatitis. These findings indicate that the spleen is a very important organ for the induction and progression of autoimmune hepatitis.

3.6 Primary Biliary Cholangitis

Primary biliary cholangitis is characterized by the presence of the most highly directed and specific autoantibody in human immunopathology: the antimitochondrial antibody and the presence of a high frequency of antigen-specific autoreactive CD4 and CD8 T cells [67, 68]. In autoimmune diseases, the germinal center may be a pathogenic hot spot for production of autoantibodies [69]. T_{FH} cells are located in germinal center where primarily drive B cells differentiate into memory B cells and form antibody-producing plasma cells [70]. Wang et al. [71] reported that Splenic T_{FH} cells ($CXCR5^+$ and $CD4^+$) increased in peripheral blood of primary biliary cholangitis than that in autoimmune hepatitis. Splenic T_{FH} cells were localized in germinal center-bearing B cell follicles in primary biliary cholangitis. Circulating ($CXCR5^+$ and $CD4^+$) T_{FH} cells persisting for a long time in blood. Upon subsequent antigenic stimulation, these memory cells may quickly form T_{FH} cells and promote germinal center responses. Uncontrolled generation of circulating T_{FH} cells may reflect germinal center dysregulation and play an important role in amplifying autoreactive B cells, promoting pathogenic autoantibody production, the onset of clinical symptoms, continued immune responsiveness, and eventually irreversible tissue damage [72]. In primary biliary cholangitis, there is a higher percentage of T_{FH} cells in antimitochondrial antibody-positive patients than antimitochondrial antibody negative patients suggesting that T_{FH} cells may be specifically involved in the production of autoantibodies [71]. In addition, they also clarified that circulating CXCR5$^+$ and CD4$^+$ T$_{FH}$ cells in patients with primary biliary cholangitis generated more IL-21 after stimulation with PMA/ionomycin and these cells induced naïve B cells to differentiate to plasmablasts in order to induce the production of immunoglobulin under the stimulation of IL-21 [71]. Levels of CXCR5$^+$ and CD4$^+$ T$_{FH}$ cells were significantly lower in ursodeoxycholic acid responders than those in nonresponders. In patients with primary biliary cholangitis, circulating CXCR5$^+$ and CD4$^+$ T$_{FH}$ cells were also decreased in number in responders to ursodeoxycholic acid treatment. In contrast, no significant changes in circulating CXCR5$^+$ and CD4$^+$ T$_{FH}$ cells was observed in nonresponders to ursodeoxycholic acid treatment. These findings suggest that CXCR5$^+$ and CD4$^+$ T$_{FH}$ cells in patients with primary biliary cholangitis interact with localized B cells to form lymphoid follicle-like structures that promote B cells to differentiate to plasmablasts, a key factor associated with the pathogenesis of primary biliary cholangitis.

Primary biliary cholangitis is usually accompanied by high IgM level in peripheral blood. The naïve B cells that are generated in the bone marrow enter the spleen through blood flow and subsequently enter the white pulp through the periarteriolar lymphoid sheath. These cells differentiated to the switched memory B cells that express IgG on cell surface and IgM memory B cells that actively produce high-affinity IgM [73, 74]. Circulating innate immune factors stimulate IgM memory B cells and increase IgM production in the spleen [75]. Kikuchi et al. [76] reported that accumulation of IgM-positive cells was observed in the CD21-positive lymph follicle in the spleen of primary biliary cholangitis patients. Toll-like receptor ligand CpG stimulated IgM memory B cells in the peripheral blood mononuclear cells of primary biliary cholangitis to produce an excessive amount of IgM [77]. From these findings, Kikuchi et al. speculate that circulating pathogen-associated molecular patterns stimulate proliferation of the IgM memory B cells and IgM overexpression in the spleen.

References

1. Lucas CE. Splenic trauma. Choice of management. Ann Surg. 1991;213(2):98–112.
2. Thacker RI, Janssen EM. Cross-presentation of cell-associated antigens by mouse splenic dendritic cell populations. Front Immunol. 2012;3:41. doi:10.3389/fimmu.2012.00041.
3. Mahnke K, Knop J, Enk AH. Induction of tolerogenic DCs: 'you are what you eat'. Trends Immunol. 2003;24(12):646–51.
4. Weiss L. Barrier cells in the spleen. Immunol Today. 1991;12(1):24–9. doi:10.1016/0167-5699(91)90108-6.
5. Li ZF, Zhang S, Huang Y, Xia XM, Li AM, Pan D, et al. Morphological changes of blood spleen barrier in portal hypertensive spleen. Chin Med J (Engl). 2008;121(6):561–5.
6. Ashraf SS, Mishra KN, Sharma AC. Static structure factor and pair correlation function of graphene. J Phys Condens Matter. 2010;22(35):355303. doi:10.1088/0953-8984/22/35/355303.
7. Ameiss K, Ashraf S, Kong W, Pekosz A, Wu WH, Milich D, et al. Delivery of woodchuck hepatitis virus-like particle presented influenza M2e by recombinant attenuated Salmonella

displaying a delayed lysis phenotype. Vaccine. 2010;28(41):6704–13. doi:10.1016/j.vaccine.2010.07.083.
8. Shah SH, Hayes PC, Allan PL, Nicoll J, Finlayson ND. Measurement of spleen size and its relation to hypersplenism and portal hemodynamics in portal hypertension due to hepatic cirrhosis. Am J Gastroenterol. 1996;91(12):2580–3.
9. Kayacetin E, Efe D, Dogan C. Portal and splenic hemodynamics in cirrhotic patients: relationship between esophageal variceal bleeding and the severity of hepatic failure. J Gastroenterol. 2004;39(7):661–7. doi:10.1007/s00535-003-1362-x.
10. Rockey D. The cellular pathogenesis of portal hypertension: stellate cell contractility, endothelin, and nitric oxide. Hepatology. 1997;25(1):2–5. doi:10.1053/jhep.1997.v25.ajhep0250002.
11. Wiest R, Groszmann RJ. Nitric oxide and portal hypertension: its role in the regulation of intrahepatic and splanchnic vascular resistance. Semin Liver Dis. 1999;19(4):411–26. doi:10.1055/s-2007-1007129.
12. Farzaneh-Far R, Moore K. Nitric oxide and the liver. Liver. 2001;21(3):161–74.
13. Inoue A, Yanagisawa M, Kimura S, Kasuya Y, Miyauchi T, Goto K, et al. The human endothelin family: three structurally and pharmacologically distinct isopeptides predicted by three separate genes. Proc Natl Acad Sci U S A. 1989;86(8):2863–7.
14. Nagasue N, Dhar DK, Yamanoi A, Emi Y, Udagawa J, Yamamoto A, et al. Production and release of endothelin-1 from the gut and spleen in portal hypertension due to cirrhosis. Hepatology. 2000;31(5):1107–14. doi:10.1053/he.2000.6596.
15. Ohara N, Futagawa S, Watanabe S, Fukasawa M, Takamori S. Clinical investigation of endothelin-1 and nitric oxide in patients with portal hypertension focusing on plasma levels and immunohistological staining of liver tissues. Hepatol Res. 2001;21(1):40–54.
16. Bosch J, Navasa M, Garcia-Pagan JC, DeLacy AM, Rodes J. Portal hypertension. Med Clin N Am. 1989;73(4):931–53.
17. Iwakiri Y, Shah V, Rockey DC. Vascular pathobiology in chronic liver disease and cirrhosis - current status and future directions. J Hepatol. 2014;61(4):912–24.
18. Grace JA, Klein S, Herath CB, Granzow M, Schierwagen R, Masing N, et al. Activation of the MAS receptor by angiotensin-(1-7) in the renin-angiotensin system mediates mesenteric vasodilatation in cirrhosis. Gastroenterology. 2013;145(4):874–84 e5. doi:10.1053/j.gastro.2013.06.036.
19. Santos RA, Simoes e Silva AC, Maric C, Silva DM, Machado RP, de Buhr I, et al. Angiotensin-(1-7) is an endogenous ligand for the G protein-coupled receptor Mas. Proc Natl Acad Sci U S A. 2003;100(14):8258–63. doi:10.1073/pnas.1432869100.
20. Heitsch H, Brovkovych S, Malinski T, Wiemer G. Angiotensin-(1-7)-stimulated nitric oxide and superoxide release from endothelial cells. Hypertension. 2001;37(1):72–6.
21. Liangpunsakul S, Ulmer BJ, Chalasani N. Predictors and implications of severe hypersplenism in patients with cirrhosis. Am J Med Sci. 2003;326(3):111–6.
22. Gielchinsky Y, Elstein D, Hadas-Halpern I, Lahad A, Abrahamov A, Zimran A. Is there a correlation between degree of splenomegaly, symptoms and hypersplenism? A study of 218 patients with Gaucher disease. Br J Haematol. 1999;106(3):812–6.
23. Tana MM, Zhao X, Bradshaw A, Moon MS, Page S, Turner T, et al. Factors associated with the platelet count in patients with chronic hepatitis C. Thromb Res. 2015;135(5):823–8. doi:10.1016/j.thromres.2015.02.010.
24. Panzer S, Seel E, Brunner M, Kormoczi GF, Schmid M, Ferenci P, et al. Platelet autoantibodies are common in hepatitis C infection, irrespective of the presence of thrombocytopenia. Eur J Haematol. 2006;77(6):513–7. doi:10.1111/j.0902-4441.2006.t01.1-EJH2888.x.
25. Kondo R, Yano H, Nakashima O, Tanikawa K, Nomura Y, Kage M. Accumulation of platelets in the liver may be an important contributory factor to thrombocytopenia and liver fibrosis in chronic hepatitis C. J Gastroenterol. 2013;48(4):526–34. doi:10.1007/s00535-012-0656-2.
26. Pinzani M, Gesualdo L, Sabbah GM, Abboud HE. Effects of platelet-derived growth factor and other polypeptide mitogens on DNA synthesis and growth of cultured rat liver fat-storing cells. J Clin Invest. 1989;84(6):1786–93. doi:10.1172/JCI114363.

27. Li Z, Zhang S, Huang C, Zhang W, Hu Y, Wei B. MicroRNAome of splenic macrophages in hypersplenism due to portal hypertension in hepatitis B virus-related cirrhosis. Exp Biol Med (Maywood). 2008;233(11):1454–61. doi:10.3181/0711-RM-321.
28. Imura S, Shimada M, Utsunomiya T, Morine Y, Ikemoto T, Mori H, et al. Impact of splenectomy in patients with liver cirrhosis: results from 18 patients in a single center experience. Hepatol Res. 2010;40(9):894–900. doi:10.1111/j.1872-034X.2010.00688.x.
29. Sugawara Y, Yamamoto J, Shimada K, Yamasaki S, Kosuge T, Takayama T, et al. Splenectomy in patients with hepatocellular carcinoma and hypersplenism. J Am Coll Surg. 2000;190(4):446–50.
30. Watanabe M, Murata S, Hashimoto I, Nakano Y, Ikeda O, Aoyagi Y, et al. Platelets contribute to the reduction of liver fibrosis in mice. J Gastroenterol Hepatol. 2009;24(1):78–89. doi:10.1111/j.1440-1746.2008.05497.x.
31. Kodama T, Takehara T, Hikita H, Shimizu S, Li W, Miyagi T, et al. Thrombocytopenia exacerbates cholestasis-induced liver fibrosis in mice. Gastroenterology. 2010;138(7):2487–98, 98 e1–7. doi:10.1053/j.gastro.2010.02.054.
32. Shi Z, Wakil AE, Rockey DC. Strain-specific differences in mouse hepatic wound healing are mediated by divergent T helper cytokine responses. Proc Natl Acad Sci U S A. 1997;94(20):10663–8.
33. Patsenker E, Schneider V, Ledermann M, Saegesser H, Dorn C, Hellerbrand C, et al. Potent antifibrotic activity of mTOR inhibitors sirolimus and everolimus but not of cyclosporine A and tacrolimus in experimental liver fibrosis. J Hepatol. 2011;55(2):388–98. doi:10.1016/j.jhep.2010.10.044.
34. van der Laan LJ, Hudson M, McPherson S, Zondervan PE, Thomas RC, Kwekkeboom J, et al. Results of a two-center study comparing hepatic fibrosis progression in HCV-positive liver transplant patients receiving cyclosporine or tacrolimus. Transplant Proc. 2010;42(10):4573–7. doi:10.1016/j.transproceed.2010.10.013.
35. Czaja MJ, Weiner FR, Takahashi S, Giambrone MA, van der Meide PH, Schellekens H, et al. Gamma-interferon treatment inhibits collagen deposition in murine schistosomiasis. Hepatology. 1989;10(5):795–800.
36. Baroni GS, D'Ambrosio L, Curto P, Casini A, Mancini R, Jezequel AM, et al. Interferon gamma decreases hepatic stellate cell activation and extracellular matrix deposition in rat liver fibrosis. Hepatology. 1996;23(5):1189–99. doi:10.1002/hep.510230538.
37. Farah IO, Mola PW, Kariuki TM, Nyindo M, Blanton RE, King CL. Repeated exposure induces periportal fibrosis in Schistosoma mansoni-infected baboons: role of TGF-beta and IL-4. J Immunol. 2000;164(10):5337–43.
38. Wynn TA. Fibrotic disease and the T(H)1/T(H)2 paradigm. Nat Rev Immunol. 2004;4(8):583–94. doi:10.1038/nri1412.
39. Tanabe K, Taura K, Koyama Y, Yamamoto G, Nishio T, Okuda Y, et al. Migration of splenic lymphocytes promotes liver fibrosis through modification of T helper cytokine balance in mice. J Gastroenterol. 2015. doi:10.1007/s00535-015-1054-3.
40. Nomura Y, Kage M, Ogata T, Kondou R, Kinoshita H, Ohshima K, et al. Influence of splenectomy in patients with liver cirrhosis and hypersplenism. Hepatol Res. 2014;44(10):E100–9. doi:10.1111/hepr.12234.
41. Akahoshi T, Hashizume M, Tanoue K, Shimabukuro R, Gotoh N, Tomikawa M, et al. Role of the spleen in liver fibrosis in rats may be mediated by transforming growth factor beta-1. J Gastroenterol Hepatol. 2002;17(1):59–65.
42. Tomikawa M, Hashizume M, Highashi H, Ohta M, Sugimachi K. The role of the spleen, platelets, and plasma hepatocyte growth factor activity on hepatic regeneration in rats. J Am Coll Surg. 1996;182(1):12–6.
43. Murata K, Shiraki K, Sugimoto K, Takase K, Nakano T, Furusaka A, et al. Splenectomy enhances liver regeneration through tumor necrosis factor (TNF)-alpha following dimethylnitrosamine-induced cirrhotic rat model. Hepatogastroenterology. 2001;48(40):1022–7.

44. Sato K, Tanaka M, Tanikawa K. The effect of spleen volume on liver regeneration after hepatectomy – a clinical study of liver and spleen volumes by computed tomography. Hepatogastroenterology. 1995;42(6):961–5.
45. Arakawa Y, Shimada M, Uchiyama H, Ikegami T, Yoshizumi T, Imura S, et al. Beneficial effects of splenectomy on massive hepatectomy model in rats. Hepatol Res. 2009;39(4):391–7. doi:10.1111/j.1872-034X.2008.00469.x.
46. Ono M, Miyamura M, Kyotani S, Saibara T, Ohnishi S, Nishioka Y. Effect of Sho-saiko-to extract on HGF and TGF-beta levels of intraorgans in liver-injured rats after partial hepatectomy. J Pharm Pharmacol. 2000;52(1):111–8.
47. Carr BI, Hayashi I, Branum EL, Moses HL. Inhibition of DNA synthesis in rat hepatocytes by platelet-derived type beta transforming growth factor. Cancer Res. 1986;46(5):2330–4.
48. Ichikawa T, Zhang YQ, Kogure K, Hasegawa Y, Takagi H, Mori M, et al. Transforming growth factor beta and activin tonically inhibit DNA synthesis in the rat liver. Hepatology. 2001;34(5):918–25. doi:10.1053/jhep.2001.29132.
49. Eipel C, Abshagen K, Ritter J, Cantre D, Menger MD, Vollmar B. Splenectomy improves survival by increasing arterial blood supply in a rat model of reduced-size liver. Transpl Int. 2010;23(10):998–1007. doi:10.1111/j.1432-2277.2010.01079.x.
50. Schirmacher P, Geerts A, Jung W, Pietrangelo A, Rogler CE, Dienes HP. The role of Ito cells in the biosynthesis of HGF-SF in the liver. EXS. 1993;65:285–99.
51. Shimizu H, Takatsuka K, Yoshida A, Yoshimatsu E, Matsui K, Iwabuchi S. Partial splenic embolization reverses insulin resistance in patients with liver cirrhosis. Intern Med. 2009;48 (10):747–51.
52. Furuichi Y, Moriyasu F, Taira J, Sugimoto K, Sano T, Ichimura S, et al. Noninvasive diagnostic method for idiopathic portal hypertension based on measurements of liver and spleen stiffness by ARFI elastography. J Gastroenterol. 2013;48(9):1061–8. doi:10.1007/s00535-012-0703-z.
53. Grannis FW. Guido Banti's hypothesis and its impact on the understanding and treatment of portal hypertension. Mayo Clin Proc. 1975;50(1):41–8.
54. Suzuki T. Application of scanning electron microscopy in the study of the human spleen: three dimensional fine structure of the normal red pulp and its changes as seen in splenomegalias associated with Banti's syndrome and cirrhosis of the liver. Nihon Ketsueki Gakkai Zasshi. 1972;35(4):506–22.
55. Maesawa C, Sakuma T, Sato T, Masuda T, Muro-oka G, Satodate R. Structural characteristic of splenic sinuses in idiopathic portal hypertension. Pathol Int. 1995;45(9):642–8.
56. Sagoh T, Itoh K, Togashi K, Shibata T, Nishimura K, Minami S, et al. Gamna-Gandy bodies of the spleen: evaluation with MR imaging. Radiology. 1989;172(3):685–7. doi:10.1148/radiology.172.3.2672093.
57. Duman DG, Dede F, Akin H, Sen F, Turoglu HT, Celikel C, et al. Colloid scintigraphy in non-alcoholic steatohepatitis: a conventional diagnostic method for an emerging disease. Nucl Med Commun. 2006;27(4):387–93. doi:10.1097/01.mnm.0000203629.15784.2e.
58. Kikuchi M, Tomita K, Nakahara T, Kitamura N, Teratani T, Irie R, et al. Utility of quantitative 99mTc-phytate scintigraphy to diagnose early-stage non-alcoholic steatohepatitis. Scand J Gastroenterol. 2009;44(2):229–36. doi:10.1080/00365520802433249.
59. Tarantino G, Conca P, Pasanisi F, Ariello M, Mastrolia M, Arena A, et al. Could inflammatory markers help diagnose nonalcoholic steatohepatitis? Eur J Gastroenterol Hepatol. 2009;21 (5):504–11. doi:10.1097/MEG.0b013e3283229b40.
60. Moriguchi S, Kato M, Sakai K, Yamamoto S, Shimizu E. Decreased mitogen response of splenic lymphocytes in obese Zucker rats is associated with the decreased expression of glucose transporter 1 (GLUT-1). Am J Clin Nutr. 1998;67(6):1124–9.
61. Miyake T, Akbar SM, Yoshida O, Chen S, Hiasa Y, Matsuura B, et al. Impaired dendritic cell functions disrupt antigen-specific adaptive immune responses in mice with nonalcoholic fatty liver disease. J Gastroenterol. 2010;45(8):859–67. doi:10.1007/s00535-010-0218-4.

62. Aoki N, Kido M, Iwamoto S, Nishiura H, Maruoka R, Tanaka J, et al. Dysregulated generation of follicular helper T cells in the spleen triggers fatal autoimmune hepatitis in mice. Gastroenterology. 2011;140(4):1322–33 e1–5. doi:10.1053/j.gastro.2011.01.002.
63. King C. New insights into the differentiation and function of T follicular helper cells. Nat Rev Immunol. 2009;9(11):757–66. doi:10.1038/nri2644.
64. Imaeda AB, Watanabe A, Sohail MA, Mahmood S, Mohamadnejad M, Sutterwala FS, et al. Acetaminophen-induced hepatotoxicity in mice is dependent on Tlr9 and the Nalp3 inflammasome. J Clin Invest. 2009;119(2):305–14. doi:10.1172/JCI35958.
65. Ikade A, Aoki N, Kido M, Iwamoto S, Nishimura H, Watanabe N et al. Progression of autoimmune hepatitis is mediated by IL-18-producing dendritic cells and hepatic CXCL9 expression in mice. Hepatology. 2014;60(1):224–36.
66. Maruoka R, Aoki N, Kido M, Iwamoto S, Nishiura H, Ikeda A, et al. Splenectomy prolongs the effects of corticosteroids in mouse models of autoimmune hepatitis. Gastroenterology. 2013;145(1):209–20 e9. doi:10.1053/j.gastro.2013.03.011.
67. Kita H, Lian ZX, Van de Water J, He XS, Matsumura S, Kaplan M, et al. Identification of HLA-A2-restricted CD8(+) cytotoxic T cell responses in primary biliary cirrhosis: T cell activation is augmented by immune complexes cross-presented by dendritic cells. J Exp Med. 2002;195(1):113–23.
68. Takahashi T, Miura T, Nakamura J, Yamada S, Yanagi M, Matsuda Y, et al. Plasma cells and the chronic nonsuppurative destructive cholangitis of primary biliary cirrhosis. Hepatology. 2012;55(3):846–55. doi:10.1002/hep.24757.
69. Zhang X, Ing S, Fraser A, Chen M, Khan O, Zakem J, et al. Follicular helper T cells: new insights into mechanisms of autoimmune diseases. Ochsner J. 2013;13(1):131–9.
70. Cannons JL, Lu KT, Schwartzberg PL. T follicular helper cell diversity and plasticity. Trends Immunol. 2013;34(5):200–7. doi:10.1016/j.it.2013.01.001.
71. Wang L, Sun Y, Zhang Z, Jia Y, Zou Z, Ding J, et al. CXCR5+ CD4+ T follicular helper cells participate in the pathogenesis of primary biliary cirrhosis. Hepatology. 2015;61(2):627–38. doi:10.1002/hep.27306.
72. Simpson N, Gatenby PA, Wilson A, Malik S, Fulcher DA, Tangye SG, et al. Expansion of circulating T cells resembling follicular helper T cells is a fixed phenotype that identifies a subset of severe systemic lupus erythematosus. Arthritis Rheum. 2010;62(1):234–44. doi:10.1002/art.25032.
73. Agematsu K, Nagumo H, Oguchi Y, Nakazawa T, Fukushima K, Yasui K, et al. Generation of plasma cells from peripheral blood memory B cells: synergistic effect of interleukin-10 and CD27/CD70 interaction. Blood. 1998;91(1):173–80.
74. Klein U, Rajewsky K, Kuppers R. Human immunoglobulin (Ig)M+IgD+ peripheral blood B cells expressing the CD27 cell surface antigen carry somatically mutated variable region genes: CD27 as a general marker for somatically mutated (memory) B cells. J Exp Med. 1998;188(9):1679–89.
75. Aranburu A, Ceccarelli S, Giorda E, Lasorella R, Ballatore G, Carsetti R. TLR ligation triggers somatic hypermutation in transitional B cells inducing the generation of IgM memory B cells. J Immunol. 2010;185(12):7293–301. doi:10.4049/jimmunol.1002722.
76. Kikuchi K, Tsuneyama K, Yamada H, Kajiyama Y, Matsumoto K, Tsunashima H, et al. Splenic lymph follicles generate immunoglobulin M-producing B cells in primary biliary cirrhosis. Hepatol Res. 2014;44(10):E253–6. doi:10.1111/hepr.12231.
77. Kikuchi K, Lian ZX, Yang GX, Ansari AA, Ikehara S, Kaplan M, et al. Bacterial CpG induces hyper-IgM production in CD27(+) memory B cells in primary biliary cirrhosis. Gastroenterology. 2005;128(2):304–12.

Chapter 4
The Brain and Liver

Yasuhiro Takikawa, Hidekatsu Kuroda, and Kei Sawara

Abstract The brain integrates numerous sources of information and stimuli from both inside and outside the body and responds to them both voluntarily and involuntarily. To maintain this function, the brain consumes a great deal of energy and oxygen through a large blood supply. The supply of blood, energy, and substances used by the neurons in the brain are strictly regulated by a principal framework of the brain, the neurovascular unit, which includes the blood-brain barrier. The information transduction of the brain nervous system is executed through the electrical conduction of membrane action potentials and chemical transmission at the synapses. Metabolic disorders, such as hypoglycemia and hyperammonemia due to liver failure, perturb the energy supply and the information transduction of the brain nervous system and cause a range of brain disorders that are represented by hepatic encephalopathy (HE). Although the precise mechanisms of HE have not been fully elucidated, noninvasive methods of examination that have been recently developed, including high-quality magnetic resonance spectroscopy and imaging, have made it possible to evaluate the metabolic changes that occur in the brain of cirrhotic patients and then reveal the accumulation of toxic substances prior to overt manifestation of HE.

Keywords Neurovascular unit • Neurotransmitter • Blood-brain barrier • Astrocyte • Glutamine • Ammonia • Hepatic encephalopathy • Acute liver failure • Liver cirrhosis

Organisms receive and integrate numerous sources of information and stimuli from both inside and outside the body and respond to them both voluntarily and involuntarily. The brain occupies the center of this information management system (nervous system) and consumes a great deal of energy and oxygen through a large blood supply to maintain this function. The information transduction of the nervous system is executed through the electrical conduction of membrane action potentials and chemical transmission at the synapses. Metabolic disorders such as

Y. Takikawa (✉) • H. Kuroda • K. Sawara
Division of Hepatology, Department of Internal Medicine, Iwate Medical University, 19-1 Uchimaru, Morioka 020-8505, Japan
e-mail: ytakikaw@iwate-med.ac.jp

H. Ohira (ed.), *The Liver in Systemic Diseases*, DOI 10.1007/978-4-431-55790-6_4

hypoglycemia and hyperammonemia due to liver failure perturb the energy supply and the information transduction of the brain nervous system and cause various brain disorders which are represented by hepatic encephalopathy (HE).

4.1 The Functional Structure of the Normal Brain

4.1.1 Cell Types and Blood Flow Regulation

The main types of cells in the brain are neurons and glial cells. The neuron is the basic functional unit of the nervous system. Glial cells are auxiliary cells that pass nutrients transported via cerebral capillaries to the neurons thereby facilitating their smooth function. Although glial cells continue to divide and proliferate throughout the entirety of their lives, cell division permanently ceases in neurons once their differentiation from neural stem cells is complete. After completing differentiation during the embryonic stage, most neurons remain viable until the death of the organism.

The human brain comprises approximately 2 % of the adult body weight but consumes about 15 % of the cardiac output and represents approximately 20 % of the body's oxygen demand [1]. A renowned feature of blood circulation in the brain, which is distinct from that in other organs, is the self-regulation function known as autoregulation [2, 3]. The regulation of cerebral blood flow (CBF) is mediated by changes in the diameter of cerebral arteries and ultimately depends on the contraction or relaxation responses of arterial smooth muscles. Aside from arterial contraction, there is also a secondary decrease in CBF due to changes that occur because of an increase in the venous pressure or passive pressure placed on the intracerebral parenchyma capillary beds and the venous vascular beds. Furthermore, among the cerebral arteries, the arteries of the pia matter and the arterioles of the intracerebral parenchyma are involved in physiologically regulating CBF. Both types of arteries have roles in maintaining the autoregulation of CBF through neurogenic regulation.

4.1.2 Neurons: Structure and Function

4.1.2.1 Dendrites, Cell Bodies, Axons, and Their Connections

The major function of neurons is to receive, integrate, and transmit information to other cells [4]. A neuron consists of three parts: dendrites, which are elongated processes that receive information from the environment or from other neurons; the cell body, which contains the nucleus; and the axon, which may be up to 1 m in length and which conducts impulses to muscles, glands, or other neurons (Fig. 4.1.). Most neurons are multipolar, containing one axon and several dendrites. Axons and

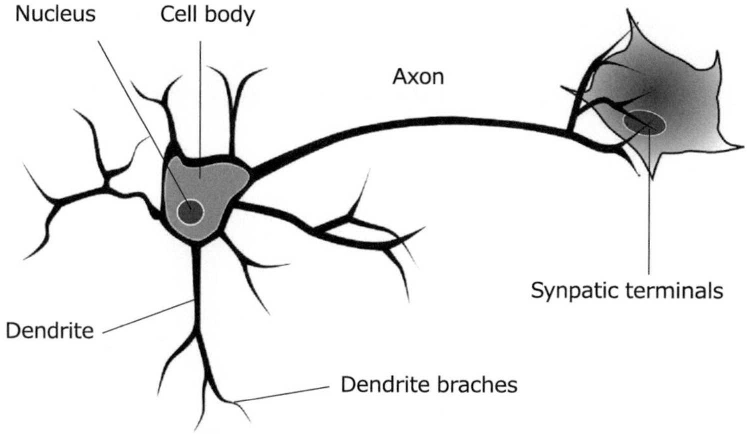

Fig. 4.1 The structure of a typical neuron. A typical neuron in a vertebrate consists of three major regions: a cell body, a dendrite, and an axon

dendrites usually branch extensively at their ends. Dendritic branching can be very complex, with the result that a single neuron may receive thousands of inputs. Axonal branching allows several target cells to simultaneously receive a message from a single neuron. Each branch of the axon terminates on the next cell at a synapse, which is a structure specialized for the transfer of information from the axon to muscle tissue, glands, or another neuron.

4.1.2.2 Synapses

A synapse is where two neurons communicate electrically or chemically [5, 6]. A chemical synapse is a small gap that exists between the axonal terminals of one neuron and the dendrites of another, into which neurotransmitters are released. At an electrical synapse, two neurons are physically connected to each other via gap junctions. Gap junctions make it possible for an electrical signal in one neuron to pass directly to another.

4.1.2.3 Signals and Impulses: The Action Potentials

The electrical signal moves through the neuron as a result of changes in the electrical charge of the axon. Normally, the axon remains in the resting potential, a state in which the interior of the neuron contains a greater number of negatively charged ions than the area outside the cell. If the electrical signal from the dendrites is strong enough that it passes a certain level or threshold, when it stimulates the segment of the axon that is closest to the cell body, the cell membrane in this first segment opens its gates, allowing positively charged Na^+, which were previously

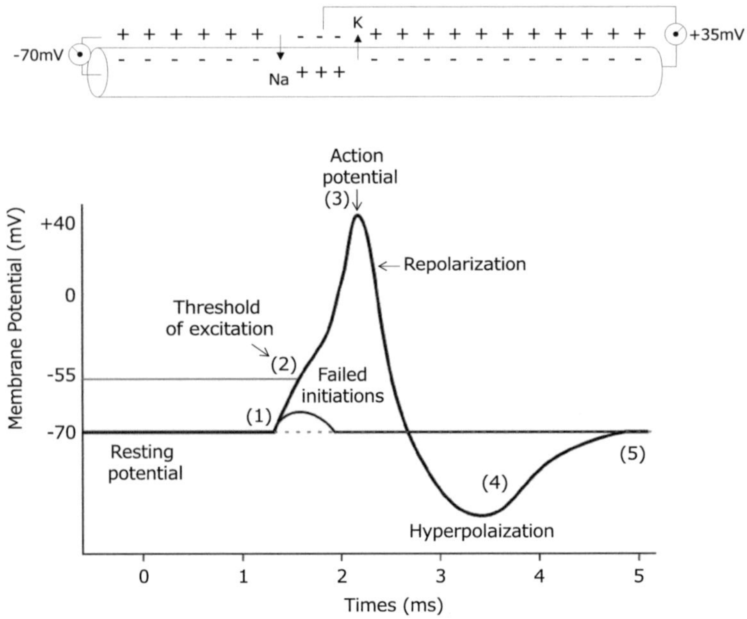

Fig. 4.2 The formation of an action potential can be divided into five steps. (1) A stimulus from a sensory cell or another neuron causes the target cell to depolarize toward the threshold potential. (2) If the threshold of excitation is reached, all of the Na^+ channels open and the membrane depolarizes. (3) At the peak action potential, the K^+ channels open, and K^+ begins to leave the cell. At the same time, the Na^+ channels close. (4) The membrane becomes hyperpolarized as K^+ ions continue to leave the cell. The hyperpolarized membrane is in a refractory period and cannot fire. (5) The K^+ channels close, and the Na^+/K^+ transporter restores the resting potential

were kept out to enter. This change in electrical charge that occurs in a neuron when a nerve impulse is transmitted is known as the action potential. Once the action potential occurs, the number of positive ions exceeds the number of negative ions in this segment, and the segment temporarily becomes positively charged. Figure 4.2 depicts the formation of an action potential.

4.1.2.4 Membrane Potentials and Ligand-Gated and Voltage-Gated Ion Channels

The membrane potentials may be altered by increasing the permeability of the membrane to another ion, which drives the resting membrane potential toward the equilibrium potential for that ion. Neurons are highly specialized to use rapid changes in the membrane potentials to generate electrical signals. This is accomplished by ligand-gated and voltage-gated ion channels which allow the passage of Na^+, K^+, Ca^{2+}, or Cl^- ions in response to electrical or chemical stimuli [6]. These channels are composed of protein complexes that are embedded in the lipid membrane to form aqueous pores to the inside of the cell. In general, the channels are selective for a particular species of ion. An array of charged amino acids within voltage-dependent channels detects changes in voltage and induces a conformational change in the channel to alter ion permeability.

4.1.2.5 Neurotransmitters

When an electrical impulse from an action potential reaches the end of the axon, it signals the terminal buttons to release neurotransmitters, such as glutamate, γ-aminobutyric acid (GABA), glycine, or acetylcholine, into the synapse. A neurotransmitter is a chemical that relays signals across the synapses between neurons. Neurotransmitters travel across the synaptic space between the terminal buttons of one neuron to the dendrites of the neighboring neurons, where they bind to specific receptors. Furthermore, different terminal buttons release different neurotransmitters, and different dendrites are particularly sensitive to different neurotransmitters. The dendrites will only respond to the neurotransmitters if they are of a shape that fit into the receptor sites on the receiving neuron. For this reason, the receptor sites and neurotransmitters are often compared to a lock and key.

4.1.3 Glial Cells

4.1.3.1 Astrocytes

Astrocytes provide a variety of metabolic, immunologic, structural, and nutritional support functions that are required for normal neuronal function. They possess numerous processes that radiate from the cell body, surrounding blood vessels and covering the surfaces of the brain and spinal cord. Astrocytes have voltage- and ligand-gated ion channels that help to regulate K^+ and Ca^{2+} concentrations within the interstitial space. Many synapses are invested with astrocytic processes, and this allows astrocytes to modulate neurotransmission by regulating extracellular concentrations of these cations. Astrocytes provide structural and trophic support for neurons through the production of extracellular matrix molecules such as laminin and through release of growth factors such as nerve growth factor, fibroblast growth factors, and brain-derived neurotrophic factor. The astrocytic foot processes in the blood vessels provide sites for the release of cytokines and chemoattractants during central nervous system (CNS) injury. The astrocytes respond to brain injury by increasing in size—and in some cases in number—through a process called reactive astrocytosis. This phenotypic change is characterized by an increase in cells expressing glial-fibrillary acidic protein and by the synthesis and release of cytokines that regulate inflammatory responses and the entry of hematogenous cells into the CNS. Astrocytes also play an important role in terminating neuronal responses to glutamate, the most abundant excitatory neurotransmitter in the brain [7]. The glutamate transporters that are present on astrocyte cell membranes remove glutamate from the synapse. Astrocytes also contain glutamine synthetase, which converts glutamate to glutamine, detoxifying the CNS of both glutamate and ammonia.

4.1.3.2 Oligodendrocytes

The main functions of oligodendrocytes are to provide support and insulation to axons in the CNS of some vertebrates, equivalent to the function performed by Schwann cells in the peripheral nervous system. The plasma membrane of oligodendrocytes in the CNS and Schwann cells in the peripheral nervous system envelops axons. For many axons, the membranes of these glial cells are wrapped layer upon layer around the axon, forming a myelin sheath. Gaps form between the myelin sheaths of neighboring glia, forming nodes of Ranvier, where a small portion of the axon is exposed to the interstitial space and where voltage-dependent Na^+ channels are clustered in the axonal membrane. Between the nodes, myelin insulates the axon from the extracellular space, allowing the efficient spread of depolarization from one node to another. This allows action potentials to propagate rapidly by jumping from node to node in a process called saltatory conduction [8].

4.1.3.3 Microglia

Although peripheral blood lymphocytes and monocytes enter from the circulation and patrol the CNS, the resident microglia function as the main immune effector cells. It appears that they are derived from bone marrow precursors of the macrophage-monocyte lineage and that they invade the CNS during the perinatal period. Microglial cells are activated by brain injury, infection, or neuronal degeneration. Activation is characterized by proliferation; migration into damaged tissue; the increased or de novo expression of surface receptors, including CD45 (leukocyte common antigen), major histocompatibility complex class I and II antigens, and immunoglobulin Fc receptors; and the secretion of several cytokines, reactive oxygen intermediates, and proteinases. This response functions to remove dead tissue and destroy invading organisms, but it may also contribute to damage of CNS, particularly in certain inflammatory and degenerative diseases the CNS.

4.1.4 The Neurovascular Unit (NVU) and the Blood-Brain Barrier (BBB)

The neural regulation of the microcirculation and metabolism is performed by the functional neurovascular unit (NVU), which is composed of vascular, astroglial, and neuronal cells.

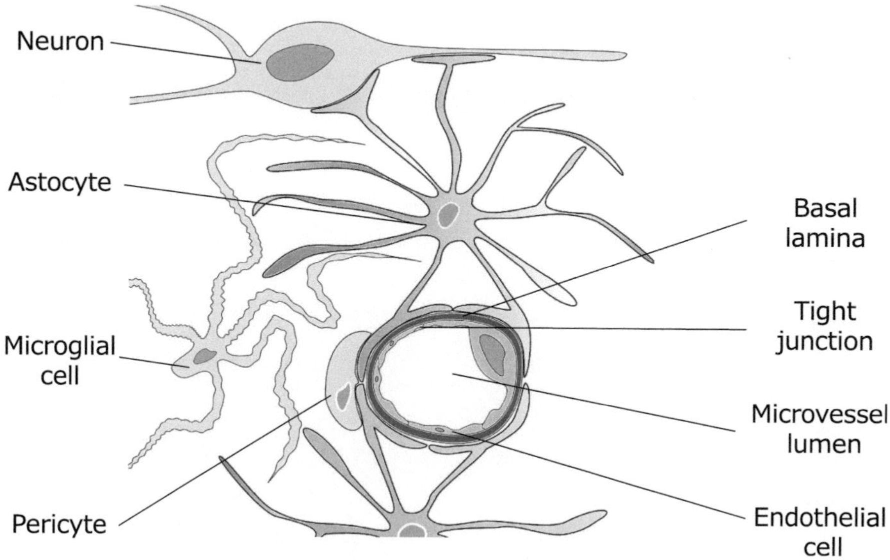

Fig. 4.3 The neurovascular unit (NVU)

4.1.4.1 NVU Structure

The NVU, which is based on neurons and brain microcirculation, comprehensively encompasses the cerebral functions and is the conceptual framework required to understand the diseases that are caused by brain ischemia. The major structural elements of the NVU include the microvasculature/endothelial cells, the neurons, and the astrocytes, which represent the glial system of the cells which acts as an intermediary between the two brain areas (Fig. 4.3) [9, 10].

4.1.4.2 Blood Flow Controlled by Astrocytes

The CBF is thought to mainly be controlled by astrocyte activation through the function of the NVU. Glutamate and K^+ released from neurons in association with enhanced nervous activity act on astrocytes to cause vascular contraction or dilatation via astrocytic foot processes, thereby regulating CBF. Currently, 50 % of the functional hyperemia that occurs alongside neural functional hyperactivity is thought to be astrocyte dependent. Synaptically released glutamate acts on both neurons and astrocytes. In neurons, glutamate attaches to N-methyl-d-aspartate (NMDA) receptors to raise neuronal Ca^{2+}, causing neuronal nitric oxide synthetase to release nitric oxide, which acts via soluble guanylate cyclase and cyclic guanosine monophosphate in smooth muscle cells to dilate blood vessels. Raised Ca^{2+} may also generate arachidonic acid (AA), which is converted to vasodilatory prostaglandins (PGs). In astrocytes, glutamate raises Ca^{2+} by activating

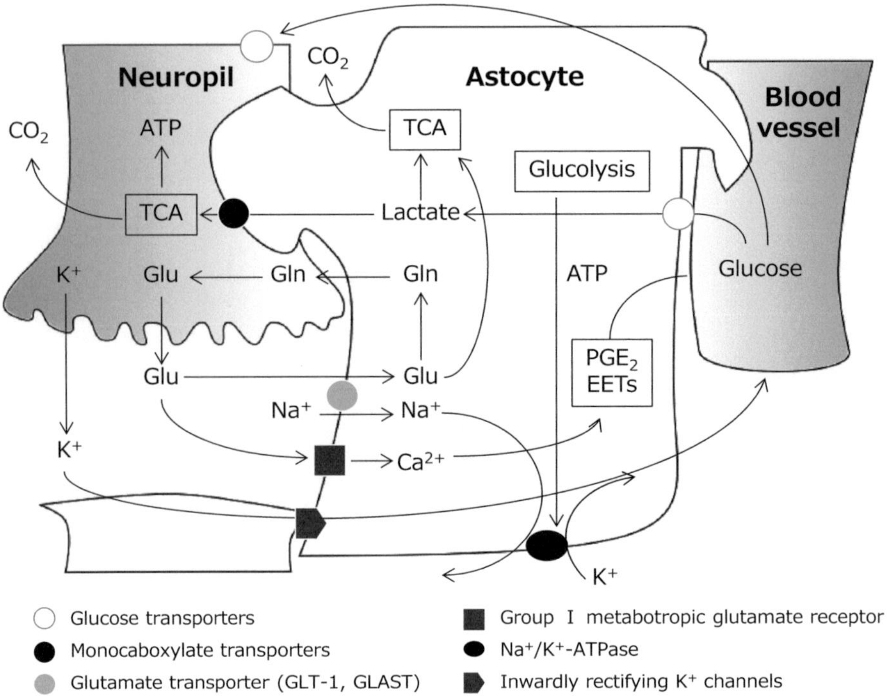

Fig. 4.4 The roles of astrocytes in the regulation of CBF in response to neuronal activation and metabolic demand

metabotropic glutamate receptors, generating AA and three types of AA metabolites. PGs and epoxyeicosatrienoic acids (EETs) in astrocytes dilate vessels, while 20-hydroxyeicosatetraenoic acid in smooth muscle constricts vessels. Voltage-dependent, Ca^+-activated K^+ or bradykinin channels are expressed highly in astrocytic foot processes, with higher densities in areas that are close to synapses and blood vessels. These channels are also activated by EETs. The activation of these channels following glutamate-induced increases in Ca^+ and EET results in the rapid efflux of K^+ into the perivascular space. Increases in extracellular K^+ can lead to vasodilation (and in higher concentrations, paradoxically, vasoconstriction) (Fig. 4.4) [11].

4.1.4.3 Metabolic Coupling Between Neurons and Astrocytes

In 1994, Pellerin and Magistretti showed that lactic acid production increases when glutamate is added to cultured astrocytes and proposed that glucose supplied through blood vessels may constitute a functional metabolic compartment between astrocytes and neurons, in which lactic acid serves as an energy substrate for neurons [12]. Glutamate is released as a result of neural activity and is absorbed

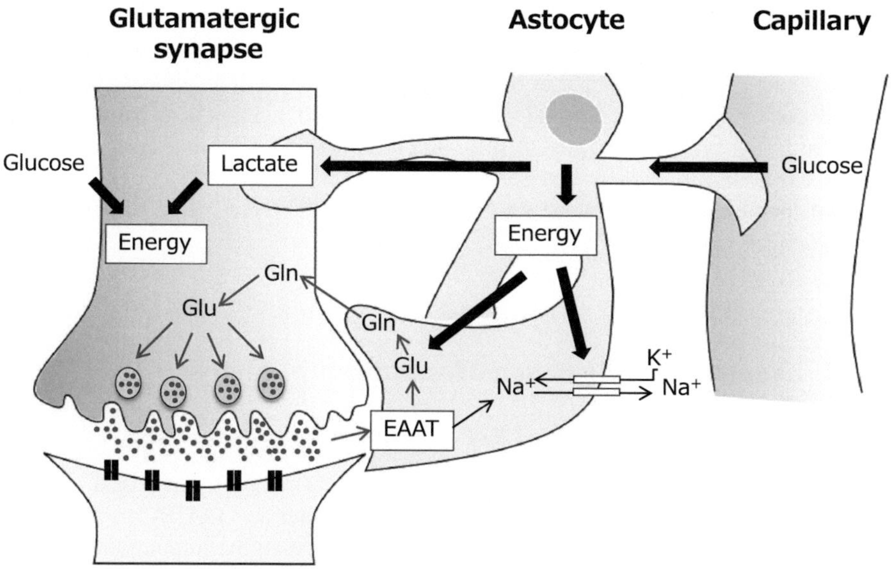

Fig. 4.5 A revised coupling between synaptic activity and glucose metabolism

via a Na^+-dependent glutamate transporter facilitated by astrocytes. The Na^+/K^+-ATPase is activated to maintain the Na^+ concentration gradient during transportation, with ATP supplied mainly from the glycolytic pathway. Lactic acid is transported from astrocytes to neurons by a monocarboxylate transporter and is then consumed as an energy substrate through the TCA cycle. Therefore, glutamate not only regulates CBF but also simultaneously acts as a signal to supply an energy substrate (Fig. 4.5) [13, 14].

4.1.4.4 Disruption of the BBB

The blood-brain barrier (BBB) restricts the transportation of substances into the brain and serves as a protection mechanism. The BBB is composed of vascular endothelial cells which are attached to each other by horizontal adhesion, mainly via tight junctions, the extracellular matrix (ECM) lying outside the endothelial cells, and the astrocytic foot processes that cover the entire capillary lying on the outside of the ECM. The breakdown of the BBB and the subsequent invasion of the brain by inflammatory cells are important pathological factors in cerebrospinal diseases. Protection of the BBB specifically means the protection of endothelial cells and also the protection of the NVUs, including the astrocytic foot processes. In NVUs, glucose is broken down into lactic acid in the astroglia. Lactic acid is then supplied to neurons, allowing the establishment of an efficient metabolic environment for ATP synthesis [15]. Furthermore, the glycolytic pathway of the astroglia reduces oxidative stress through the pentose phosphate pathway [16]. In addition, in fatty acid metabolism, lactic acid is used as a substrate for the synthesis of ketone bodies (KB) in the astroglia and has been suggested to serve as an energy substrate for neurons [17]. The possibilities of using the KB substrate as an alternative energy source during ischemic neuronal damage and of enhancing the neuroprotective effect of KBs have been suggested, although their significance under physiological conditions remains unclear. Overall, the BBB restriction may be regarded as a cellular metabolic compartment for NVU protection wherein astrocytes appear to play a central role.

4.1.5 Neurotransmitters and Mechanisms of Signal Transmission

Neurotransmitters are endogenous chemicals that transmit signals across a synapse from one neuron to another "target" neuron. Glutamate and GABA are the main excitatory and inhibitory neurotransmitter, respectively, in the mammalian cortex. Changes in glutamate and GABA metabolism play important roles in the control of cortical excitability.

4.1.5.1 Membrane Potentials, Ion Channels, and Gating

An action potential arises primarily from voltage-dependent changes in membrane permeability to Na^+ and K^+. If a depolarizing stimulus raises the membrane potential to approximately −45 mV, voltage-gated Na^+ channels open, allowing an influx of Na+ and further depolarization toward the equilibrium potential for sodium (+50 mV). The nearby areas of the membrane are depolarized to the threshold for Na^+ channel activation, propagating a wave of depolarization from the initial site. The resting potential is restored quickly by a combination of events. First, the Na^+ channels close rapidly and remain in an inactive state until the membrane potential returns to a lower level for several milliseconds. The voltage-dependent K^+ channels open as the membrane potential peaks, speeding the efflux of K^+ from the cells and driving the membrane potential back to the equilibrium potential for K^+. The K^+ channels are also inactivated but more slowly than Na^+ channels, and this may transiently hyperpolarize cells. Plasma membrane ion exchangers and ion pumps then counteract the ion fluxes and eventually restore the resting state.

Neurons transmit signals chemically to other cells at the synapses. Presynaptic and postsynaptic cells are electrically isolated from each other and separated by a narrow synaptic cleft. Signaling across the cleft occurs through the release of neurotransmitters from the terminal of the presynaptic neuron. Most neurotransmitters are stored in membrane-bound synaptic vesicles and are released into the synaptic cleft by Ca^{2+}-dependent exocytosis. The depolarization of the nerve terminal opens the voltage-gated Ca^{2+} channels, stimulating the influx of Ca^{2+} and the release of neurotransmitter. Neurotransmitter diffuses across the cleft and bind to receptors on ligand-gated ion channels, which are concentrated on the postsynaptic membrane. This produces local permeability changes, altering the membrane potential of the postsynaptic cell. If the response is depolarizing, then an action potential may be generated if there are enough voltage-gated Na^{+} channels located nearby and if the membrane potential has been raised to the threshold for their activation. Receptor-gated ion channels are highly selective for a particular neurotransmitter and for the type of ions that they allow to pass, which determine whether they generate excitatory or inhibitory responses.

4.1.5.2 Glutamate and Na^{+} or Ca^{2+} Ion Channels

Glutamate is a powerful excitatory neurotransmitter that is released by nerve cells in the brain. It opens the cation channels to allow the influx of Na^{+} or Ca^{2+} and generates a depolarizing excitatory postsynaptic potential [18]. Glutamate is responsible for sending signals between nerve cells and plays an important role in learning and memory under normal conditions.

Glutamate is released from vesicles in presynaptic terminals by a Ca^{2+}-dependent mechanism. The glutamate concentration within the vesicle is thought to be ~100 mmol/L; the release of a single vesicle produces an excitatory postsynaptic potential that is primarily related to the activation of α-amino-3-hydroxy-5-methyl-4-isoxazolepropionic acid receptor.

4.1.5.3 GABA and Glycine and Cl^{-} Ion Channels

GABA and glycine are arguably the most important inhibitory neurotransmitters in the brain and brainstem/spinal cord, respectively. GABA is used at the great majority of fast inhibitory synapses in virtually every part of the brain [19]. Many sedative/tranquilizing drugs act by enhancing the effects of GABA, which is synthesized from glutamate in a reaction catalyzed by glutamate decarboxylase (GAD).

Glycine is the major inhibitory neurotransmitter in the brainstem and spinal cord, where it participates in a variety of motor and sensory functions [20]. Glycine is also present in the forebrain, where it has recently been shown to function as a co-agonist at the NMDA subtype of glutamate receptor. Glycine promotes the actions of glutamate, the major excitatory neurotransmitter. Thus, glycine underlies both inhibitory and excitatory functions within the CNS.

Inhibitory neurotransmitters such as GABA and glycine open the Cl^{-} channels and generate an inhibitory postsynaptic potential, keeping the postsynaptic membrane near the equilibrium potential for Cl^{-} (ECl = −70 mV).

4.1.5.4 Second Messengers, cAMP, and PKC

Not all neurotransmitter receptors are associated with ion channels; many receptors are coupled to cellular enzymes that regulate levels of intracellular second messengers to modulate the function of ion channels and many other cell proteins. A major mechanism by which the second messengers regulate ion channels is through the promotion of the phosphorylation of channel subunits. For example, the binding of the neurotransmitter norepinephrine to β-adrenergic receptors activates the enzyme adenylyl cyclase and stimulates the production of cyclic adenosine monophosphate (cAMP). The cAMP, in turn, activates a cAMP-dependent protein kinase that can phosphorylate voltage-gated Ca^{2+} channels. In many cases, this increases the duration of time that the channel remains open once it is activated, resulting in an increased influx of Ca^{2+} through the channel. Other neurotransmitter receptors, such as α_1-adrenergic, muscarinic cholinergic, or metabotropic glutamate receptors, are coupled to the enzyme phospholipase C, which catalyzes the hydrolysis of the membrane lipid phosphatidylinositol-4,5-bisphosphate. The binding of a neurotransmitter to the receptor activates phospholipase C to produce two second messengers: 1,2-diacylglycerol and inositol-1,4,5 trisphosphate. Diacylglycerol activates several enzymes of the protein kinase C (PKC) family, some of which phosphorylate ion channels either enhance or suppress their function. Inositol-1,4,5 trisphosphate binds an intracellular receptor that is itself a calcium ionophore, allowing release of calcium from intracellular stores into the cytosol. This calcium signal activates several calcium-dependent enzymes, including phosphatases and kinases that can alter the phosphorylation state and function of several ion channels and other cell proteins.

4.2 Hepatic Encephalopathy (HE)

4.2.1 The Concept and Classification of Hepatic Encephalopathy

HE is a generic term (syndrome) for neuropsychiatric symptoms that are mainly observed with consciousness disorders that repeatedly occur during the course of serious, acute, and chronic hepatic disorders. It includes consciousness disorders that range from mild disorders to severe disorders that result in a deep coma. HE is largely classified into the three types: type A or HE associated with acute liver failure (ALF) with coma, type B or HE associated with portal-systemic bypass without intrinsic hepatocellular disease, and type C or HE associated with cirrhosis and portal hyper tension or portal-systemic shunts. In addition, type C is further divided into several subcategories and subdivisions according to the severity, duration, and clinical course, as shown in Table 4.1 [21]. In the subcategory of cirrhosis type, minimal HE (MHE) is defined as a state with subtle abnormalities

Table 4.1 HE-type nomenclature subcategory subdivisions

Type	Nomenclature	Subcategory	Subdivisions
A (Acute) type	Encephalopathy associated with acute liver failure		
B (Bypass) type	Encephalopathy associated with portal-systemic bypass and no intrinsic hepatocellular disease		
C (Cirrhosis) type	Encephalopathy associated with cirrhosis and portal hypertension/or portal-systemic shunts	Episodic HE	Precipitated
		Persistent HE mild	Spontaneous[a]
		Minimal HE	Recurrent
			Mild
			Severe
			Treatment dependent

[a]Without recognized precipitating factors

that are only detected by the use of specific neuropsychometric and/or neurophysiological tools in cirrhosis patients with otherwise normal neurological examination results. MHE is clinically indicated by a lack of awareness and cognitive impairment and has been reportedly observed as a complication in approximately 30 % of cirrhosis patients [22]. MHE should be determined as a stage prior to overt encephalopathy, but it has not yet been clarified. However, there are reports including that overt HE corresponding of grade II or higher occurred in 23 % of cases within 6 months of initial diagnosis of MHE [23]. The diagnostic significance of MHE is to evaluate the decline in quality of life (QOL) [24], impairment of driving skills [25], the poor prognosis associated with cirrhosis [26], and other factors.

4.2.2 Diagnosis and Grade

In Japan, mental state diagnoses are made based on the Inuyama classification system. In contrast, Western countries base their diagnoses on the West Haven criteria (Table 4.2). In the clinical setting, however, it is difficult to diagnose and differentiate grade 0 to I. Amodio et al. suggested a method using the West Haven with a quantitative neuropsychological tests to diagnose grades I–IV [27, 28] (Table 4.3).

The following criteria are said to be required for an accurate diagnosis of)MHE: (1) an evaluation of QOL, including changes in the behavioral patterns of daily life, such as appetite, sleep, and physical activity; (2) an evaluation of mental state such as memory, concentration, cognition, and consciousness; (3) a quantitative neuropsychological testing; and (4) the presence of speech disorders, such as a lisp, along with an evaluation of cognitive activity disorders, such as reaction time, and space

Table 4.2 West Haven criteria for the semiquantitative grading of mental state

Grade 0	No abnormality detected
Grade I	Trivial lack of awareness
	Euphoria or anxiety
	Shortened attention span
	Impaired performance of addition
Grade II	Lethargy or apathy
	Minimal disorientation for time or place
	Subtle personality change
	Inappropriate behavior
	Impaired performance of subtraction
Grade III	Somnolence to semistupor but responsive to verbal stimuli
	Confusion
	Gross disorientation
Grade IV	Coma (unresponsive to verbal or noxious stimuli)

Table 4.3 Suggested modification of the West Haven criteria for the grading of the mental state of patients with cirrhosis

Grade	Proposed operative definition
I	Not able to complete TMT-A [a] in 120 s
	(Individuals with ≥5 years of education) or naming ≤7 animals in 120 s
	Orientated in time and space
II	Disorientated in time: (≥3 items incorrect)
	Day of the week
	Day of the month
	The month
	The year
	Orientated in place
III	Disorientated in place: (≥2 items incorrect)
	State/country
	Region/county
	City
	Place
	Floor/ward
	Disorientated in time and reduction of Glasgow score (8–14)
IV	Coma, unable to test mental state
	Unresponsive to pain stimuli
	(Glasgow score <8)

recognition [27]. However, it is difficult to perform such a comprehensive diagnosis in everyday clinical practice; thus, the early objective diagnosis of slight abnormalities in neurological function is generally attempted with a combination of quantitative neuropsychological tests (Table 4.4). Moreover, attempts have been made to use 3.0 Tesla magnetic resonance imaging (MRI) and magnetic resonance

Table 4.4 Clinical examinations for the diagnosis of minimal hepatic encephalopathy

Quantitative neuropsychological tests
WAIS (Wechsler adult intelligence scale)
Number connection test A (NCT-A), number connection test B (NCT-B)
Digit symbol test (DST), block design test (BDT), etc.
Electrophysiology tests
Electroencephalogram (EEG)
Evoked potentials (EP), P300 wave
Flicker frequency test (CFF test)
Noninvasive brain functional imaging and spectroscopy
Magnetic resonance imaging (MRI, functional MRI)
Magnetic resonance spectroscopy (MRS)
Positron-emission tomography (PET)

analysis (MRS) for the minimally invasive detection of metabolic disturbances in the brain from increases in glutamine and declines in myoinositol in the brain [29].

4.2.3 Pathogenic Mechanism

Although it is difficult to explain the pathogenic activity of HE via a single mechanism, toxic substances derived from the intestinal tract are believed to be the greatest pathogenic factor. With hepatic failure or portosystemic shunts, it is believed that toxic substances that are derived from intestinal tract and which should be detoxified in the liver flow into the systemic circulation and pass the BBB, thereby inhibiting brain function (Fig. 4.6).

The representative neurotoxic substance which is derived from the intestinal tract is ammonia. Most studies on ammonia investigate the toxicity mechanism. Some of the proposed mechanisms include (1) the inhibitory effects on the blood-brain barrier, the transport system, and amino acid metabolism; (2) the inhibitory effects on energy metabolism, glycometabolism, and blood flow; (3) the inhibitory effects on the neurotransmitting action; and (4) the effects on morphological changes in astrocytes. Moreover, in addition to these neurotoxicities, it is believed that ammonia causes a range of conditions including cerebral edema, pseudo-neurotransmitter and amino acid imbalance, and abnormalities in GABA and benzodiazepine (BZ) receptor complex, which work in combination, leading to the onset of encephalopathy.

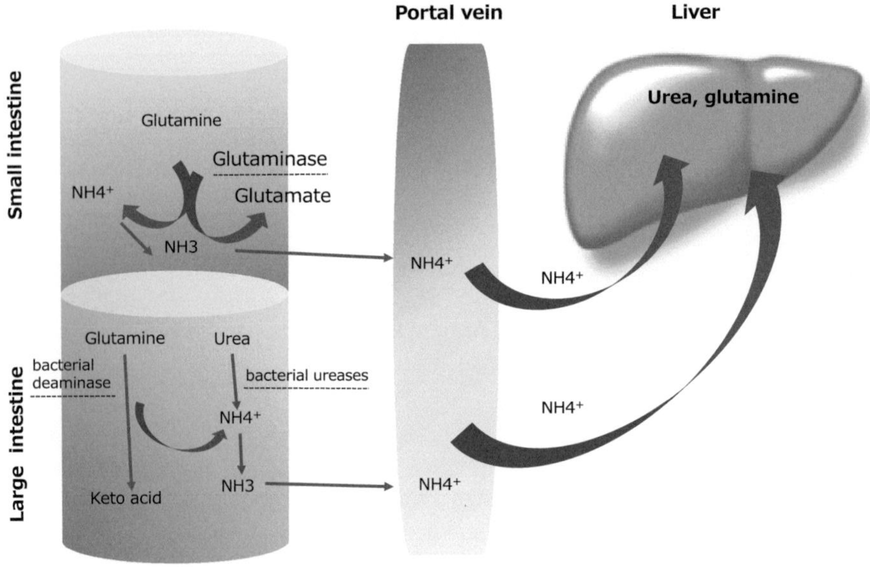

Fig. 4.6 Ammonia metabolism in the intestinal tract with the portal vein and liver

4.2.3.1 Neurotoxicity of Ammonia

Disturbance of the BBB, Transport System, and Amino Acid Metabolism

Ammonia inside the brain is metabolized by the conversion of glutamate into glutamine by glutamine synthetase in astrocytes. Within the astrocytes, ammonia processing causes a decline in glutamate (Fig. 4.7). Furthermore, it is believed that the glutaminase inhibitory effect, due to ammonia, is involved in the decline of glutamate inside the brain. Glutamate is an excitatory synaptic transmitter, and it is believed that hyperammonemia and the decline in glutamate that accompanies ammonia processing are the primary causes of encephalopathy.

Simple diffusion due to the configuration of gas is considered regarding the migration of ammonia into the brain tissue [30]; however, ammonia permeability into the BBB is said to be promoted in chronic hepatic failure. Astrocytes produce inflammatory cytokines such as tumor necrosis factor (TNF), interleukin-1 (IL-1), interleukin-6 (IL-6), etc., and these are said to increase the vascular permeability of vascular endothelial cells, thereby promoting the inflow of ammonia into the astrocytes [31].

Moreover, in cerebral cortexes with chronic hepatic failure, it is believed that increased glutamine resulting from ammonia detoxification inhibits glutamine synthetase by providing feedback, thereby disabling the detoxification of ammonia, and subsequently further accelerating the increase in ammonia level [32]. That is, it is believed that when hyperammonemia is observed in chronic hepatic failure and cirrhosis cases, the activity of ammonia metabolism-related enzymes has already

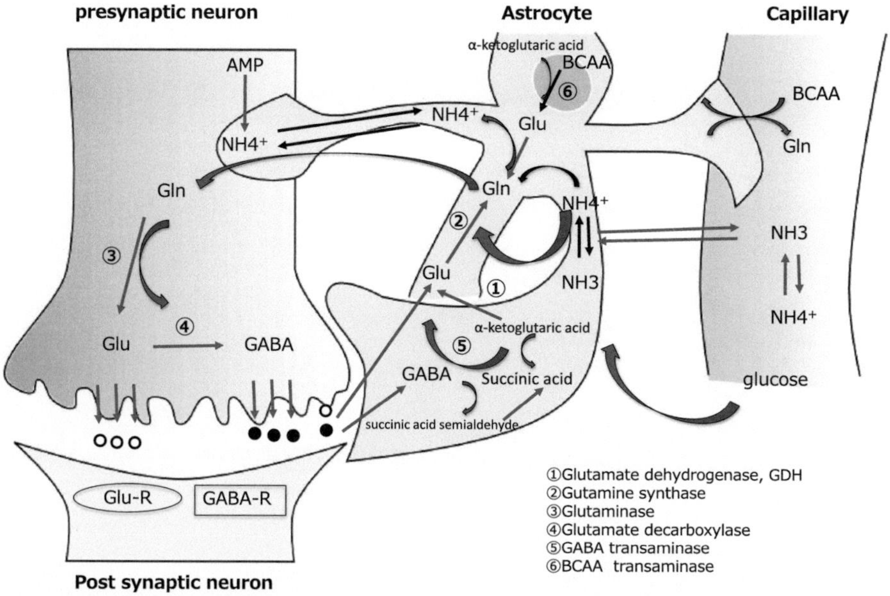

Fig. 4.7 Ammonia metabolism in the brain

reached its maximum, with a state induced in which ammonia metabolism cannot be efficiently controlled.

Disturbance of Energy Metabolism, Glucose Metabolism, and Blood Flow

It has been proven by both experimental and clinical studies that hyperammonemia inhibits energy metabolism, glucose metabolism, and blood flow inside the brain [33, 34]. This trend is particularly strong in the reticular activating system and cerebral cortex and is believed to be involved in consciousness disorders and higher cortical dysfunction in HE.

Regarding the effects of hyperammonemia on energy metabolism, it is surmised that the malate shuttle, which is a pathway for supplying nicotinamide adenine dinucleotide (NADH), which is produced in the glycolytic pathway to the oxidative phosphorylation system inside the mitochondria, is suppressed by ammonia. In this way, a decline in the adenosine triphosphate (ATP) level and the ATP/adenosine diphosphate (ADP) ratio along with an increase in NADH/nicotinamide adenine dinucleotide ($NAD^{+)}$ ratio in the brain is said to occur. Moreover, a mechanism has been considered in which α−ketoglutarate, which is the matrix of the tricarboxylic acid (TCA) cycle, becomes amidated to process excessive ammonia, which is converted to glutamate and glutamine, thereby decreasing the matrix of the TCA cycle and decreasing the production of ATP (Fig. 4.8) [35, 36].

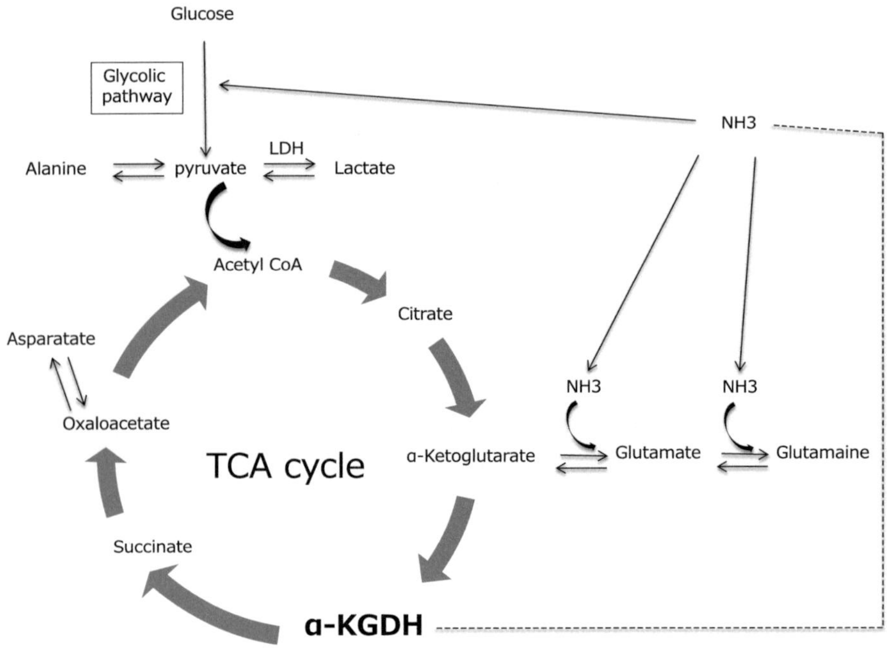

Fig. 4.8 The potential effect of ammonia on glucose metabolism. A schematic representation of the potential effects of ammonia on glucose metabolism. Ammonia stimulates the amidation of glutamine synthetase and possibly α-ketoglutarate (*solid arrows*) leading to the increased synthesis of glutamine. Ammonia has also been shown to inhibit the enzyme α-ketoglutarate dehydrogenase α-KGDH (*dashed line*) and to enhance the activity of glycolytic enzymes

In a clinical study, 2-deoxy-2-[fluorine-18]fluoro-D-glucose computed tomography (FDG PET) indicated a decrease in glycometabolism in the cerebral cortex of cirrhosis patients. This, in combination with decreased blood flow in the cerebral cortex, was suggested in the evaluation of cerebral blood flow using ^{15}O-water [37].

Disturbance of Neurotransmitters

It has been proven by experimental studies that ammonia promotes the transmission of the inhibitory system in the synapses of the brain, thereby inhibiting excitatory transmission [38]. Inhibitory postsynaptic potential (IPSP) is caused by an inhibitory transmitter (GABA or glycine), which affects the receptors of GABA or glycine and opens the Cl^- channels of the receptors. It has been confirmed by an experimental study that the ammonia load causes postsynaptic inhibition to make the equilibrium potential of IPSP close to the resting membrane potential [39]. Excitatory postsynaptic potential (EPSP) is generated by excitatory neurotransmitters (glutamate and asparagine), which affect their receptors, thereby increasing permeability with respect to Na^+, K^+ ions. Ammonia is said to electrictrophysiologically inhibit the transmission of EPSP.

The Effects of Astrocyte and Neuron Morphology

In addition to supporting cells in the central nervous system, astrocytes play a role in forming neurovascular units with nerve cells and vascular structures, thereby functioning as part of the BBB and supporting the metabolism of nerve cells. Norenberg et al. [40] loaded encephalopathy-inducing substances, mainly ammonia, in astrocyte culture media, and observed the resulting morphological change. The authors reported the occurrence of Alzheimer type II changes in the astrocytes, which were characterized by an expanded and vacuolated nucleus, increased chromatin of the cell border, the protrusion of the nucleolus, and swelling. Moreover, Gregorios et al. [41] observed the effect of ammonia on the morphology of astrocytes under light and electron microscopy and proved that the degree of change in the astrocytes was affected by the duration of exposure to ammonia. Moreover, it is believed that the abovementioned permeability of the BBB resulted in further migration of ammonia into the astrocytes, thereby further aggravating the swelling of astrocytes.

It was suggested that the morphological changes and the swelling of astrocytic lead to the dysfunction of the astrocytes and, further, the decline in the function of the neurovascular unit. Based on these findings, it is believed that the onset of encephalopathy occurs due to gliopathy.

4.2.3.2 Effects of Ammonia on Cerebral Edema

Cerebral edema and increased intracranial pressure are very serious and life-threatening complications that are observed in patients with acute hepatic failure. The onset of cerebral edema is considered to be caused by a vasogenic factor due to the disruption of the BBB and abnormal ionic exchanges in the neuron and the astrocyte cell membrane [42]. As noted previously, it is believed that ammonia both promotes the permeability of the BBB and increases glutamine which is produced through the metabolism of ammonia. It is believed that glutamine has a strong osmotic pressure effect and that is involved in the increase the volume of fluid in the brain. The increased glutamine in the brain has also been confirmed in patients with minimal HE that abnormalities in substance metabolism occur within the brain in the early stages after the onset of encephalopathy [29].

4.2.3.3 Pseudo-neurotransmitters, Amino Acid Imbalance, γ-Aminobutyric Acid, and Abnormalities in GABA and BZ

During hepatic encephalopathy branched chain amino acids (BCAA) are ,consumed by the muscles via the metabolism of ammonia; as a result, an imbalance of amino acids in the blood, particularly decreases in BCAA and increases in the aromatic amino acids (AAA), is observed [43]. The migration of AAA in the brain via the BBB competes with BCAA. It is thus hypothesized that excessive AAA migrates inside the brain during HE. As a result, the presence of excessive AAA inside the brain inhibits the generation of norepinephrine, dopamine, and other catecholamines (which are neurotransmitters) and instead promotes the production of β-hydroxide sympathomimetic amines (which are pseudo-neurotransmitters), such as octopamine, β-phenylethanolamine, and serotonin. This process is believed to be one of the causes of HE. Moreover, Schafer et al. [44] proposed that GABA, an inhibitory neurotransmitter in the central nerves, that is generated in the intestinal tract migrates inside the systemic circulation via portal-systemic shunts and is transported inside the brain, thereby inhibiting neurotransmission through the activation of GABA agonistic neurons. In subsequent studies, it was clarified that GABA receptors bond with benzodiazepine (BZ) in addition to GABA. That is, it is believed that GABA receptors are a complex of receptors for a range of substances including GABA, BZ, and barbiturates, which is linked through a Cl^- channel. Inhibitory signals are transmitted when the Cl^- channel opens as a result of GABA or BZ bonding to the receptors. Through this mechanism, many substances (in addition to GABA itself) such as endogenous GABA-like substances and BZ-like substances are assumed to activate GABA neurons [45]. Recently, it has been hypothesized that neuro-steroids, the level of which increase due to inflammation and oxidative stress, ultimately activate the GABA and BZ receptor systems [46].

4.2.4 *Treatment*

The fundamental causes of HE including acute or chronic hepatocyte dysfunction and portosystemic shunts are not easily resolved by medical therapy alone. Chronic HE develops when some additional triggers overlie these fundamental causes, such as constipation, a high-protein diet, and gastrointestinal bleeding, which are the therapeutic targets of medical treatment.

Moreover, while there is room for discussion regarding the choice of active therapeutic intervention with respect to MHE, when cases are believed to be in the stage prior to overt encephalopathy, it is important that any improvements should be carefully considered if hyperammonemia is observed.

4.2.4.1 Synthetic Disaccharides (Lactulose and Lactitol)

Synthetic disaccharides are administered with the object of inhibiting the production and absorption of ammonia in the intestinal tract. Synthetic disaccharides are led to the large intestine without being absorbed by the small intestine. Due to β-galactosidase, which is produced by enteric bacteria, lactulose is hydrolyzed to galactose and fructose, while lactitol is hydrolyzed to galactose and sorbitol, ultimately becoming organic acids (e.g., lactic acid, acetic acid). The following factors are believed to have a role in the decline of ammonia: (1) the inhibited growth of urease-producing bacteria accompanying decreased pH in the large intestine that occurs due to the production of organic acids suc, (2) the ionization of ammonia (NH3) to $NH4^{+}$ due to the decreased pH in the large intestine, which results in decreased absorption from the intestinal tract membrane, and (3) the promotion of intestinal movement due to the production of organic acids and the increase in water content and the shortening of the transit time of the intestinal tract content due to osmotic diarrhea.

4.2.4.2 Minimally Absorbed Antibiotics

Minimally absorbed antibiotics are administered with the objective of inhibiting the growth of gram-negative bacillus, which is an ammonia-producing bacterium that is found inside the intestinal tract, along with inhibiting the breakdown of glutamine in the small intestine.

Rifaximin, which is a rifamycin antimicrobial, is widely used for the treatment of HE. It has been shown to achieve a greater improvement of HE and hyperammonemia than lactitol. Moreover, with absorptivity of $<0.4\,\%$, it is not absorbed from the gastrointestinal tract into the blood, and it is associated with few side effects [47].

4.2.4.3 BCAA

Ammonia is metabolized in the process of generating glutamine from α-ketoglutarate and glutamate in the brain and skeletal muscles. This results in BCAA becoming conjugatively oxidized. Therefore, in cirrhosis and hyperammonemia, a vicious cycle occurs in which the serum BCAA concentration declines due to the promotion of BCAA consumption, thereby encouraging hyperammonemia. Furthermore, decline in serum BCAA promotes the transition of AAA inside the brain, where it causes an imbalance of amino acids, leading to an increase in the levels of pseudo-neurotransmitters. For these reasons, HE is treated with the oral and intravenous administration of a BCAA preparation.

4.2.4.4 Zinc

Ornithine transcarbamylase (OTC) is a zinc enzyme in the urea cycle. The liver acts as the principal organ in the metabolism of ammonia. Zinc is also involved in maintaining ammonia metabolism, through its promotion of the activation of glutamine synthetase of the skeletal muscles. Most of the ammonia that migrates inside the liver is processed via the urea cycle, with residual ammonia in the blood processed by glutamine synthetase. It is known that zinc is depleted during cirrhosis and that ammonia metabolism declines due to the reduced activity of the two enzymes. There are reports [48] which suggest that encephalopathy was improved by the oral administration of zinc acetate or zinc sulfate preparations, along with report [49] which indicates that the concomitant administration of synthetic disaccharides (as mentioned above) is effective in combination with BCAA granules.

4.2.4.5 Benzodiazepine Receptor Antagonist (Flumazenil)

Regarding HE, the administration of GABA-BZ receptor antagonist (flumazenil) has been attempted based on a report [44] which mentions the abnormalities that have been observed in the GABA-BZ receptor complex (see Sect. 4.2.3.2.), although its clinical effectiveness is still controversial [50].

4.2.4.6 Probiotics

The usefulness of probiotic preparations on MHE has been reported [51], with improvement in neuropsychiatric function event-related potential (P300) and ammonia concentration in the blood observed in patients who underwent treatment with a probiotic preparation alone and patients who used probiotics in combination with lactulose. Probiotics affect the intestinal flora inside the intestinal tract, causing a decline in the pathogenesis of urease-producing bacteria and thereby decreasing the production of toxic substances that are derived from the intestinal tract, in particular, ammonia.

4.2.4.7 Carnitine

Carnitine (CA) is a vitamin-like substance that plays an essential role in supplying fatty acids (long chain) inside the mitochondria when burning fat in vivo and producing energy. Cirrhosis is considered to be a state of CA deficiency because of insufficient absolute intake due to a protein-restricted diet, declined biosynthesis due to hepatocellular dysfunction, and declined internal storage due to declined skeletal muscle mass. The metabolic disturbance of CA is related to disorders in the urea cycle and TCA cycle in the mitochondria; such a decline may therefore ultimately lead to hyperammonemia. Malaguamera et al. [52] carried out a randomized, controlled, double-blind trial on HE patients and observed a significant improvement in the ammonia concentration in the blood along with improvement in cognitive function in 88 % of patients who received CA.

References

1. Hall JE. Guyton and hall textbook of medical physiology. 12th ed. New York: Saunders; 2011.
2. Paulson OB, Strandgaard S, Edvinsson L. Cerebral autoregulation. Cerebrovasc Brain Metab Rev. 1990;2(2):161–92.
3. Bruyn GW, Klawans HL, Vinken PJ, Vinken PJ, Klawans HL. Handbook of clinical neurology: vascular diseases v. 53: vascular diseases, vol 53 (Handbook of clinical neurology-revised Edition). 1st ed. Amsterdam: Elsevier Science Ltd; 1989.
4. Hammer GD, McPhee SJ. Pathophysiology of disease: an introduction to clinical medicine. 7th ed. New York: McGraw-Hill; 2014.
5. Schacter DL, Gilbert DT, Wegner DM. Psychology. 2nd ed. New York: Worth Publishers; 2011.
6. Purves D, Augustine GJ, Fitzpatrick D, Hall WC, LaMantia A-S, McNamara JO, White LE. Neuroscience. 4th ed. Sunderland: Sinauer Associates; 2007.
7. Santello M, Volterra A. Synaptic modulation by astrocytes via Ca2+-dependent glutamate release. Neuroscience. 2009;158(1):253–9.
8. Kettenmann H, Ransom BR. Neuroglia. 3rd ed. New York: Oxford University Press; 2012.
9. Zlokovic BV. The blood-brain barrier in health and chronic neurodegenerative disorders. Neuron. 2008;57(2):178–201.
10. Guo S, Lo EH. Dysfunctional cell-cell signaling in the neurovascular unit as a paradigm for central nervous system disease. Stroke. 2009;40(3 Suppl):S4–7.
11. Takahashi S, Abe T. Roles of astrocytes in the regulation of CBF in response to neuronal activation and metabolic demand. Cereb Blood Flow Metab Online J. 2005;17:150–5.
12. Pellerin L, Magistretti PJ. Glutamate uptake into astrocytes stimulates aerobic glycolysis: a mechanism coupling neuronal activity to glucose utilization. Proc Natl Acad Sci U S A. 1994;91(22):10625–9.
13. Valeur N, Clemmensen P, Saunamäki K, Grande P, DANAMI-2 investigators. The prognostic value of pre-discharge exercise testing after myocardial infarction treated with either primary PCI or fibrinolysis: a DANAMI-2 sub-study. Eur Heart J. 2005;26(2):119–27.
14. Magistretti PJ, Pellerin L, Rothman DL, Shulman RG. Energy on demand. Science. 1999;283 (5401):496–7.
15. Takahashi S, Abe T, Izawa Y, Iizumi T, Suzuki N. Roles of blood-brain barrier in neurovascular unit and cellular metabolic compartment. Cereb Blood Flow Metab Online J. 2013;24(2):75–82.
16. Takahashi S, Izawa Y, Suzuki N. Astroglial pentose phosphate pathway rates in response to high-glucose environments. ASN Neuro. 2012;4(2):71–88.
17. Guzmán M, Blázquez C. Is there an astrocyte-neuron ketone body shuttle? Trends Endocrinol Metab. 2001;12(4):169–73.
18. Meldrum BS. Glutamate as a neurotransmitter in the brain: review of physiology and pathology. J Nutr. 2000;130(4S Suppl):1007S–15.
19. Watanabe M, Maemura K, Kanbara K, Tamayama T, Hayasaki H. GABA and GABA receptors in the central nervous system and other organs. Int Rev Cytol. 2002;213:1–47.
20. López-Corcuera B, Geerlings A, Aragón C. Glycine neurotransmitter transporters: an update. Mol Membr Biol. 2001;18(1):13–20.

21. Ferenci P, Lockwood A, Mullen K, Tarter R, Weissenborn K. Hepatic encephalopathy-definition, nomenclature, diagnosis and quantification; final report of the working party at the 11th World Congress of Gastroenterology, Vienna, 1998. Hepatology. 2002;35(3):716–21.
22. Kato A, Tanaka H, Kawaguchi T, et al. Nutritional management contributes to improvement in minimal hepatic encephalopathy and quality of life in patients with liver cirrhosis: a preliminary, prospective, open-label study. Hepatol Res. 2013;43(5):452–8.
23. Kaneta H, Kato A, Suzuki K. Clinical manifestation of subclinical hepatic encephalopathy in patients with non-alcoholic cirrhosis. Hepatol Jpn. 1994;35:167–71.
24. Groeneweg M, Quero JC, De Bruijin I, et al. Subclinical hepatic encephalopathy impairs daily functioning. Hepatology. 1998;28(1):45–9.
25. Schomerous H, Hamster W, Blunck H, et al. Latent portosystemic encephalopathy. I. Nature of cerebral functional defects and their effect on fitness to drive. Did Dis Sci. 1981;26(7):622–30.
26. Das A, Dhiman RK, Saraswat VA, et al. Prevalence and natural history of subclinical hepatic encephalopathy in cirrhosis. J Gastroenterol Hepatol. 2001;16(5):531–5.
27. Amodio P, Montagnese S, Gatta A, et al. Characteristics of minimal hepatic encephalopathy. Metab Brain Dis. 2004;19(3–4):253–67.
28. Kato A, Kato M, Ishii H, et al. Development of quantitative neuropsychological tests for diagnosis of subclinical hepatic encephalopathy in liver cirrhosis patients and establishment of diagnostic criteria- multicenter collaborative study in Japanese. Hepatol Res. 2004;30(2):71–8.
29. Kooka Y, Sawara K, Endo R, et al. Brain metabolism in minimal hepatic encephalopathy assessed by 3.0-Tesla magnetic resonance spectroscopy. Hepatol Res. 2015;46:269–76.
30. Phelpes ME, Hoffman EJ, Raybaund C. Factors which affect cerebral uptake and retention of ^{13}NH3. Stroke. 1977;8(6):694–702.
31. Tranah TH, Vijay GK, Ryan JM, Shawcross DL. Systemic inflammation and ammonia in hepatic encephalopathy. Metab Brain Dis. 2013;28(1):1–5.
32. Schenker S. Hepatic encephalopathy. In: Butterworth RF, Pomier Layrargues G, editors. The present and the future. Hepatic encephalopathy, experimental biology and medicine, vol. 22. Clifton: Humana Press; 1989. p. 3–24.
33. Hindfelt B, Plum F, Duffy TE. Effect of acute ammonia intoxication on cerebral metabolism in rats with portacaval shunts. J Clin Invest. 1977;59(3):386–96.
34. Bessaman SP, Bessaman AN. The cerebral and peripheral uptake of ammonia in liver disease with an hypothesis for the mechanism of hepatic coma. J Clin Invest. 1955;34(4):622–8.
35. Butterworth RF, Vaquero J. In: Aris I, Alter H, Boyer J, Cohen D, Feusto N, Shafritz D, Wollkoff A, editors. Hepatic encephalopathy: the liver: biology and pathology. 5th ed. Hoboken: Wiley; 2009.
36. Lai JC, Cooper AJ. Brain alpha-ketoglutarate dehydrogenase complex: kinetic properties, regional distribution, and effects of inhibitors. J Neurochem. 1986;47(5):1376–86.
37. Lockwood AH, Yap EW, Rhoades HM, Wong WH. Altered cerebral blood flow and glucose metabolism in patients with liver disease and minimal encephalopathy. J Cereb Blood Flow Metab. 1991;11(2):331–6.
38. Lux HD. Ammonium and chloride extrusion. Hyperpolarizing synaptic inhibition in spinal motoneurons. Science. 1971;173(3996):555–7.
39. Raabe WA. Neurophysiology of ammonia intoxication. In: Butterworth RF, Pomier Layrargues G, editors. Hepatic encephalopathy, experimental biology and medicine, vol. 22. Clifton: Humana Press; 1989. p. 49–77.
40. Norenberg MD. A light and electron microscopic study of experimental portal-systemic (ammonia) encephalopathy. Progression and reversal of the disorder. Lab Investig. 1977;36 (6):618–27.
41. Gregorios JB, Mozes LW, Norenberg LO, Norenberg MD. Morphologic effects of ammonia on primary astrocyte cultures. I. Light microscopic studies. J Neuropathol Exp Neurol. 1985;44(4):397–403.
42. Swain M, Butterworth RF, Blei AT. Ammonia and related amino acids in the pathogenesis of brain edema in acute ischemic liver failure in rats. Hepatology. 1992;15(3):449–53.

43. O'Keefe SJ, Abraham R, El-Zayadi A, Marshall W, Davis M, Williams R. Increased plasma tyrosine concentrations in patients with cirrhosis and fulminant hepatic failure associated with increased plasma tyrosine flux and reduced hepatic oxidation capacity. Gastroenterology. 1981;81(6):1017–24.
44. Schafer DF, Jones EA. Hepatic encephalopathy and the gamma-aminobutyric-acid neurotransmitter system. Lancet. 1982;1(8262):18–20.
45. Fischer JE, Baldessarini RJ. False neurotransmitters and hepatic failure. Lancet. 1971;2 (7715):75–80.
46. Ahboucha S, Butterworth RF. The neurosteroid system: implication in the pathophysiology of hepatic encephalopathy. Neurochem Int. 2008;52:575–87.
47. Bass NM, Mullen KD, Sanyal A, et al. Rifaximin treatment in hepatic encephalopathy. N Engl J Med. 2010;362(12):1071–81.
48. Katayama K, Saito M, Sawara K, et al. Effect of zinc on liver cirrhosis with hyperammonemia: a preliminary randomized, placebo-controlled double-blind trial. Nutrition. 2014;30 (11–12):1409–14.
49. Takuma Y, Nouso K, Makino K, et al. Clinical trial: oral zinc in hepatic encephalopathy. Aliment Pharmacol Ther. 2010;32(9):1080–90.
50. Barbaro G, Di Lorenzo G, Soldini M, et al. Flumazenil for hepatic coma in patients with liver cirrhosis: an Italian multicentre double-blind, placebo-controlled, crossover study. Eur J Emerg Med. 1998;5:213–8.
51. Sharma P, Sharma BC, Puri V, Sarin SK. An open-label randomized controlled trial of lactulose and probiotics in the treatment of minimal hepatic encephalopathy. Eur J Gastroenterol Hepatol. 2008;20(6):506–11.
52. Malaguarnera PG, Elvira R, et al. Effects of L-carnitine in patients with hepatic encephalopathy. World J Gastoenterol. 2005;11:7197–202.

Chapter 5
Glucose Metabolism and Liver

Shigeatsu Hashimoto

Abstract Liver is a main organ to regulate energy metabolism, nutrients production, storage and supply to the whole body. Glucose is the essential energy source for the whole body organs, especially for brain which has no ability to synthesize glucose and store glycogen or utilize non-glucose nutrients. Liver plays pivotal role to regulate glucose metabolism by precise regulation of glycogenolysis and gluconeogenesis, which are controlled not only by endocrine system, insulin and its counterregulatory hormones, but also by neuronal network, autonomic nervous system and brain. Recent development of molecular biology and gene analysis has revealed the precise molecular mechanism of hepatic carbohydrate metabolism and regulatory system by endocrine system, insulin or glucagon signaling pathway and those hormone-induced transcription of effector molecules, CREB, FoxO1, ChREBP, SREBPs, PGC1 or several kinds of enzymes. Recent studies also revealed that organ-to-organ network medicated autonomic neural system plays important roles in hepatic glucose metabolism.

Energy controlling system of carbohydrate metabolism by the liver and organ-to-organ network is excellent to starvation, however dose not adapt to the persistent satiety. Excessive energy intake causes hepatic dysregulation of glucose and lipid metabolism which promote insulin resistance, diabetes mellitus or non-alcoholic fatty liver disease.

Keywords Glycolysis • Glycogenolysis • Gluconeogenesis • Insulin • Counterregulatory hormones • Insulin resistance • Non-alcoholic fatty liver disease

5.1 Introduction

Liver is a main organ to regulate energy metabolism, nutrients production, storage and supply to the whole body. Glucose is the energy source for the whole body organs, especially for brain which has no ability to synthesize glucose and store

---

S. Hashimoto (✉)
Radiation Medical Science Center for the Fukushima Health Management Survey, Fukushima Medical University, 1, Hikarigaoka, Fukushima 960-1295, Japan
e-mail: raijinsh@fmu.ac.jp

H. Ohira (ed.), *The Liver in Systemic Diseases*, DOI 10.1007/978-4-431-55790-6_5

glycogen or utilize non-glucose nutrients. Hypoglycemia easily causes central nervous system dysfunction, consciousness loss and consequent death. Therefore, maintenance of plasma glucose concentration is essential for survival. Liver plays pivotal role to regulate glucose metabolism, which are preciousely controlled by endocrine system, insulin and its counterregulatory hormones, such as glucagon, adrenalin, glucocorticoids or growth hormone. This elegant system has been acquired by a very long process of evolution suffering from starvation. Glucose metabolism in the liver has a close association inevitably with lipid metabolism, as an efficient energy storage system with a large amount more than glycogen.

The carbohydrate metabolism in the liver changes dramatically in feeding time and fasting. Liver intakes glucose and synthesizes glycogen and lipids by insulin upon feeding. In fasting time, liver conversely produces glucose from stored nutrients, supplies and oxidizes lipids by glucagon and other counter regulatory hormones.

Recent development of molecular biology and gene analysis has revealed the precise molecular mechanism of hepatic carbohydrate metabolism and regulatory system by endocrine system, insulin or glucagon signaling pathway and those hormone-induced transcription of effector molecules or enzymes. Effective combination usage of gene manipulation, physiology or metabolome analysis has given us further discovery and integrated understanding of the hepatic glucose and lipid metabolism, its interaction and regulation under physiological or pathological state. For example, existence of hyperglycemia requires not only insulin deficiency but also glucagon excess [1]. As well as the endocrine system, organ-to-organ network medicated autonomic neural system, such as hepatic-neural [2], or gut-hepatic interaction [3], plays an important role in hepatic glucose metabolism.

These energy controlling system of carbohydrate metabolism is excellent to starvation, however dose not adapt to the persistent satiety which we have not experienced in the history of the evolution and results in a pandemic of diabetes mellitus, dysregulation of glucose metabolism, caused by insulin insufficiency and/or insulin resistance, and inappropriate secretion or action of counter regulatory hormone, such as glucagon, which causes insufficient control of hepatic glucose uptake and production, consequent increase of hepatic glucose output and hyperglycemia.

5.2 Glucose Homeostasis in Liver

5.2.1 Mechanisms Involved in Glucose Homeostasis of the Basal State

Basal glucose disposal is approximately 2.0 mg/kg/min [4], which is exactly equal to the endogenous glucose production rate. In the basal (10–12 h overnight fast state, post absorptive state), about 75 % of total glucose use occurs in insulin independent tissues. About 50 % of all glucose disposal used in brain, 25 % in the splanchnic area and remaining 25 % in insulin dependent tissues, muscle or adipose tissue [4]. Liver produces about 85 % of endogenous glucose, and kidneys produce the remaining 15 %. Glycogenolysis and gluconeogenesis contribute equally to the basal hepatic glucose production rate.

Following glucose uptake after eating, plasma glucose concentration increases, and consequently insulin secretion is stimulated. Increase in plasma glucose and high concentration of insulin stimulate hepatic glucose uptake and suppress hepatic endogenous glucose production. Liver uptakes about 60 % of glucose in the portal vein with hepatocyte glucose uptake via GLUT2, which is non-insulin dependent and has high Km (glucose affinity is low) [5]; therefore it works only under high glucose concentration.

Mechanism of the increase in hepatic glucose metabolism is caused by phosphorylation of glucose, glycogen synthesis, activation of pentose phosphate pathway, increment in glycolysis and suppression of gluconeogenesis.

5.2.1.1 Hepatic Glucose Uptake (Fig. 5.1)

Glucose is transported into hepatocyte via glucose transporter (GLUT) 2 [6], which facilitates glucose diffusion into the cell in accordance with the concentration gradient. GLUT2 is a high-capacity, low-affinity (Km > 10 mM) isoform relative to other members of this family [5]. GLUT2 transports glucose into the hepatocyte only when extracellular glucose concentration is high (10 mM), but can do large amount of glucose. Transported glucose into the hepatocyte is phosphorylated by glucokinase (GK, hexokinase IV) as a first step of glucose metabolism pathway, yielding glucose-6-phophate. GK has a high capacity and low affinity (Km > 5 mM) like GLUT2, relatively compared with other members of this enzyme family. GK is active when plasma glucose concentration is higher than its Km, and its activity remains while glucose is abundant because it is not inhibited by its product, glucose-6-phosphate [7]. In addition of kinetic feature of hepatic GK, its activity is also regulated by GK regulatory protein (GKRP) [7], a physiological inhibitor of GK, and insulin. GK is inactive and locates associated with GKRP in the nucleus during fasting. Ingestion of glucose after eating stimulates translocation of GK from the nucleus to the cytosol and activation with dissociation of GK from GKRP. And insulin increases GK gene expression with a modest enzyme activity [8]. Therefore, glucose uptake by hepatocyte occurs only during absorption phase depending on glucose concentration gradient because of kinetic features of GLUT2 and GK expressed in hepatocyte [7].

Phosphorylation of Glucose Glucose-6-phosphate (G-6-P) produced from glucose by GK, one of the glycolytic intermediates, is a key molecule. G-6-P stands on the cross road of the hepatic glucose metabolism, of which starting point to glycolysis, glycogenesis or pentose monophosphate pathway. Conversion of

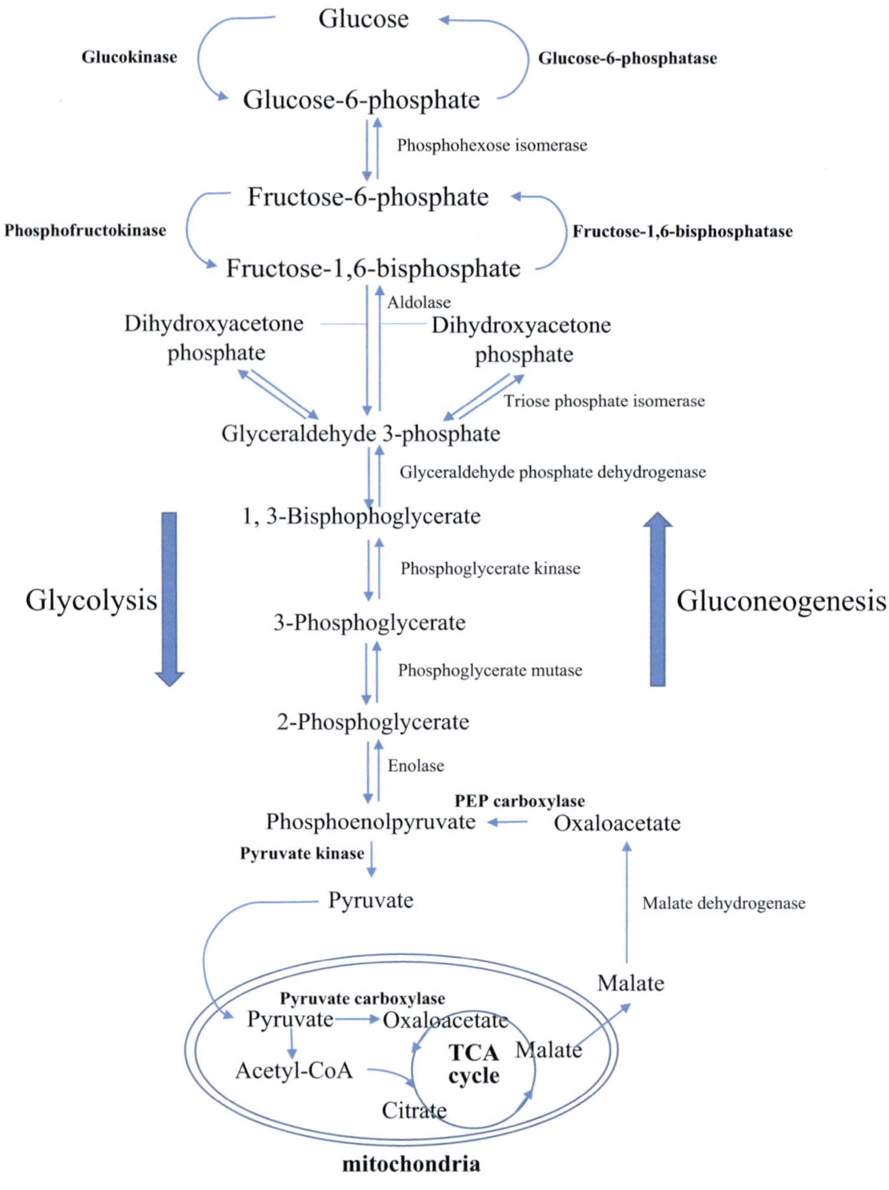

Fig. 5.1 Glycolysis and gluconeogenesis pathway

glucose to glucose-6-phosphate is regulated by reciprocal actions of GK and glucose-6-phophatase (G-6-Pase) [9]. GK is not inhibited allosterically by G-6-P, but is regulated inhibitorily by GKRP, as described above. Fructose-6-phophate, yielded from G-6-P by phosphoglucoisomerase, stimulates translocation of GK to the nucleus from the cytosol and inactivates GK with association of GKRP

[10]. Conversely, GK is activated not only by increased intracellular glucose concentration but also by fructose-1-phophate [11], which is the derivative from fructose generated by hepatic fructokinase, with stimulation of GK dissociation with GKRP. In this way, the nutritional state of the liver cells alters the GK activity and also GK gene expression. The transcription of the GK-gene is turned on by insulin [12] and turned off by glucagon/cyclic AMP (cAMP), which mediated repression is dominant mechanism for the regulation of glucokinase gene transcription in the hepatocyte. Insulin may act by relieving the gene from repression via increase in Akt-activated SREBP-1c, which binds to the SREBP-responsive elements of GK promoter and its expression [13].

G-6-Pase enzyme complex is located in the endoplasmic reticulum and catalyzes the hydrolysis of G-6-P [14], as the opposing reaction of GK, to phosphate group and free glucose, which is exported from the hepatocyte via membrane glucose transporter and used for homeostasis of plasma glucose level. Only organ which expressed G-6-Pase, such as the liver and kidney unlike other organs, can make glucose to release into circulation. G-6-Pase is a rate-limiting enzyme for the hepatic glucose output.

G-6-Pase activity is affected by nutrition intake with the changes in hormone secretion or glucose itself. G-6-Pase activity is accelerated by starvation [15, 16] and diabetes [17] associated with a 2–4-fold increase in G-6-Pase mRNA. Glucocorticoid, cAMP and elevation of glucose concentration also increase in G-6-Pase expression. Conversely, insulin decreases in G-6-Pase expression [15].

Glycogen Synthesis Glycogen synthesis begins with conversion of G-6-P to glucose-1-phosphate (G-1-P) by phosphoglucomutase. After that, G-1-P was converted to uridine 5'-diphosphate-glucose by UDP-glucose pyrophosphorylase. Finally, UDP-glucose is added to no reducing end of glycogen chain or to glycogenin to start a new chain for growing glycogen molecule by glycogen synthase, which is rate-limiting step of glycogen synthesis. Glycogen synthase is activated allosterically associated with G-6-P and UDP-glucose.

Glycogen synthase is regulated by phosphorylation/dephosphorylation event. Glycogen synthase is modified by phosphorylation of its serine residues [18], on which occurred by different kinases, such as glycogen synthase kinase (GSK) 3β or protein kinase A (PKA). Glycogen synthase activity is generally suppressed by phosphorylation, which is occurred by PKA induced by glucagon receptor activation or GSK3β phosphorylation. Suppression of GSK3β activity, namely glycogen synthase reactivation, is occurred by insulin mediated via Akt phosphorylation of GSK3β [19]. And insulin also activates glycogen synthase by dephosphorylation of it via the protein phosphatase (PP) 1 activation [18], which is primary phosphatase involved by insulin action. PP1 is composed of several subunits, one of which is a member of the PP1 binding protein family targeting glycogen and organizing the phosphatase activity of enzymes involved in the glycogen metabolism. G_L is one of the proteins targeting glycogen and is expressed primarily in the liver. G_L can bind glycogen and PP1, and determines the localization of PP1 to glycogen particle in the hepatocyte [20].

5.2.1.2 Hepatic Glucose Output

Liver maintains the plasma glucose concentration during fasting condition by the glycogenolysis and gluconeogenesis; the former supplies rapidly glucose by breaking down glycogen and the latter supplies it relative slowly by converting non-carbohydrate precursor molecules, such as lactate, glycerol and amino acids, to glucose.

Glycogenolysis The main glycogen storage organs in a whole body are liver and muscle, the former stores approximately 100 g of glycogen (300 mM of glucose), the latter is 300 g of it [21]. Hepatic glycogen is used for the maintenance of fasting blood glucose concentration, while glycogen in the muscles is used for an energy source during the first ten minutes of skeletal muscular exercise.

Glycogenolysis, that is degradation of glycogen, converts stored glycogen into glucose. Glycogenolysis is not the reverse of glycogenesis, but is a separate pathway. Initiation of the glycogenolytic process is the removal of one glucose residue from the non-reducing termini of the glycogen molecule, which is composed of three steps of reaction caused by two enzymes, glycogen phosphorylase and glycogen debranching enzyme. Glycogenolysis is catalyzed by the active glycogen phosphorylase, which is rate limiting step of glycogenolysis [22], the phosphorolytic cleavage of the α-1,4-glycosidic bonds of the glucose polymer to yield G-1-P. The terminal glucosyl residues from the outermost chains of the glycogen molecule are removed sequentially until approximately four glucose residues remain on either side of $1 \rightarrow 6$ branches. There are different isozymes of glycogen phosphorylase in liver, muscle and brain encoded by different genes. Glycogen phosphorylase requires pyridoxal phosphate as its coenzyme [23]. The debranching enzyme has two catalytic sites in a single polypeptide chain. One is a glucan transferase that transfers a trisaccharide unit from one branch to the other, exposing $1 \rightarrow 6$ branch point. The other is a 1,6-glucosidase that catalyzes hydrolysis of $1 \rightarrow 6$ glycoside bond to liberate free glucose. Further phosphorylase action can then proceed. The combined action of phosphorylase and these other enzymes leads to the complete breakdown of glycogen. The terminal glycosyl residues from the outermost chain of the glycogen molecule are removed sequentially until approximately four glucose residues remain on either side $1 \rightarrow 6$ branches and are resulted in cleavage product of limit dextrin which is not able to degrade furthermore by glycogen phosphorylase.

G-1-P yielded by glycogen phosphorylase is converted to G-6-P by phosphoglucomutase in cytosol. The reaction catalyzed by phosphoglucomutase is reversible, so that G-6-P can be formed from glucose 1-phophate. In liver, glucose-6-phophate is translocated to endoplasmic reticulum by G-6-P translocase [21]. In liver, but not muscle, G-6-Pase catalyzes hydrolysis of G-6-P, yielding glucose that in exported, leading to an increase in the blood glucose concentration. This reaction sustains until initiation of glucose production with gluconeogenesis.

Gluconeogenesis Gluconeogenesis is the metabolic pathway to synthesize glucose from non-carbohydrate three carbon substrates such as glycolytic end products of pyruvate and lactate, glucogenic amino acids which are converted oxaloacetate, and glycerol. Liver produces about 85–90 % of endogenous glucose, and kidneys produce the remaining 10–15 %. After overnight fasting, glycogenolysis and gluconeogenesis contribute equally to the basal hepatic glucose production rate in human. As the fasting time becomes longer, endogenous glucose production is kept constant because the proportion of gluconeogenesis is increased to compensate reduced glycogenolysis as glycogen consumption. Liver stores about 100 g of glucose as glycogen. After 48 h fasting in human, hepatic glycogen is depleted, and total glucose production depends on gluconeogenesis.

Gluconeogenesis is essential reversal of glycolysis, but not merely reversal, because those would be endergonic and glycolysis has some irreversible enzymatic steps (Fig.5.1). To produce one glucose molecule from pyruvate, it requires at least 11 steps of enzymatic reaction. Seven of these reactions are reversible, and they are catalyzed by glycolytic enzymes such as aldolase and triose-phosphate isomerase. However, remaining four reactions are irreversible. These opposing reactions of irreversible steps are required the enzymes to be separated with catalyzing reaction of glycolysis, of which steps are important points of transcriptional and post-transcriptional control of gluconeogenesis. These irreversible steps are conversion of glucose/G-6-P, fructose-6-phosphate (F-6-P)/fructose-1,6-bisphosphate (F-1,6-BP) and phosphoenolpyruvate (PEP)/pyruvate. Opposing phosphorylation and dephosphorylation of glucose and fructose-6-phosphate were catalyzed by GK/G-6-BPase and phosphofructokinase (PFK)/fructose-1,6-bisphosphatase (FBPase)1, respectively. The conversion of phosphoenolpyruvate (PEP) to pyruvate is catalyzed by L-pyruvate kinase (PK), however requires additional steps to synthesize PEP from pyruvate. Among the three irreversible reaction mentioned above, FBPase1 activity is inhibited allosterically associated with AMP [24] and fructose-2,6-bisphosphate (F-2,6-BP) [25], a product of F-1,6-BP. AMP and F-2,6-BP activate PFK-1 catalyzing reverse reaction of FBPase1. In other words, increase in F-2,6-BP and AMP enhances glycolysis; in the contrary decrease in those enhances gluconeogenesis. Enzyme activities of G-6-Pase converting from G-6-P to glucose and PEPCK from oxaloacetate to PEP, catalyzing the other two non-reversible reactions, are regulated not with allosteric manner but with expression level of those.

Gluconeogenesis begins pyruvate transportation into the mitochondria matrix with mitochondrial pyruvate carrier (MPC) [26]. Pyruvate in the mitochondria was carboxylated into the four carbon oxaloacetate by mitochondria enzyme, pyruvate

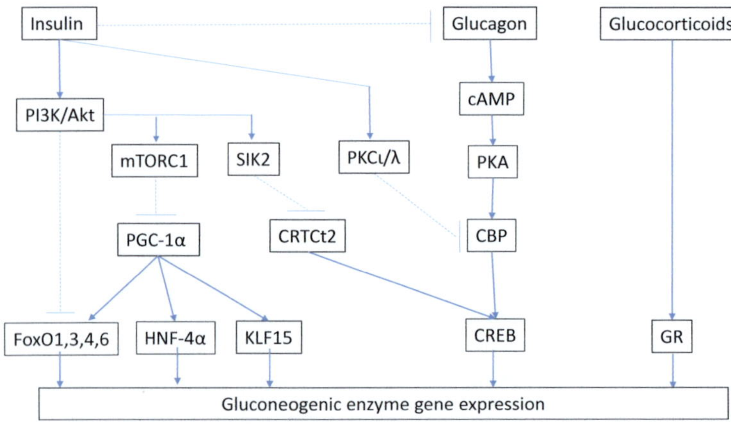

Fig. 5.2 Hormonal regulatory mechanism of transcription of gluconeogenic enzyme genes

carboxylase [27]. Following reduction of oxaloacetate to malate by malate dehydrogenase with oxidation NADH to NAD^+, malate is transported out of mitochondria to cytosol via malate transporter. In the cytosol, the malate is oxidized to yield oxaloacetate by cytosolic malate dehydrogenase with generation of an NADH. Alternatively, mitochondrial oxaloacetate transaminated to asparate with amino group is donated by glutamate. The asparate is transported to cytosol via asparate/glutamate transporter. Cytosolic asparate is transaminated back to oxaloacetate and then converted PEP by PEPCK. PEP is converted to F-1,6-BP via six steps with common enzymes of glycolysis.

Conversion of F-1,6-BP to F-6-P is catalyzed by FBPase, which is different from the enzyme, phosphofructokinase, catalyzing reverse reaction of glycolysis because this step is ATP-consuming irreversible reaction. F-6-P is converted to G-6-P by phosphohexose isomerase of common glycolysis enzyme. Hydrolytic reaction of G-6-P to glucose catalyzed by the G-6-Pase is a final step of gluconeogenesis.

Transcriptional Regulation to Gluconeogenic Enzyme Genes (Fig. 5.2)

Gluconeogenesis plays pivotal role to maintain plasma glucose levels during fasted state. Nutritional state changes glucoregulatory hormones, insulin and its counter-regulatory hormones, glucagon or glucocorticoids. Those hormones regulate gluconeogenic enzyme gene expression, PEPCK, FBPase and the G-6-Pase subunit by affecting promotor regions of the genes via several transcription factors, cAMP responsive element (CRE)-binding protein (CREB) [28] and Fork head box O1 (FoxO1) [29–31], co-activator, peroxisome proliferator-activated receptor γ (PPARγ) coactivator (PGC)-1α [32] or nuclear receptors, GR [33] and hepatic nuclear factor (HNF)-4α [34, 35].

PEPCK mRNA is increased and stabilized under fasting condition in response to glucagon [27] or glucocorticoids, those pathways act synergistically but the underlying mechanism is not same. Glucagon binds its own G-protein coupled receptor on the hepatocyte and stimulates cAMP production [36], which activates PKA. PKA translocates into the nucleus and phosphorylates CREB at serine residue 133. CREB binds to the CRE in the PEPCK promoter area. Phosphorylated CREB binding to its CRE site forms the assembly of its co-activator, the CREB binding protein (CBP), and initiates transcription. Co-activator, cAMP-regulated transcriptional co-activator (CRTC2) also potentiates transcription by CREB [37]. Phosphorylated CRTC2 by salt-induced kinase (SIK) is inactive form [38]. CRTC2 is dephosphorylated by PKA via SIK inhibition or calcineurin (CN) [38]. Dephosphorylated CRTC2 translocated into nucleus and then exerts the function as a co-activator, promoting transcription of CREB target genes [39].

Glucocorticoids bind cytosolic glucocorticoid receptor (GR) and translocate into the nucleus. Glucocorticoid-GR binds to a glucocorticoid response element (GRE) in the PEPCK promoter [33]. GR/GRE complex formation recruits multicomponent regulatory complex and enhances PEPCK gene expression.

PGC-1α plays important role to regulate energy metabolism through binding of PPARγ [40]. In the liver, PGC-1α expression is very low under fed condition; however, fasting dramatically increases its expression by glucagon and catecholamines via the stimulation of cAMP pathway and the CREB transcription factor. PGC-1α increases PEPCK expression via co-activation of a variety of transcription factors, such as HNF-4α [34, 35], FoXO1 [29, 30], Kruepel-like factor 15 [41] or GR [33]. In addition to these activation mechanisms with expression control, PGC-1α regulates PEPCK activity by post-translational mechanism of deacetylation with SIRT1 [41].

In contrast, insulin secreted under fed condition represses transcription of gluconeogenic enzymes, which is achieved via activation of Akt/PKB signal and the consequent disruption of interactions between certain transcription factors/coactivators and their positive response elements in the promoters of those genes. These repressive effects of insulin on gluconeogenic enzymes expression surpass the action of cAMP or glucocorticoid. These insulin actions are mediated via several pathways. FoxO1 is one of the important factors responsible for this mechanism of insulin [29].

FoxO1 have positive and negative effects on gene expression. Under the condition of low level of insulin, FoxO1 locates in the nucleus and binds directly to DNA target sites. Thereby FoxO1 stimulates the transcription of target genes which interact with and modulate the function of other transcription factors and co-activators important for the regulation of gene expression in the liver. Akt activation by insulin via PI3K induces FoxO1 phosphorylation and its exportation from the nucleus into the cytosol [42]. FoxO1 dissociation from the promoter area of PEPCK or G-6-Pase causes repression of these gluconeogenic enzymes.

Insulin exerts another direct mechanism of gene repression of glyconeogenic enzymes through CBP phosphorylation [43]. As mentioned above, phosphorylated CREB by PKA stimulated with cAMP initiates transcription of gluconeogenic enzymes genes associated with CBP. Insulin phosphorylates CBP at the serine residue 436 [42], which decreases in transcriptional activity as a coactivator of CREB. Therefore, insulin suppresses the gene expression of gluconeogenic enzymes by the inhibition of AMP transcriptional signals via CBP phosphorylation of serine residue.

Indirect Action of Insulin on Gluconeogenesis In addition to the direct effect, insulin acts indirectly on the hepatic gluconeogenesis mediated through extrahepatic action. Insulin suppresses glucagon secretion from the pancreatic α cells [44], one of the most important factors of gluconeogenesis. The gluconeogenic substrate determines hepatic glucose production. Insulin decreases the substrate supply for gluconeogenesis, such as glycerol, lactate, pyruvate and glucogenic amino acids. Insulin suppresses lipolysis through the activation of Akt, resulting in the inhibition of PKA of the main positive effector of lipolysis, and then glycerol supply to the liver is decreased. Insulin acts as an anabolic hormone for protein metabolism and decreases the release of amino acids. Mechanisms of anabolic effect of insulin are different for each organ, in which insulin exerts via promoting protein synthesis or via suppressing protein degradation. Insulin increases hepatic albumin production, which may be result of insulin action to affect protein turnover in the liver. However, its mechanism has not been fully resolved in human. Mechanism of insulin anabolic action on skeletal muscle, containing half of body protein, has not been also resolved. Insulin stimulates amino acid uptake and transportation into the skeletal muscle with regulation of its transporter mRNA and protein expression via Akt-mTORC1 pathway [45] and via ATF4 [46].

Recently, it has been revealed that the hypothalamus is the important insulin target organ which affects hepatic glucose production [47]. The activation of insulin signaling in the arcuate nucleus of the hypothalamus [48] without increase in systemic insulin levels decreases blood glucose levels via a substantial inhibition of endogenous glucose production. Insulin acts on K_{ATP} channel in the arcuate nucleus to control hepatic glucose production [49] by decreasing glucose-6-phosphate and phosphoenolpyruvate kinase expression in the liver. This effect is mediated by the activation of efferent vagal fibers, which innervate the liver [2].

Regulation of Amino Acid Catabolic Enzyme Genes in Response to Proteolysis Following lactate, alanine, glutamine and other gluconeogenic amino acids (threonine, serine, glutamate and glycine) are important gluconeogenic precursors and they account for approximately 40 % of gluconeogenic substrate. Under fasting condition, decrease of plasma insulin stimulates protein catabolism and is resulted in increase of amino acid supply. Gluconeogenic amino acids are converted to pyruvate, and thereafter they are used for gluconeogenesis. These reactions are catalyzed by alanine aminotransferase 1,4-hydroxyphenylpuruvate dioxygenase and proline dehydrogenase, which are activated by glucagon/cAMP signal via transcription factor KLF15 under fasting condition [30].

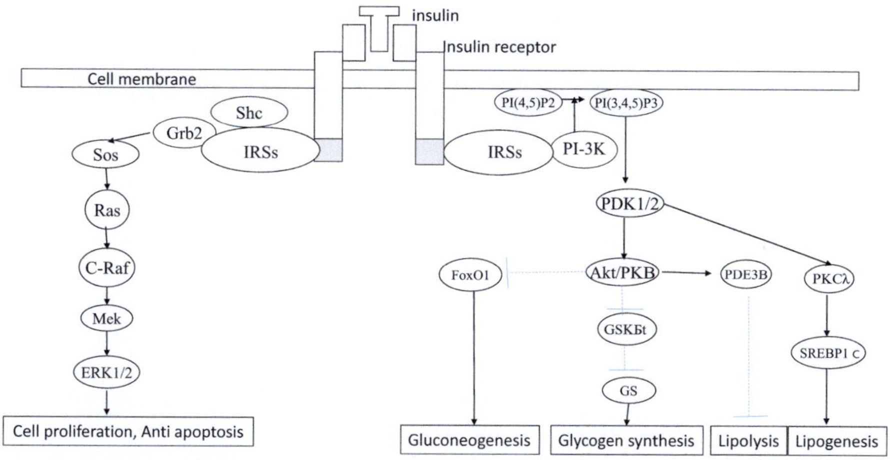

Fig. 5.3 Insulin signaling pathway

5.2.2 Hormonal Regulation of Hepatic Glucose Metabolism

5.2.2.1 Inulin and Insulin Sensitizing Hormones

Insulin (Fig. 5.3)

Insulin signaling begins with tyrosine phosphorylation of the insulin receptor and insulin receptor substrate molecules. Three major steps in insulin signal transduction are insulin receptor/receptor substrate binding, PI-3 kinase and Akt/protein kinase B, those exert divergence of activated pathways affecting multiple cellular functions, such as metabolism, proliferation and many other functions [50]. Insulin exerts a wide variety of its actions by the direct effect on gene transcription via its signaling mechanisms or and by indirect effects on glucose or lipid substrate metabolism or on interaction between counter-regulatory hormones.

Insulin receptor molecule is a transmembrane glycoprotein, which is a heterotetramer consisting of two α- and two β- subunits. The 135 kDa α-subunits is a ligand biding domain and locates outside the cell binding to 95 kDa β-subunits, which span the membrane and have tyrosine kinase activity [51]. Insulin binds extracellular α-subunits and causes conformational change of α-subunits; subsequently ATP can bind to intracellular domain of β-subunits. Following insulin binding, there occurs autophosphorylation of one β-subunit catalyzed by a specific domain in the other β-subunit within the same heterotetramer. Autophosphorylation of this kinase makes it more active and accelerates phosphate transfer to other tyrosine sites within the same receptor. Ligand-dependent stimulation of the β-subunit tyrosine kinase activity plays a decisive role to propagate the insulin signaling. The β-subunits have also serine and threonine residue, of which phosphorylation within the insulin receptor also occurs following insulin binding, and can diminish receptor tyrosine kinase activity. This is a regulatory feedback mechanism and can induce insulin resistance under pathophysiologic conditions.

Following insulin binding and autophosphorylation of insulin receptor, the next step is phosphorylation of the tyrosine residue of insulin receptor substrate (IRS) [51, 52]. IRS has no enzymatic activity, but has three important functional domains capable of interaction with other proteins, an N-terminal pleckstrin homology (PH) domain, an intermediate phosphotyrosine-binding (PTB) domain and a carboxy-terminal region containing the multiple tyrosine and serine phosphorylation sites. The PH domain helps position the insulin receptor for coupling with IRS, and PTB domain recognizes phosphotyrosine in the motif of asparagine-proline-any amino acid-phosphotyrosine which exists in insulin receptor. PTB domain binds directly to β-subunit with phosphorylated tyrosine residue and provides phosphorylation of tyrosine residues in their COOH-terminal domains.

There are six insulin receptor substrate proteins (IRS-1, IRS-2, IRS-3, IRS-4, IRS-5 and IRS-6) [53]. IRS-1 [52] and IRS-2 [54] are expressed in a wide range of tissues, including muscle, fat, liver and pancreatic islets, and their relative levels are different for each tissue. IRS-3 is expressed in adipose tissue, fibroblasts and liver cells [53]; IRS-4 is in brain, thymus and embryonic kidney [55]. IRS-5 is ubiquitously expressed but most abundant in kidney and liver. IRS-6 is expressed highest in skeletal muscle. To investigate each IRS function, some of knockout mice model have been developed. IRS-1 knockout mice had growth retardation and insulin resistance, however unexpectedly they did not develop overt diabetes [56]. On the other hand, IRS-2 knockout mouse showed insulin resistance and overt diabetes mellitus with impaired insulin secretion due to reduced βcell mass [57]. IRS-3 has not been detected in the human genome. IRS-4 null mice also appear normal, but have infertility. In bioluminescence resonance energy transfer experiments, interaction between IRS-5 and insulin receptor was not observed, while interaction with IRS-6 was not enhanced by insulin. In addition, IRS-5 and IRS-6 showed very weak phosphorylation levels. These results suggest that IRS-5 and IRS-6 are poor substrates for the insulin receptor. It has been questioned their relevance to insulin action, because both isoforms show very weak affinity for the insulin receptor. Therefore, IRS-1 and IRS-2 play pivotal roles in glucose homeostasis among the IRS isoforms, and IRS-1 functions as the principal IRS in skeletal muscle, and that IRS-2 predominates in liver and β cells where insulin action is required for normal β-cell growth and development. IRS-2, unlike other IRS proteins, contains another region interacting with the insulin receptor kinase of the phosphorylated regulatory loop, which is designated as the kinase regulatory loop binding domain (KRLB). This KRLB domain has been thought to restrict tyrosine phosphorylation of IRS-2 [58]; however it has not been clarified whether the presence of the KRLB can explain the differences in phenotype between IRS-1 and IRS-2 knockout mice model. While it has not fully clarified the molecular mechanism of variety of insulin actions of each organ, the difference in expression of IRS-1 and IRS-2 of each cells constituting organ might be involved in diversity of insulin action of each organ.

SHC protein is also a substrate of the insulin receptor. Following insulin biding to its receptor, SHC is phosphorylated and interacts with SH-2 domain-containing proteins through their tyrosine phosphorylation sites. SHC binding to the Grb-2 can activate Ras/MAP kinase signaling pathway which stimulates cell proliferation.

After phosphorylation of IRS tyrosine residue, SH2-containing proteins recognize their target of phosphotyrosine motifs and bind to IRS proteins. Some kinds of SH2-contaning protein have tyrosine kinase activity, such as PI-3 kinase, Fyn (tyrosine kinase), Csk (tyrosine kinase) or phosphotyrosine phosphatase activity, SHIP-2, and have function of adapter proteins such as Grb-2, Crk, APS and Nck. These SH2-containig adaptor proteins have also SH3 domains and can bind to proline-rich consensus sequence (PXXP). The adapter proteins bind to the receptor substrates via their SH2 domains and connect with other proteins with their SH3 domains. The SH3-bound proteins act as downstream signaling molecules with its catalytic subunits and transduce the insulin signal. These docking proteins possess their own different enzymatic activities which activate specific downstream molecules. These protein–protein interactions define the specificities of insulin signal transduction. Insulin receptor substrates provide the first divergent step of insulin signal transduction pathways activating metabolic pathway via PI-3 kinase and the mitogenic pathway via Ras/MAP kinase.

Adiponectin Adiponectin is an adipocyte-derived hormone and acts as an insulin sensitizing adipocytokine through regulating glucose levels and fatty oxidation [59], which is different from other adipocytokines, such as TNFα or free fatty acid (FFA) increasing insulin resistance. Adiponectin improves liver insulin sensitivity by the inhibition of expression of gluconeogenic enzymes, PEPCK and G-6-Pase and lipogenic molecule, sterol regulatory element-binding protein 1c (SREBP1c) via adiponectin receptor 1 (AdiopoR1)-AMPK pathway and by stimulation of βoxidation in the liver via AdipoR2-PPARα pathway [60]. Adiponectin can mediate the metabolic effects of FGF21 on glucose homeostasis and insulin sensitivity [61]. On the other hand, secretion of adiponectin is decreased along with the enlargement of adipocytes in the visceral obesity, leading to insulin resistance.

Fibroblast Growth Factor Fibroblast growth factor 19 (FGF19) secreted from small intestine promotes postprandial glycogen synthesis which is independent of the activity of either insulin or the protein kinase Akt [62]. FGF19 stimulates the ERK/RSK pathway by activating its receptors FGFR4 and β-klotho, and activated RSK phosphorylates and inactivates GSK-3, which negatively regulates glycogen synthase, thereby activate glycogen synthase.

FGF21 is an important metabolic hormone secreted mainly from the liver in the fast state acts as a metabolic hormone with pleiotropic effects on regulating glucose and lipid homeostasis and insulin sensitivity. FGF21 is induced directly by PPARα in liver or stimulated by the secretion of it by glucagon in response to fasting or starvation and then stimulates lipolysis in white adipose tissue and ketogenesis in liver [63]. FGF21 improves insulin sensitivity via the stimulation of expression and secretion of adiponectin from adipose tissue with regulating glucose and lipid metabolism.

5.2.2.2 Counterregulatory Hormones

The major counterregulatory hormones are glucagon, epinephrine, glucocorticoids and growth hormone. The former hormones act quickly and shortly, and the latter acts slowly and generally more long-lasting. These hormones increase blood glucose concentration by hepatic glucose output through the stimulation of glycogenolysis and gluconeogenesis and by inhibition of various metabolic actions of insulin, such as glucose uptake inhibition of peripheral tissues.

Glucagon Glucagon acts through binding to specific receptors to activate adenylate cyclase and to increase the intracellular production of cAMP. Liver is a major target organ of glucagon. Glucagon acts as a major counterregulatory hormone by antagonizing the suppressive effects of insulin on glucose production and by stimulating glucose production. The main effect of glucagon on the liver is increase in glucose output with inhibition of glycogen synthesis and stimulation of hepatic glycogenolysis and gluconeogenesis. Glucagon stimulates glycogenolysis by the activation of glycogen phosphorylase via phosphorylation of glycogen phosphorylase kinase by PKA and also stimulates gluconeogenesis by the increase of gene transcription of PEPCK and G-6-Pase via serine phosphorylation of CREB by cAMP/PKA pathway. CRTC2 is a critical CREB coactivator and is regulated by SIK2 via phosphorylation [37], of which CRTC2 is translocated from the nucleus to the cytoplasm, ubiquitinated and degraded. PKA promotes dephosphorylation of CRTC2 and inhibits CRTC2 degradation [38]. PKA activates calcineurin by the stimulation of the Ca^{2+} release from ER to cytoplasm via activation of inositol-1,4,5-triphosphate receptors and dephosphorylates and stabilizes CRTC2. Glucagon also increases the stability and gluconeogenic activity of CRTC2 via acetylation of CRTC2 by p300/CBP. Another pathway of CREB/CRTC2 is Ca^{2+}/CaMKII pathway for glucagon stimulated gluconeogenesis. Glucagon stimulates Ca^{2+} release from the ER in hepatocytes via PKA-mediated phosphorylation of IP3R. CaMKII activated by Ca^{2+} promotes nuclear translocation and activation of FoxO1 via p38 MAPK activation and increases gluconeogenesis as described above. Acetylation of FoXO1 by p300/CBP is negatively controlled its binding ability to the promoters of target genes. Glucagon promotes deacetylation and activation of FoxO1 at the promoters of target genes by Class I HDAC3 recruitment via nuclear translocation of Class IIa HDACs (4/5/7) with its phosphorylation [37].

In this way, basal glucagon maintains hepatic glucose production during a prolonged fast by stimulation of gluconeogenesis and glycogenolysis.

Another effect of glucagon on the liver is the stimulation of ketogenesis, which depends on the flux of FFA into the liver and glucagon/insulin ratio. During fast condition, increase of intracellular cAMP derived by elevated glucagon/insulin ratio reduces glycolysis and activities of acetyl-CoA carboxylase via decrease of amount of mRNA for SREBP1c and intracellular malonyl-CoA concentration. Decrease of intracellular malonyl-CoA concentration suppresses fatty acid synthesis and reduces carnitine acyltransferase activity, resulting in conversion of fatty acids into acetoacetate and 3-hydroxybutyrate. Under starvation, lipolysis and ketogenesis by glucagon are crucial for energy source.

Growth Hormone (GH). GH acts as counterregulatory hormone by the stimulation of gluconeogenesis. GH binds to its cognate receptor of GH (GHR) and regulates signal transducer and activator of transcription 5 (STAT5) through recruitment of intracellular activation of JAK2. GH causes STAT5 phosphorylation and nuclear translocation, and then STAT5 binds to the promotor area of the PEPCK and stimulates its expression. GH-induced STAT5 phosphorylation increases pyruvate dehydrogenase kinase 4 (PDK4) [64], which conserves substrate for gluconeogenesis via inhibition of pyruvate dehydrogenase complex.

Glucocorticoid-Glucocorticoid Receptor Complex Cortisol is a member of glucocorticoids and has permissive effects on insulin. In the early state of fasting, cortisol opposes insulin by direct stimulation of gluconeogenesis and glycogenolysis via activation of glycogen phosphorylase in corporation with adrenalin. On the other hand, cortisol stimulates hepatic glycogenesis in the late state of fasting. Cellular action of cortisol is attributed to their binding to intracellular glucocorticoid receptor (GR), a member of the nuclear receptor family. Until ligand binding, GR resides in the cytoplasm in a complex with chaperones heat shock protein (HSP) 90 and HSP70 and co-chaperones HSP40 and p23. Upon cortisol binding to GR, receptor-ligand complex translocates to the nucleus and activates gluconeogenic genes PEPCK, G-6-Pase, FBPase and pyruvate carboxylase in the liver [32]. Deacetylase, HDAC6 plays pivotal role to ligand-induced nuclear translocation of GR via activation of HSP90 and promotion of GR-HSP90 complex assembly [65]. GR binds to STAT5 which promotes GH-stimulated gluconeogenesis, as described above. Additionally, elevated transcription factor Yin Yang 1 [66] in the fasted condition positively regulates gluconeogenesis via GR upregulation.

5.3 Lipid Metabolism in the Liver/Transcriptional Regulation to Lipogenic Enzyme Genes (Fig. 5.4)

To control energy balance, under enough carbohydrate condition, liver synthesizes and stores glycogen and lipids from nutrients absorbed into hepatocytes in postprandial state and, under fasting condition, provides them by glycolysis or oxidation of lipids as energy sources for other organs. Therefore, hepatic glucose metabolism interacts with lipid metabolism each other.

In fed condition, ingestion of carbohydrate and consequent insulin secretion promote lipogenesis. Glycolysis is closely related to lipogenesis because pyruvate

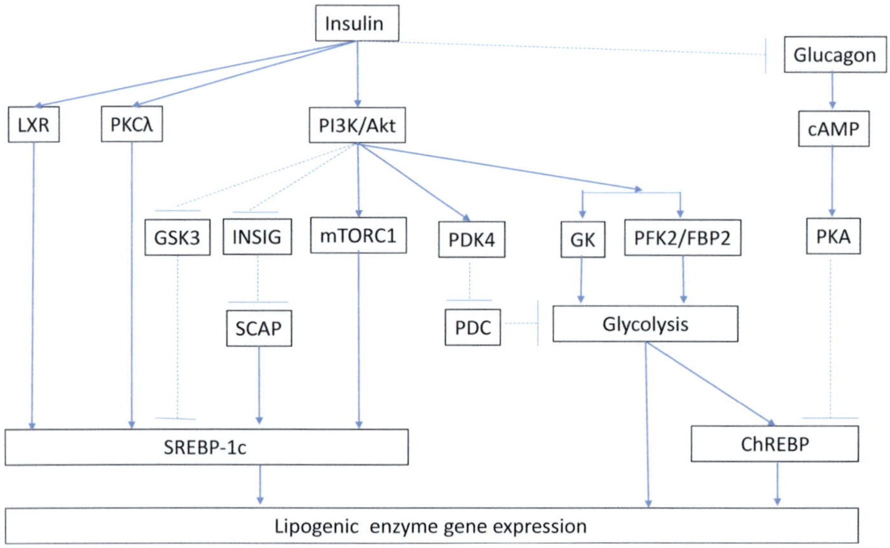

Fig. 5.4 Hormonal regulatory mechanism of transcription of lipogenic enzyme genes

as a glycolytic product is a main carbon source for lipogenesis. Glucose taken into the liver is metabolized to acetyl-CoA, via production of pyruvate in the mitochondria through glycolysis. Acetyl-CoA is carboxylated by acetyl-CoA carboxylase (ACC), biotin dependent enzyme, to produce malonyl-CoA. Malonyl-CoA is not only used with NADPH by fatty acid synthase (FAS) to synthesize palmitic acid, a 16-carbon fatty acid, but also suppresses β oxidation of fatty acids via inhibition of carnitine palmitoyltransferase 1, which is rate-limiting enzyme for β oxidation located on the mitochondrial outer membrane. Palmitic acid is elongated by fatty acyl-CoA elongase (Elovls) to produce long chain fatty acids which carbon atom number is bigger than 16.

Lipogenesis is controlled by the transcription of glycolytic and lipogenic genes, which are regulated by multiple transcription factors and coregulators. Carbohydrate response element binding protein (ChREBP) is a glucose responsive basic helix–loop–helix leucine zipper transcription factor (bHLH-Zip). Glucose controls ChREBP function via increase in expression and transactivation activity, phosphorylation-dependent upregulation of nuclear translocation and DNA binding [67]. ChREBP stimulates the expression of a glycolytic gene and liver pyruvate kinase gene *(L-PK)* and also stimulates the expression of lipogenic genes, such as malic enzyme to generate NADPH, ATP citrate lyase gene (*ACL*), *ACC*, *FAS*, stearoyl-CoA desaturase 1 gene (*SCD1*) and *Elovls* [68].

Another important transcription factor is sterol regulatory element-binding proteins (SREBP) family. SREBPs (SREBP-1a, -1c and -2) also belong to the bHLH-Zip family of transcription factors which act as master regulators for lipid metabolism by directly activating gene expression of enzymes to synthesize fatty acids, triglycerides, phospholipids and cholesterol. SREBP-1c and SREBP-2 are expressed predominantly in the liver; the former enhances transcription of genes required for fatty acid synthesis but not cholesterol synthesis, in contrast, the latter enhances those of cholesterol synthesis [69]. SREBPs are regulated at transcriptional and post-transcriptional level. Post-transcriptional regulation is the sterol-mediated suppression of SREBP processing. SREBPs locate on the endoplasmic reticulum (ER) membrane forming dimer with SREBP cleavage-activating protein (SCAP), which has cholesterol sensing domain and plays a role of a cholesterol sensor in the ER [70]. SCAP mediates SREBPs translocation from ER to Golgi apparatus [71]. In the presence of sterols in the ER, SREBP-SCAP complex remains on the ER membrane binding to insulin-induced gene (INSIG)-1 or -2 protein with interaction between sterol sensing domain (SSD). In the absence of sterols, SCAP dissociates with INSIG-1 or -2. SREBP-CAPS complex then leaves from ER for the Golgi apparatus to be processed. They are cleaved sequentially by the site-1 protease (S1P) and S2P yielding bHLH-Zip, which is translocated into the nucleus, thereafter shows transcriptional activity. Insulin stimulates SREBP-1 activation via suppression of inhibitory molecule of SREBP-1, INSIG 2 and lipin 1. INSIG2 in the liver is downregulated by insulin, thereby SREBP-SCAP complex move to the Golgi apparatus to be processed for activation. Insulin also stimulates SREBP-1c activation with promoting lipin 1 phosphorylation and cytoplasmic translocation from nucleus by mTORC1 through PI3/Akt pathway [72, 73]. Another mechanism of SREBP activation through Akt is inhibition of GSK3, which phosphorylates SREBP1c to degrade through ubiquitin-proteasome pathway.

Transcription of SREBP-1c is controlled by main three factors, LXR [74], insulin [72] and glucagon [75]. Fasting reduces the expression of lipogenic enzyme genes, on the other hand, refeeding markedly upregulates those expressions in the liver as well as in the adipose tissue. SREBP1c expression in NAFLD has been revealed to be higher than normal control [75]. In the liver cell line, LXR activation by oxysterol upregulates the expression of SRBP1c. These facts indicate that cholesterol upregulates SREBP-1c via LXR activation in the liver, which is independent and different from SREBP2 regulation suppressed by cholesterol. Insulin induces SREBP expression via PI3K-PKCλ pathway in the liver [76]. Conversely, glucagon decreases mRNA for SREBP-1c.

PPARγ is one of the nuclear receptors and is considered to be one of the master regulators of adipocyte differentiation and adipogenesis. PPARγ stimulates adipogenic and lipogenic genes, such as adipose differentiation-related protein (ADRP), adipocyte fatty acid-binding protein 4, SREBP-1, FAS and ACC. Levels of hepatic PPARγ expression are low in normal body fat composition. Under fasted condition, hepatic PPARγ expression is suppressed by CREB via stimulating the expression of the Hairy Enhancer of Split (HES-1) gene [77], a transcriptional repressor. However, PPARγ expression is demonstrated to increase in hepatic steatosis of animal models. Several kinds of transcriptional factors have been reported to stimulate PPARγ expression. Promotor area of PPARγ gene has CCAAT/enhancer-binding proteins (C/EBPs) recognition elements [78]. C/EBPs

(C/EBPα, β and δ) are basic leucine zipper family of transcription factors, which form homo- and hetero-dimers to bind to their consensus sequences on target genes to stimulate adipogenesis. Recent study revealed that C/EBPβ binds to PPARγ promoter region earlier than other transcription factors in the early phase of adipogenesis.

5.4 Interaction Between Liver, Gut and Central Nervous System

5.4.1 Liver-Brain Interaction

Liver plays the important role to sense the absorbed nutrients from the gut via portal vein and originates signals to the brain to regulate systemic metabolism. Food ingestion increases portal vein glucose level, and those signals encoded by hepato-portal glucose sensor are transmitted via afferent vagal nerve fibers to the nucleus of the solitary tract in the hindbrain [79], thereafter feeding is suppressed and hepatic glucose uptake and insulin secretion from pancreatic β cell are increased. Infusion of long-chain fatty acids into the portal vein activates vagal afferent nerve, which transmits hepatic signals to the central nervous system (CNS). Liver steatosis caused by liver-specific overexpression of PPARγ2 reduces peripheral adiposity with increase of lipolysis, which is abolished by hepatic vagal afferent denervation [80]. CNS increases circulating levels of epinephrine and norepinephrine and accelerates hepatic glucose production by the activation of sympathetic efferent nerve to the adrenal glands and the liver. These findings indicate that liver transmits nutritional information to the CNS via afferent vagal nerve, CNS, in turn, regulates hepatic glucose metabolism via efferent nerve activation.

Several hormones can affect hypothalamus and regulate liver glucose metabolism.

Insulin action on CNS also regulates hepatic energy metabolism indirectly by activating its cognate receptor signaling in the hypothalamus. Insulin stimulates the PI 3-kinase/Akt pathway in the brain [49], which in turn causes downregulation of GSK-3β in the liver and increases glycogen synthesis [81]. Hypothalamic insulin signals suppress hepatic glucose production via activation of insulin receptor/PI3kinase/K_{ATP} channels pathway [49]. These signals are transmitted to the liver via vagal innervation to suppress hepatic gluconeogenic enzymes expression, such as PEPCK and G-6-Pase, thereby decreases hepatic glucose output. Agouti-related peptide expressing neurons of the arcuate nucleus is thought to be responsive to transmit hypothalamic insulin action. Another mechanism of suppressive effect of hepatic glucose production by hypothalamic insulin action is promotion of IL-6 production of hepatic Kuepfer cell. Increased IL-6 activates hepatic STAT3 [82, 83], which suppresses PEPCK and G-6-Pase expression.

Leptin derived from adipocyte has pleotropic effects on food intake and body weight but also regulates liver energy metabolism. Leptin suppresses glycogenolysis and gluconeogenesis by inhibition of G-6-Pase and PEPCK expression in the liver which required hypothalamic leptin signaling through its cognate receptor/STAT3 pathway [84].

Hypothalamus, as well as liver, acts as sensor of plasma nutrients of glucose, amino acids and lipids and suppresses hepatic glucose production by stimulating hepatic efferent vagal branch outflow [85] via hypothalamic K_{ATP} channel activation.

5.4.2 Gut-Liver Interaction

Gastrointestinal (GI) system connects closely to the liver with portal vein circulation. Therefore, GI system affects hepatic glucose metabolism directly by the absorbed nutrients and secreted GI hormone, or indirectly via CNS. Duodenum acts as a lipid sensor for long-chain fatty acyl coenzyme A (LCFA-CoA) increased by lipid ingestion to the upper intestine and transmits its nutritional signal via afferent vagal nerve fibers to the nucleus of the solitary tract in the hindbrain [3], which in turn suppresses hepatic glucose production via vagal efferent nerve innervated to the liver. Duodenal nutritional signal is thought to be transmitted to the vagal afferent nerve by binding of cholecystokinin (CCK) released from duodenal mucosa to the CCK- A receptor on the vagal nerve end to decrease hepatic glucose production [86], which is the gut-brain-liver axis.

Gut microbiota interact with host human energy balance and glucose metabolism.

Contents and calorie of diet alter composition of gut microbiota. High fat diet promotes imbalance of gut microbiota, which increases energy extraction and monosaccharide via short chain fatty acids (SCFAs) production from the indigestible dietary polysaccharide by hydrolysis and fermentation, fatty acid storage in adipocyte by the suppression of fasting-induced adipocyte factor and inhibition of fatty acid oxidation in the liver by AMPK inhibition, resulting in liver energy storage as fat [87, 88]. Alteration of microbiota composition induced by a diet rich in lipids promotes intestinal permeability and increases plasma lipopolysaccharides (LPS), leading to low-grade inflammation and elevation of inflammatory cytokines. Increased hepatic lipogenesis and low-grade inflammation induces insulin resistance in the liver.

In this way, hepatic glucose metabolism is regulated by the communication between liver, gut and the CNS. CNS integrates nutrient information from peripheral sites, such as the liver or intestine, and sends signals to modulate hepatic glucose and lipid metabolism through the afferent autonomic nerve fibers.

5.4.3 Adipose Tissue-Liver Interaction

Adipose tissue affects liver glucose and lipid metabolism by supplying liver with free fatty acids (FFAs) and glycerol and by releasing several kinds of adipocytokines. TG stored in the adipocyte is hydrolyzed by adipose triglyceride lipase (ATGL) to FFAs and diacylglycerol (DG), which is further hydrolyzed to monoacylglycerol (MG), and MG was hydrolyzed to glycerol by MG lipase. These hydrolyzed products are released from adipocyte to portal vein. Glycerol is taken into the liver through aquaporin 9 and converted to glycerol-3-phosphate (Glycerol-3-P) by glycerol kinase, resulting in use for gluconeogenesis. FFAs are taken into the liver though CD36 and fatty acid transporter proteins (FATP) and are esterified with glycerol-3-P to generate TG. FFAs increase insulin resistance with serine phosphorylation of insulin receptor and IRS substrate by PKC activation that diminishes its tyrosine kinase activity [89], which is resulted in disturbance of the PI-3 kinase pathway.

5.5 Disturbance of the Glucose Metabolism in the Liver-Obesity, Liver Steatosis and Type2 Diabetes

5.5.1 Hepatic Insulin Resistance

Insulin resistance is defined as the inability of a quantity of exogenous or endogenous insulin to increase tissue glucose uptake and suppress hepatic glucose production in an individual as much as it does in a normal population. Insulin resistance in peripheral tissues characterizes obesity and T2DM, and is involved in the pathogenesis of diabetes. Insulin resistance causes disturbance of postprandial glucose uptake and suppression of glucose output in the liver.

Visceral obesity is caused by excessive calorie intake and/or lack of exercise and is characterized by adipocyte hypertrophy, ectopic lipids deposition and chronic low-grade inflammation. In visceral adipose tissue of obesity, resident T cell population is changed, and M1 macrophages, the inflammatory M1 phenotype, with expression of the CD11c marker are infiltrated and localized around necrotic adipocytes and form crown-like structures. Production of pro-inflammatory cytokines, such as tumor necrosis factor (TNF) α, IL-1β or IL-6, is increased in those adipose tissue.

Regarding insulin signal transduction, insulin resistance is caused by two major impaired stages of insulin signal transduction. One is at the stage of the tyrosine residue phosphorylation of insulin receptor and its receptor substrate, and the other is at the stage involving a glucose transport into the cell. Under insulin resistance state, insulin-stimulated tyrosine phosphorylation of both insulin receptor and IRS were reduced.

In visceral obesity, insulin sensitivity is decreased in adipocytes and accelerated lipolysis, which is resulted in increased plasma FFA. FFA promotes serine phosphorylation of insulin receptor and IRS that diminishes its tyrosine kinase activity via activation of PKC isoforms which act as serine/threonine kinase. Serine-threonine phosphorylation of IRS disturbs its association with the insulin receptor and with PI-3 kinase, resulting in desensitization of the PI-3 kinase pathway. Classical and novel PKC isoforms are activated by increase of intracellular diacylglycerol due to hyperinsulinemia and elevated plasma FFA, and atypical PKC isoform, PKCζ, is activated by insulin via PI3 kinase pathway.

Increased TNFα released from visceral adipose tissue promotes phosphorylation of serine residue (serine^{312} in human) within the PTB domain of IRS-1 via activation of serine kinase, c-Jun terminal kinase (JNK). Serine phosphorylation of IRS-1 causes conformational change of it and decreases IRS-1 binding to insulin receptor, thereby diminishes the tyrosine residue phosphorylation and inhibits insulin signaling.. In this way, insulin-stimulated tyrosine phosphorylation of both insulin receptor and IRS were reduced, and association of PI-3 kinase with IRS and Akt phosphorylation is decreased. TNFα also activates IκB kinase β (IKKβ), which also acts as serine kinase and phosphorylates serine residues of IRS and insulin receptor, thereby diminishes insulin signaling. IKKβ also activates nuclear transcription factor kappa-B (NF-κB) via phosphorylation of IκB, which causes NF-κB dissociation from the IκB and translocation to the nucleus. NF-κB activates multiple genes involved in inflammatory reactions, innate immunity or stress response, which products can enhance insulin resistance. As a result, transcription of the glucokinase gene turned on by insulin is suppressed, that is one of the reasons for decrease in hepatic glucose uptake under condition of insulin resistance.

In the liver, IRS-2 is the main mediator of insulin signaling and control insulin sensitivity. Transcription of IRS-2 is regulated by FoxO1 [90]. The IRS-2 promoter is activated by forkhead proteins through an insulin response element (IRE). Obesity or fatty liver is associated with hyperinsulinemia caused by increased insulin secretion from β cell or insulin clearance in the liver. Insulin phosphorylates Akt via PI3 kinase activation. Phosphorylated Akt causes nuclear exclusion of FoxO1 by its phosphorylation. FoxO1 phosphorylation is irreversible reaction and phosphorylated FoxO1 is ubiquitinated and degraded. Increased FoxO1 exclusion from the nucleus by sustained hyperinsulinemia represses transcription of IRS-2 and inhibits hepatic insulin signaling.

SREBPs are transcription factors that regulate genes involved in lipid synthesis, as described above. SREBP-1c is the predominant isoform in most adult non-dividing metabolic tissues such as liver and adipose. The SREBP-1c promoter is autoregulated by SREBPs and stimulated by both insulin signaling and liver X receptor (LXR). In non-alcoholic fatty liver disease in human, insulin signaling via IRS-1 causes the upregulation of SREBP1-c, following a decrease of IRS-2. SREBPs directly repress transcription of IRS-2. IRS-2 promoter has IRE where forkhead proteins can bind and positively regulate IRS-2 expression. Nuclear SREBPs effectively replace and interfere in the binding to these transactivators, resulting in inhibition of the downstream PI3K/Akt pathway, thereby glycogen synthesis is decreased. Disturbance of Akt activation by insulin resistance decreases FoxO1 phosphorylation and its exportation from the nucleus, allowing FoxO1 retaining in nucleus and decrease in dissociation from the promoter area of PEPCK or G-6-Pase, results in increase of the expression of these gluconeogenic enzymes [68], as described above.

Hyperinsulinemia induces ubiquitin-mediated degradation of IRS-1 and IRS-2 by suppressor of cytokine signaling (SOCS) proteins [91]. IRS can be induced proteasomal degraded by post-translational modification of O-linked N-acetylglucosamine adducts (O-GlcNAc) on serine/threonine residues under hyperglycemic conditions [91], or by S-nitrosylation as a consequence of nitric oxide generation [92].

References

1. Unger RH, Cherrington AD. Glucagonocentric restructuring of diabetes: a pathophysiologic and therapeutic makeover. J Clin Invest. 2012;122(1):4–12. doi:10.1172/JCI60016.
2. Uno K, Katagiri H, Yamada T, Ishigaki Y, Ogihara T, Imai J, et al. Neuronal pathway from the liver modulates energy expenditure and systemic insulin sensitivity. Science. 2006;312:1656–9.
3. Wang PY, Caspi L, Lam CK, Chari M, Li X, Light PE. Upper intestinal lipids trigger a gut-brain-liver axis to regulate glucose production. Nature. 2008;452(7190):1012–16. doi:10.1038/nature06852.
4. Ferrannini E, Smith JD, Cobelli C, Toffolo G, Pilo A, DeFronzo RA. Effect of insulin on the distribution and disposition of glucose in man. J Clin Invest. 1985;76:357–64.
5. Waeber G, Thompson N, Haefliger JA, Nicod P. Characterization of the murine high Km glucose transporter GLUT2 gene and its transcriptional regulation by glucose in a differentiated insulin-secreting cell line. J Biol Chem. 1994;269:26912–19.
6. Agius L. Glucokinase and molecular aspects of liver glycogen metabolism. Biochem J. 2008;414:1–18. doi:10.1042/BJ20080595.
7. Tiedge M. Lenzen S Effects of glucose refeeding and glibenclamide treatment on glucokinase and GLUT2 gene expression in pancreatic B-cells and liver from rats. Biochem J. 1995;308 (Pt 1):139–44.
8. Sibrowski W, Seitz HJ. Rapid action of insulin and cyclic AMP in the regulation of functional messenger RNA coding for glucokinase in rat liver. J Biol Chem. 1984;259:343–6.
9. van Schaftingen E, Gerin I. The glucose-6-phosphatase system. Biochem J. 2002;362 (Pt 3):513–32.
10. Chu CA, Fujimoto Y, Igawa K, Grimsby J, Grippo JF, Magnuson MA, et al. Rapid translocation of hepatic glucokinase in response to intraduodenal glucose infusion and changes in plasma glucose and insulin in conscious rats. Am J Physiol Gastrointest Liver Physiol. 2004;286:G627–34.
11. Davies DR, Detheux M, Van Schaftingen E. Fructose 1-phosphate and the regulation of glucokinase activity in isolated hepatocytes. Eur J Biochem. 1990;192:283–9.
12. Nouspikel T, Iynedjian PB. Insulin signalling and regulation of glucokinase gene expression in cultured hepatocytes. Eur J Biochem. 1992;210:365–73.
13. Kim SY, Kim HI, Kim TH, Im SS, Park SK, Lee IK, et al. SREBP-1c mediates the insulin-dependent hepatic glucokinase expression. J Biol Chem. 2004;279:30823–9.

14. Nordlie RC, Arion WJ. Evidence for the common identity of glucose 6-phosphatase, inorganic pyrophosphate, and pyrophosphate –glucose phosphotransferase. J Biol Chem. 1964;239:1680–5.
15. Argaud D, Zhang Q, Pan W, Maitra S, Pilkis SJ, Lange AJ. Regulation of rat liver glucose-6-phosphatase gene expression in different nutritional and hormonal states: gene structure and 5'-flanking sequence. Diabetes. 1996;45:1563–71.
16. Minassian C, Zitoun C, Mithieux G. Differential time course of liver and kidney glucose-6 phosphatase activity during long-term fasting in rat correlates with differential time course of messenger RNA level. Mol Cell Biochem. 1996;155:37–41.
17. Liu Z, Barrett EJ, Dalkin AC, Zwart AD, Chou JY. Effect of acute diabetes on rat hepatic glucose-6-phosphatase activity and its messenger RNA level. Biochem Biophys Res Commun. 1994;205:680–6. doi:10.1006/bbrc.1994.2719.
18. Yang SD, Chang SY, Soderling TR. Characterization of an autophosphorylation-dependent multifunctional protein kinase from liver. J Biol Chem. 1987;262:9421–7.
19. Patel S, Doble BW, MacAulay K, Sinclair EM, Drucker DJ, Woodgett JR. Tissue-specific role of glycogen synthase kinase 3beta in glucose homeostasis and insulin action. Mol Cell Biol. 2008;20:6314–28. doi:10.1128/MCB.00763-08.
20. Gasa R, Jensen PB, Berman HK, Brady MJ, DePaoli-Roach AA, Newgard CB. Distinctive regulatory and metabolic properties of glycogen-targeting subunits of protein phosphatase-1 (PTG, GL, GM/RGl) expressed in hepatocytes. J Biol Chem. 2000;275:26396–403.
21. Landau BR, Wahren J, Chandramouli V, Schumann WC, Ekberg K, Kalhan SC. Contributions of gluconeogenesis to glucose production in the fasted state. J Clin Invest. 1996;98:378–85.
22. Sutherland EW, Robison GA. The role of cyclic AMP in the control of carbohydrate metabolism. Diabetes. 1969;18:797–819.
23. Holm L, Sander C. Evolutionary link between glycogen phosphorylase and a DNA modifying enzyme. EMBO J. 1995;14:1287–93.
24. Erion MD, Dang Q, Reddy MR, Kasibhatla SR, Huang J, Lipscomb WN. Structure-guided design of AMP mimics that inhibit fructose-1,6-bisphosphatase with high affinity and specificity. J Am Chem Soc. 2007;129:15480–90.
25. Pilkis SJ, el-Maghrabi MR, Claus TH. Fructose-2,6-bisphosphate in control of hepatic gluconeogenesis. From metabolites to molecular genetics. Diabetes Care. 1990;13:582–99.
26. Tang BL. The mitochondrial pyruvate carrier and metabolic regulation. Cell Biol. 2014;3:111–17. doi:10.4236/cellbio.2014.34011.
27. Groen AK, van Roermund CW, Vervoorn RC, Tager JM. Control of gluconeogenesis in rat liver cells. Flux control coefficients of the enzymes in the gluconeogenic pathway in the absence and presence of glucagon. Biochem J. 1986;237:379–89.
28. Herzig S, Long F, Jhala US, Hedrick S, Quinn R, Bauer A, et al. CREB regulates hepatic gluconeogenesis through the coactivator PGC-1. Nature. 2001;413:179–83. doi:10.1038/35093131.
29. Oh KJ, Han HS, Kim MJ, Koo SH. CREB and FoxO1: two transcription factors for the regulation of hepatic gluconeogenesis. BMB Rep. 2013;46:567–74. doi:10.5483/BMBRep.2013.46.12.248.
30. Puigserver P, Rhee J, Donovan J, Walkey CJ, Yoon JC, Oriente F, et al. Insulin-regulated hepatic gluconeogenesis through FOXO1-PGC-1alpha interaction. Nature. 2003;423:550–5.
31. Gray S, Wang B, Orihuela Y, Hong EG, Fisch S, Haldar S, Cline GW, Kim JK, Peroni OD, Kahn BB, Jain MK. Regulation of gluconeogenesis by Krüppel-like factor 15. Cell Metab. 2007;5:305–12. doi:10.1016/j.cmet.2007.03.002.
32. Yoon JC, Puigserver P, Chen G, Donovan J, Wu Z, Rhee J, et al. Control of hepatic gluconeogenesis through the transcriptional coactivator PGC-1. Nature. 2001;413:131–8. doi:10.1038/35093050.
33. Imai E, Miner JN, Mitchell JA, Yamamoto KR, Granner DK. Glucocorticoid receptor-cAMP response element-binding protein interaction and the response of the phosphoenolpyruvate carboxykinase gene to glucocorticoids. J Biol Chem. 1993;268:5353–6.

34. Hall RK, Sladek FM, Granner DK. The orphan receptors COUP-TF and HNF-4 serve as accessory factors required for induction of phosphoenolpyruvate carboxykinase gene transcription by glucocorticoids. Proc Natl Acad Sci U S A. 1995;92:412–16.
35. Rhee J, Inoue Y, Yoon JC, Puigserver P, Fan M, Gonzalez FJ, et al. Regulation of hepatic fasting response by PPARgamma coactivator-1alpha (PGC-1): requirement for hepatocyte nuclear factor 4alpha in gluconeogenesis. Proc Natl Acad Sci U S A. 2003;100:4012–17. doi:10.1073/pnas.0730870100.
36. Habegger KM, Heppner KM, Geary N, Bartness TJ, DiMarchi R, Tschöp MH. The metabolic actions of glucagon revisited. Nat Rev Endocrinol. 2010;6(12):689–97. doi:10.1038/nrendo.2010.187.
37. Luo Q, Viste K, Urday-Zaa JC, Senthil Kumar G, Tsai WW, Talai A, et al. Mechanism of CREB recognition and coactivation by the CREB-regulated transcriptional coactivator CRTC2. Proc Natl Acad Sci U S A. 2012;109:20865–70. doi:10.1073/pnas.1219028109.
38. Henriksson E, Säll J, Gormand A, Wasserstrom S, Morrice NA, Fritzen AM, et al. SIK2 regulates CRTCs, HDAC4 and glucose uptake in adipocytes. J Cell Sci. 2015;128:472–86. doi:10.1242/jcs.153932.
39. Altarejos JY, Montminy M. CREB and the CRTC co-activators: sensors for hormonal and metabolic signals. Nat Rev Mol Cell Biol. 2011;12:141–51. doi:10.1038/nrm3072.
40. Puigserver P, Wu Z, Park CW, Graves R, Wright M, Spiegelman BM. A cold-inducible coactivator of nuclear receptors linked to adaptive thermogenesis. Cell. 1998;92:829–39. doi:10.1016/S0092-8674(00)81410-5.
41. Takashima M, Ogawa W, Hayashi K, Inoue H, Kinoshita S, Okamoto Y, et al. Role of KLF15 in regulation of hepatic gluconeogenesis and metformin action. Diabetes. 2010;59 (7):1608–15. doi:10.2337/db09-1679.
42. Brunet A, Bonni A, Zigmond MJ, Lin MZ, Juo P, Hu LS, et al. Akt promotes cell survival by phosphorylating and inhibiting a Forkhead transcription factor. Cell. 1999;96:857–68. doi:10.1016/S0092-8674(00)80595-4.
43. He L, Sabet A, Djedjos S, Miller R, Sun X, Hussain MA, et al. Metformin and insulin suppress hepatic gluconeogenesis through phosphorylation of CREB binding protein. Cell. 2009;137 (4):635–46. doi:10.1016/j.cell.2009.03.016.
44. Leung YM, Ahmed I, Sheu L, Gao X, Hara M, Tsushima RG, et al. Insulin regulates islet alpha-cell function by reducing KATP channel sensitivity to adenosine 5'-triphosphate inhibition. Endocrinology. 2006;147:2155–62. doi:10.1210/en.2005-1249.
45. Vander Haar E, Lee SI, Bandhakavi S, Griffin TJ, Kim DH. Insulin signalling to mTOR mediated by the Akt/PKB substrate PRAS40. Nat Cell Biol. 2007;9:316–23. doi:10.1038/ncb1547.
46. Adams CM. Role of the transcription factor ATF4 in the anabolic actions of insulin and the anti-anabolic actions of glucocorticoids. Biol Chem. 2007;282:16744–53. doi:10.1074/jbc.M610510200.
47. Könner AC, Janoschek R, Plum L, Jordan SD, Rother E, Ma X, et al. Insulin action in AgRP-expressing neurons is required for suppression of hepatic glucose production. Cell Metab. 2007;5(6):438–49. doi:10.1016/j.cmet.2007.05.004.
48. Niswender KD, Morrison CD, Clegg DJ, Olson R, Baskin DG, Myers Jr MG, et al. Insulin activation of phosphatidylinositol 3-kinase in the hypothalamic arcuate nucleus: a key mediator of insulin-induced anorexia. Diabetes. 2003;52(2):227–31. doi:10.2337/diabetes.52.2.227.
49. Pocai A, Lam TK, Gutierrez-Juarez R, Obici S, Schwartz GJ, Bryan J, et al. Hypothalamic K (ATP) channels control hepatic glucose production. Nature. 2005;434:1026–31. doi:10.1038/nature03439.
50. Kadowaki T, Ueki K, Yamauchi T, Kubota N. SnapShot: insulin signaling pathways. Cell. 2012;148:624, 624.e1. doi:10.1016/j.cell.2012.01.034.

51. Kasuga M, Hedo JA, Yamada KM, Kahn CR. The structure of insulin receptor and its subunits. Evidence for multiple nonreduced forms and a 210,000 possible proreceptor. J Biol Chem. 1982;257:10392–9.
52. Sun XJ, Rothenberg P, Kahn CR, Backer JM, Araki E, Wilden PA, et al. Structure of the insulin receptor substrate IRS-1 defines a unique signal transduction protein. Nature. 1991;352:73–7. doi:10.1038/352073a.
53. Lavan BE, Lane WS, Lienhard GE. The 60-kDa phosphotyrosine protein in insulin-treated adipocytes is a new member of the insulin receptor substrate family. J Biol Chem. 1997;272:11439–43.
54. Sun XJ, Wang LM, Zhang Y, Yenush L, Myers Jr MG, Glasheen E, et al. Role of IRS-2 in insulin and cytokine signalling. Nature. 1995;377:173–7. doi:10.1038/377173a.
55. Lavan BE, Fantin VR, Chang ET, Lane WS, Keller SR, Lienhard GE. A novel 160-kDa phosphotyrosine protein in insulin-treated embryonic kidney cells is a new member of the insulin receptor substrate family. J Biol Chem. 1997;272:21403–7.
56. Tamemoto H, Kadowaki T, Tobe K, Yagi T, Sakura H, Hayakawa T, et al. Insulin resistance and growth retardation in mice lacking insulin receptor substrate-1. Nature. 1994;372:182–6. doi:10.1038/372182a.
57. Kubota N, Tobe K, Terauchi Y, Eto K, Yamauchi T, Suzuki R, et al. Disruption of insulin receptor substrate 2 causes type 2 diabetes because of liver insulin resistance and lack of compensatory beta-cell hyperplasia. Diabetes. 2000;49:1880–9.
58. Wu J, Tseng YD, Xu CF, Neubert TA, White MF, Hubbard SR. Structural and biochemical characterization of the KRLB region in insulin receptor substrate-2. Nat Struct Mol Biol. 2008;15:251–8. doi:10.1038/nsmb.1388.
59. Yamauchi T, Kamon J, Minokoshi Y, Ito Y, Waki H, Uchida S, et al. Adiponectin stimulates glucose utilization and fatty-acid oxidation by activating AMP-activated protein kinase. Nat Med. 2002;8:1288–95. doi:10.1038/nm788.
60. Yamauchi T, Nio Y, Maki T, Kobayashi M, Takazawa T, Iwabu M, et al. Targeted disruption of AdipoR1 and AdipoR2 causes abrogation of adiponectin binding and metabolic actions. Nat Med. 2007;13:332–9. doi:10.1038/nm1557.
61. Lin Z, Tian H, Lam KS, Lin S, Hoo RC, Konishi M, et al. Adiponectin mediates the metabolic effects of FGF21 on glucose homeostasis and insulin sensitivity in mice. Cell Metab. 2013;17:779–89. doi:10.1016/j.cmet.2013.04.005.
62. Kir S, Beddow SA, Samuel VT, Miller P, Previs SF, Suino-Powell K, et al. FGF19 as a postprandial, insulin-independent activator of hepatic protein and glycogen synthesis. Science. 2011;331:1621–4. doi:10.1126/science.1198363.
63. Inagaki T, Dutchak P, Zhao G, Ding X, Gautron L, Parameswara V, et al. Endocrine regulation of the fasting response by PPARalpha-mediated induction of fibroblast growth factor 21. Cell Metab. 2007;5:415–25. doi:10.1016/j.cmet.2007.05.003.
64. Kim YD, Kim YH, Tadi S, Yu JH, Yim YH, Jeoung NH, et al. Metformin inhibits growth hormone-mediated hepatic PDK4 gene expression through induction of orphan nuclear receptor small heterodimer partner. Diabetes. 2012;61:2484–94. doi:10.2337/db11-1665.
65. Kovacs JJ, Murphy PJ, Gaillard S, Zhao X, Wu JT, Nicchitta CV, et al. HDAC6 regulates Hsp90 acetylation and chaperone-dependent activation of glucocorticoid receptor. Mol Cell. 2005;18:601–7. doi:10.1016/j.molcel.2005.04.021.
66. Lu Y, Xiong X, Wang X, Zhang Z, Li J, Shi G, et al. Yin Yang 1 promotes hepatic gluconeogenesis through upregulation of glucocorticoid receptor. Diabetes. 2013;62:1064–73. doi:10.2337/db12-0744.
67. Yu Y, Maguire TG, Alwine JC. ChREBP, a glucose-responsive transcriptional factor, enhances glucose metabolism to support biosynthesis in human cytomegalovirus-infected cells. Proc Natl Acad Sci U S A. 2014;111:1951–6. doi:10.1073/pnas.1310779111.
68. Ido-Kitamura Y, Sasaki T, Kobayashi M, Kim HJ, Lee YS, Kikuchi O, et al. Hepatic FoxO1 integrates glucose utilization and lipid synthesis through regulation of Chrebp O-glycosylation. PLoS ONE. 2012;7(10):e47231. doi:10.1371/journal.pone.0047231.

69. Rawson RB. The SREBP pathway--insights from Insigs and insects. Nat Rev Mol Cell Biol. 2003;4:631–40. doi:10.1038/nrm1174.
70. Yellaturu CR, Deng X, Park EA, Raghow R, Elam MB. Insulin enhances the biogenesis of nuclear sterol regulatory element-binding protein (SREBP)-1c by posttranscriptional down-regulation of Insig-2A and its dissociation from SREBP cleavage-activating protein (SCAP) SREBP-1c complex. Biol Chem. 2009;284:31726–34. doi:10.1074/jbc.M109.050914.
71. Sun LP, Seemann J, Goldstein JL, Brown MS. Sterol-regulated transport of SREBPs from endoplasmic reticulum to Golgi: Insig renders sorting signal in Scap inaccessible to COPII proteins. Proc Natl Acad Sci U S A. 2007;104:6519–26. doi:10.1073/pnas.0700907104.
72. Yecies JL, Zhang HH, Menon S, Liu S, Yecies D, Lipovsky AI, et al. Akt stimulates hepatic SREBP1c and lipogenesis through parallel mTORC1-dependent and independent pathways. Cell Metab. 2011;14:21–32. doi:10.1016/j.cmet.2011.06.002.
73. Peterson TR, Sengupta SS, Harris TE, Carmack AE, Kang SA, Balderas E, et al. mTOR complex 1 regulates lipin 1 localization to control the SREBP pathway. Cell. 2011;146:408–20. doi:10.1016/j.cell.2011.06.034.
74. Yoshikawa T, Shimano H, Amemiya-Kudo M, Yahagi N, Hasty AH, Matsuzaka T, et al. Identification of liver X receptor-retinoid X receptor as an activator of the sterol regulatory element-binding protein 1c gene promoter. Mol Cell Biol. 2001;21:2991–3000. doi:10.1128/MCB.21.9.2991-3000.2001.
75. Kohjima M, Higuchi N, Kato M, Kotoh K, Yoshimoto T, Fujino T, et al. SREBP-1c, regulated by the insulin and AMPK signaling pathways, plays a role in nonalcoholic fatty liver disease. Int J Mol Med. 2008;21:507–11. doi:10.3892/ijmm.21.4.507.
76. Matsumoto M, Ogawa W, Akimoto K, Inoue H, Miyake K, Furukawa K, et al. PKClambda in liver mediates insulin-induced SREBP-1c expression and determines both hepatic lipid content and overall insulin sensitivity. J Clin Invest. 2003;112:935–44. doi:10.1172/JCI18816.
77. Herzig S, Hedrick S, Morantte I, Koo SH, Galimi F, Montminy M. CREB controls hepatic lipid metabolism through nuclear hormone receptor PPAR-gamma. Nature. 2003;426:190–3. doi:10.1038/nature02110.
78. Farmer SR. Regulation of PPARgamma activity during adipogenesis. Int J Obes (Lond). 2005;29 Suppl 1:S13–16. doi:10.1038/sj.ijo.0802907.
79. Yi CX, la Fleur SE, Fliers E, Kalsbeek A. The role of the autonomic nervous liver innervation in the control of energy metabolism. Biochim Biophys Acta. 2010;1802:416–31. doi:10.1016/j.bbadis.2010.01.006.
80. Schadinger SE, Bucher NL, Schreiber BM, Farmer SR. PPARgamma2 regulates lipogenesis and lipid accumulation in steatotic hepatocytes. Am J Physiol Endocrinol Metab. 2005;288:E1195–205. doi:10.1152/ajpendo.00513.2004.
81. Ramnanan CJ, Saraswathi V, Smith MS, Donahue EP, Farmer B, Farmer TD, et al. Brain insulin action augments hepatic glycogen synthesis without suppressing glucose production or gluconeogenesis in dogs. J Clin Invest. 2011;121(9):3713–23. doi:10.1172/JCI45472.
82. Inoue H, Ogawa W, Asakawa A, Okamoto Y, Nishizawa A, Matsumoto M, et al. Role of hepatic STAT3 in brain-insulin action on hepatic glucose production. Cell Metab. 2006;3:267–75. doi:10.1016/j.cmet.2006.02.009.
83. Myers Jr MG. Role reversal: brain insulin and liver STAT3. Cell Metab. 2006;3(4):231–2. doi:10.1016/j.cmet.2006.03.003.
84. Buettner C, Pocai A, Muse ED, Etgen AM, Myers Jr MG, Rossetti L. Critical role of STAT3 in leptin's metabolic actions. Cell Metab. 2006;4:49–60. doi:10.1016/j.cmet.2006.04.014.
85. Bernal-Mizrachi C, Xiaozhong L, Yin L, Knutsen RH, Howard MJ, Arends JJA, et al. An afferent vagal nerve pathway links hepatic PPARα activation to glucocorticoid-induced insulin resistance and hypertension. Cell Metab. 2007;5:91–102. doi:10.1016/j.cmet.2006.12.010.
86. Moran TH, Norgren R, Crosby RJ, McHugh PR. Central and peripheral vagal transport of cholecystokinin binding sites occurs in afferent fibers. Brain Res. 1990;526:95–102. doi:10.1016/0006-8993(90)90253-8.

87. Lau E, Carvalho D, Freitas P. Gut Microbiota: association with NAFLD and metabolic disturbances. Biomed Res Int. 2015;2015:979515. doi:10.1155/2015/979515.
88. Festi D, Schiumerini R, Eusebi LH, Marasco G, Taddia M, Colecchia A. Gut microbiota and metabolic syndrome. World J Gastroenterol. 2014;20:16079–94. doi:10.3748/wjg.v20.i43.16079.
89. Pereira S, Park E, Mori Y, Haber CA, Han P, Uchida T, et al. FFA-induced hepatic insulin resistance in vivo is mediated by PKCδ, NADPH oxidase, and oxidative stress. Am J Physiol Endocrinol Metab. 2014;307:E34–46. doi:10.1152/ajpendo.00436.2013.
90. Kamagate A, Kim DH, Zhang T, Slusher S, Gramignoli R, Strom SC, et al. FoxO1 links hepatic insulin action to endoplasmic reticulum stress. Endocrinology. 2010;151:3521–35. doi:10.1210/en.2009-1306.
91. Klein AL, Berkaw MN, Buse MG, Ball LE. O-linked N-acetylglucosamine modification of insulin receptor substrate-1 occurs in close proximity to multiple SH2 domain binding motifs. Mol Cell Proteomics. 2009;8:2733–45. doi:10.1074/mcp.M900207-MCP200.
92. Shinozaki S, Choi CS, Shimizu N, Yamada M, Kim M, Zhang T, et al. Liver-specific inducible nitric-oxide synthase expression is sufficient to cause hepatic insulin resistance and mild hyperglycemia in mice. J Biol Chem. 2011;286:34959–75. doi:10.1074/jbc.M110.187666.

Chapter 6
Lipid Metabolism and the Liver

Munechika Enjoji, Motoyuki Kohjima, and Makoto Nakamuta

Abstract Generally, lipid metabolism in liver hepatocytes can be summarized by three processes: (1) acquisition of lipids, including uptake of lipids and fatty acids, and fatty acid synthesis (de novo lipogenesis); (2) lipid storage, including triglyceride synthesis and the formation of lipid droplets; and (3) lipid consumption, including fatty acid degradation (lipolysis), β-oxidation, and the secretion of very low-density lipoproteins. Many liver diseases are accompanied by disorders in lipid metabolism, with the latter often involving the clinical condition of these patients. This chapter summarizes current understanding of hepatic lipid metabolism, including cholesterol and phospholipid metabolism, and associated factors. In addition, we make reference to metabolic disturbance in some liver diseases.

Keywords Lipid metabolism • Fatty acid • Triglyceride • Cholesterol • Phospholipid

6.1 Introduction

The liver is the central organ in lipid metabolism. Hepatocytes take up fatty acids (FAs) mainly from two sources: the hydrolysis of esterified FAs in triglycerides (TGs), which are transported by gut-derived chylomicrons during the postprandial period, and nonesterified free FAs, which are derived from lipolysis of adipose tissue during fasting periods. In addition, hepatocytes possess the ability to synthesize FAs

---

M. Enjoji (✉)
Department of Clinical Pharmacology, Faculty of Pharmaceutical Sciences, Fukuoka University, 8-19-1 Nanakuma, Jonan-ku, Fukuoka 814-0180, Japan

Clinical Research Institute, National Hospital Organization Kyushu Medical Center, Fukuoka, Japan
e-mail: enjoji@adm.fukuoka-u.ac.jp

M. Kohjima • M. Nakamuta
Clinical Research Institute, National Hospital Organization Kyushu Medical Center, Fukuoka, Japan

Department of Gastroenterology, National Hospital Organization Kyushu Medical Center, Fukuoka, Japan

H. Ohira (ed.), *The Liver in Systemic Diseases*, DOI 10.1007/978-4-431-55790-6_6

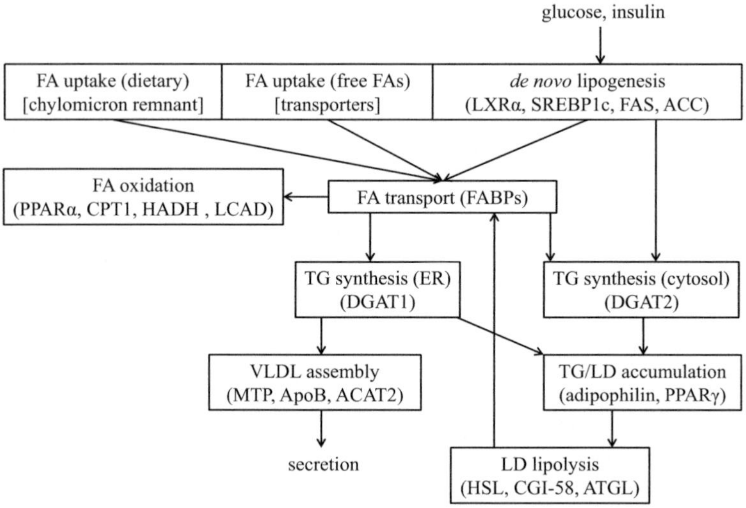

Fig. 6.1 Schematic of the FA/TG metabolic pathway in hepatocytes. Abbreviations: *FA* fatty acid, *LXR* liver X receptor, *SREBP* sterol regulatory element-binding protein, *FAS* fatty acid synthase, *ACC* acetyl-CoA carboxylase, *PPAR* peroxisome proliferator-activated receptor, *CPT* carnitine palmitoyl acyl-CoA transferase, *HADH* hydroxyacyl-CoA dehydrogenase, *LCAD* long-chain acyl-CoA dehydrogenase, *FABP* fatty acid-binding protein, *TG* triglyceride, *ER* endoplasmic reticulum, *DGAT*, *VLDL* very low-density lipoprotein, *MTP* microsomal triglyceride transfer protein, *ApoB* apolipoprotein B, *ACAT* acyl-CoA:cholesterol acyltransferase, *LD* lipid droplet, *HSL* hormone-sensitive lipase, *CGI* comparative gene identification, *ATGL* adipose triglyceride lipase

from excess glucose (de novo lipogenesis) and to hydrolyze TGs into FAs (lipolysis). These FAs, derived from various sources, are used for many important cellular events, such as the synthesis of cellular membranes and intracellular signaling pathways. In addition, FAs can be oxidized to produce acetyl-CoA and ATP, and in the synthesis/reconstruction of TGs, which are stored in lipid droplets (LDs) or secreted into plasma as very low-density lipoprotein (VLDL) particles. VLDL particles can deliver secreted TGs to adipose tissue for storage and to muscle as a source of energy. A schematic of the FA/TG metabolic pathways in hepatocytes is presented in Fig. 6.1. Additionally, the liver plays an important role in cholesterol and phospholipid metabolism. Although the regulation of these events is complex and, in some parts, still unclear, TG/LD accumulation in the cytoplasm of hepatocytes arises from an imbalance between lipid acquisition and consumption.

6.2 FA and TG Metabolism

6.2.1 Lipid Uptake

Hepatocyte uptake of FA was thought to occur through passive diffusion because of the hydrophobicity of FAs. However, recent studies indicate that the transport of FAs, particularly long-chain FAs, is regulated by translocases and transporters

[1]. The rate of FA uptake from plasma into hepatocytes depends on the plasma FA level as well as the hepatocellular capacity for FA uptake. In the fasting state, a reduction in insulin levels stimulates TG hydrolysis in adipose tissue. FAs are thereby released and transported to the liver. The process of FA uptake depends on the number and activity of transporter proteins expressed on the sinusoidal plasma membrane of the hepatocytes. Adipose differentiation-related protein (ADRP), also called adipophilin or perilipin-2, is thought to play a role in FA uptake [2], and the ability to import FAs is impaired in adipophilin-deficient livers [3]. Other plasma membrane transporters of FAs include the fatty acid transporter proteins (FATPs), caveolins, fatty acid translocase (FAT)/CD36, and fatty acid-binding protein (FABP) [4]. FATP2 and FATP5 are highly expressed in the liver, while hepatic FAT/CD36 expression is normally weak.

Dietary fats are packed into chylomicrons in enterocytes and hydrolyzed and release FAs, of which approximately 20 % are delivered to the liver [5]. Lipoprotein lipase (LPL), an enzyme that hydrolyzes TG-rich lipoproteins, is synthesized mainly in the muscle and adipose tissue and transported to capillary endothelial cells. LPL degradation of TGs in chylomicrons results in their conversion into chylomicron remnants, which are imported into hepatocytes by remnant receptors through apoE on the surface of the remnants. In the liver, FAs derived from peripheral tissue or diet, as well as endogenously synthesized FAs, can be used for: (1) energy and ketone body production via mitochondrial β-oxidation, (2) esterification into TGs and storage in LDs, or (3) TG synthesis and VLDL formation with apolipoprotein B (apoB) for secretion into the circulation [6].

6.2.2 *De novo Lipogenesis*

De novo lipogenesis of FAs occurs in the cytosol. Under physiological conditions, excess glucose stimulates FA and TG synthesis in hepatocytes. The synthesized TGs are stored in LDs or secreted into the blood as VLDL. In the liver, various nuclear transcription factors and enzymes are involved in de novo lipogenesis, with the rate of lipogenesis regulated primarily at the transcriptional level [4, 7]. Liver X receptor α (LXRα), which is activated by endogenous oxysterols as ligands, is an inducer of sterol regulatory element-binding protein 1c (SREBP1c) and carbohydrate-responsive element-binding protein (ChREBP). SREBP1c is a key transcription factor regulating FA synthesis, which upregulates several lipogenic genes, including those encoding acetyl-CoA carboxylase 1 (ACC1) and fatty acid synthase (FAS). ACC1 and FAS are enzymes that directly enhance the process of FA synthesis. ACC1 converts acetyl-CoA to malonyl-CoA, and FAS catalyzes palmitate synthesis from acetyl-CoA and malonyl-CoA. Although ChREBP is important for glucose-induced expression of glycolytic genes, it can also stimulate lipogenic genes together with SREBP1c. In the postprandial state, elevated serum glucose and insulin levels activate ChREBP and SREBP1c, respectively, resulting in the promotion of de novo lipogenesis. Insulin stimulates lipogenesis, and SREBP1c is activated by insulin receptor substrates (IRSs), while IRSs suppress FA oxidation through the inhibition factor, forkhead box protein A2

[8–11]. Reduction in expression of the *Srebp-1* gene markedly reduces hepatic lipogenesis but has no effect on VLDL secretion or the amount of white adipose tissue [12, 13].

Conversely, activation of AMP-activated protein kinase (AMPK), a marker of cellular energy stores, suppresses the expression of SREBP1c and inhibits lipogenesis, while stimulating FA oxidation [14, 15]. AMPK is activated by increased levels of cellular AMP and FA, as well as by the effect of adiponectin and peroxisome proliferator-activated receptor γ (PPARγ). Farnesoid X receptor (FXR), a bile acid receptor, and forkhead transcription factor 1 (FoxO1) also show anti-lipogenic effects. A nuclear hormone receptor FXR, which is regulated by bile acids, is a master regulator of lipid and glucose homeostasis in the liver [16]. FXR activation results in downregulation of SREBP1c and LXRα [4] and leads to reduction of TG levels in the liver by [17]: (1) reducing FA synthesis through the reduction of SREBP1c and LXRα expression; (2) enhancing PPARα expression, which promotes β-oxidation; (3) increasing TG clearance; and (4) increasing TG storage in adipose tissue. Activation of FXR can also reduce circulating VLDL levels via FXR-mediated increase in VLDL receptor expression in peripheral tissues [18]. FoxO1 is a transcription factor with an important role in lipid metabolism, in addition to its involvement in glycogenolysis and gluconeogenesis. That is, FoxO1 inhibits SREBP1c expression and suppresses the expression of genes directly involved in FA synthesis, including ACC1 and FAS [19].

The endocannabinoid (EC) system has also been associated with the stimulation of hepatic lipogenesis, as demonstrated by the CB1-mediated effect. The combinated activation of SREBP1c-mediated de novo lipogenesis, reduction of β-oxidation, and decreased VLDL excretion is thought to contribute to CB1-mediated steatogenesis [20–22]. However, under physiological conditions, cannabinoid receptors (CB1 and CB2) are only slightly expressed, suggesting that the EC system may be silent. In contrast, the expression of CBs and/or ECs, such as anandamide, is commonly enhanced in acute and chronic liver injuries. That is, the lipogenetic effect through the EC system may become apparent only in diseased or injured livers. Our group reported that HCV infection activates the EC system and precedes steatosis [23].

6.2.3 Intracellular FA Transport

The FABPs display high affinity binding to hydrophobic ligands such as saturated and unsaturated long-chain FAs. As well as functioning as plasma membrane transporters for FAs, cytoplasmic FABPs enhance the solubility of FAs and transport FAs to specific enzymes and cellular compartments. Namely, FAs are transported to mitochondria and peroxisomes for oxidation, to endoplasmic reticulum (ER) for TG formation, to LDs for storage, and to the nucleus for regulation of gene expression [24].

6.2.4 β-Oxidation

The β-oxidation of FAs occurs within the mitochondria and peroxisomes. In general, short-, medium-, and long-chain FAs are oxidized within mitochondria, while toxic and very long-chain FAs are oxidized within peroxisomes [4]. Carnitine palmitoyl acyl-CoA transferase 1 (CPT1), which mediates the transfer of FAs into mitochondria from cytosol, is a rate-limiting enzyme in mitochondrial β-oxidation. Although short- and medium-chain FAs pass the mitochondrial membrane without being activated, long-chain FAs shuttled across the membrane must be activated by CPT1. The degradation of activated FAs by acyl-CoA-synthetase to acyl-CoA is indispensable for enabling FAs to cross membranes and enter organelles. CPT1 activity is inhibited by interaction with malonyl-CoA, an early intermediate of de novo lipogenesis [7]. During the process of β-oxidation within the mitochondria, acyl-CoA is processed to acetyl-CoA, which enters the tricarboxylic acid cycle or is converted into ketone bodies.

In the liver, PPARα is a pivotal positive regulator of FA oxidation and the formation of ketone bodies. Specifically, PPARα upregulates the expression of genes involved in mitochondrial and peroxisomal β-oxidation, such as hydroxyacyl-CoA dehydrogenase (HADH), long-chain acyl-CoA dehydrogenase (LCAD), and CPT1, while PPARα activation inhibits or reduces hepatic fat storage [25, 26].

6.2.5 TG Construction

TGs are synthesized primarily in the liver, adipose tissue, and small intestine as a major nontoxic energy storage form. In the liver, synthesized TGs are either stored in cytoplasmic LDs or secreted as VLDL particles. Acyl-CoA:diacylglycerol acyltransferases (DGATs) are membrane-bound enzymes that catalyze the final step of TG synthesis from diacylglycerol (DAG) and fatty acyl-CoA. DGAT1 and DGAT2 are unrelated proteins, both of which have DGAT activity. Recently, the roles of DGAT1 and DGAT2 in TG synthesis and VLDL secretion were elucidated in model mice overexpressing DGAT1 and DGAT2 [27]. DGAT1 was located in the lumen of the ER and promoted VLDL secretion. In contrast, DGAT2-overexpressing mice showed increased liver TG content but VLDL secretion was not affected. These results indicate that DGAT1, but not DGAT2, plays a role in VLDL synthesis, whereas increased DGAT2 activity induces LD formation (steatosis). In vitro DGAT1 and DGAT2 expression assays showed small LDs around the cell periphery in DGAT1-expressing cells, whereas numerous large cytosolic LDs were observed in DGAT2-expressing cells [28]. Another in vitro experiment suggested that DGAT1 and acyl-CoA:cholesterol acyltransferase 2 (ACAT2) may coordinately participate in VLDL formation within the ER lumen [29]. These findings suggest that DGAT2 plays a major role in cytosolic lipid accumulation (LD formation), whereas DGAT1 plays a role in VLDL assembly.

6.2.6 VLDL Assembly and Secretion

Regulation of VLDL assembly and secretion is a complex process [30–32]. High levels of FA substrates for TG biosynthesis can increase hepatic VLDL assembly. ApoB; microsomal triglyceride transfer protein (MTP), which includes a rate-limiting enzyme playing a key role in VLDL assembly; and an adequate supply of lipids were found to be necessary for efficient VLDL assembly. ApoB, which can associate with neutral lipids from cellular stores, provides the structural framework for the assembly of VLDL in the liver, with the rate of apoB synthesis controlling the overall rate of VLDL production. Usually, each apoB-containing lipoprotein particle contains a single molecule of apoB. MTP is particularly important for the translocation of full-length apoB100 and transfers lipid components to apoB, facilitating apoB secretion. MTP also appears to be required for VLDL maturation, being found in the Golgi apparatus in addition to the ER. MTP induces greater TG incorporation into apoB-containing lipoproteins, leading to larger VLDL particles. Additionally, MTP can transfer cholesteryl ester from the ER, where it is synthesized by ACATs, onto nascent VLDLs.

VLDLs transport FAs from the liver to adipose and other peripheral tissues. Because adipose tissues receive fat from VLDLs and chylomicrons, an increase in blood VLDL levels may be one cause of obesity. Nascent VLDLs released from the liver contain apoB100, apoC, apoE, cholesterol, cholesteryl esters, and TGs. Circulating VLDLs will come into contact with LPL on the capillary endothelial cells. ApoC-II on lipoproteins can activate LPL, which hydrolizes TGs into FAs and glycerol. High-density lipoprotein also transfers cholesteryl esters to VLDLs in exchange for phospholipids and TGs via cholesteryl ester transfer protein (CETP). As more TGs are removed from the VLDLs owing to the action of LPL and CETP enzymes, the composition of the VLDLs changes, resulting in their conversion into intermediate-density lipoprotein (IDL) [33]. IDL is imported into hepatocytes via apoE and converted to low-density lipoprotein (LDL) by hepatic triglyceride lipase. LDL can remove TGs from VLDLs for storage or energy production, with two-thirds of LDL in the blood imported into various cells via apoB100 combining with a LDL receptor (LDLR).

The autonomic nervous input to the liver appears to have a role in hepatic lipid, as well as carbohydrate, metabolism. Increased sympathetic activity stimulates VLDL secretion, which is mediated via the secretion of noradrenaline at sympathetic nerve endings in the liver. Sympathetic outflow to the liver is activated during fasting and inhibited during feeding. Fasting also stimulates the release of neuropeptide Y (NPY) at the level of the paraventricular nucleus, and these neurons are connected to the sympathetic nervous system [34]. After intracerebroventricular infusion of NPY, hepatic mRNA expression of CPT1 decreased and mRNA expression of ADP-ribosylation factor increased, indicating decreased β-oxidation and increased VLDL assembly [35]. The parasympathetic nervous system is activated postprandially to inhibit VLDL secretion by the liver, thereby promoting the storage of TGs. A model showing the regulation of VLDL secretion by the autonomic nervous system has been formulated [36]. In the basal state, there is a basal sympathetic tone with low parasympathetic activity. In the fasted state, sympathetic activity is increased to stimulate VLDL secretion, thereby mobilizing TGs, while parasympathetic activity remains low. In the fed state, VLDL secretion is inhibited by increased parasympathetic activity and reduced sympathetic activity, favoring the storage of TGs.

6.2.7 LD Formation

LDs are considered dynamic and tightly regulated, metabolically active cell organelles that store intracellular lipids. LDs are present in virtually all types of cells and consist of a TG core with a phospholipid monolayer containing amphiphilic structural proteins. Among these LD-associated proteins are those of the PAT family, such as perilipin, adipophilin, and TIP47, which are crucial for the formation, maintenance, and modification of LDs. Perilipin is thought to be expressed mainly in adipocytes, whereas adipophilin and TIP47 are expressed nearly ubiquitously. Adipophilin is thought to be a general marker for the lipid load of non-adipogenic cells, and transcription of the adipophilin gene is upregulated by all three PPARs (α, γ, and δ) [37].

Although LDs were thought to form between the leaflets of the ER membrane, a different mechanism has been proposed [38], which LD biogenesis takes place at specialized cup-shaped regions of the ER and the LD is cupped by closely apposed ER membrane outside the ER. Adipophilin clusters in the cytoplasmic leaflet of the ER adjacent to the forming LD appear to transfer lipids from the ER to the droplet surface. Incorporation of adipophilin into LDs may also occur directly from the ER rather than from the cytoplasm.

PPARγ is a master transcriptional regulator of adipogenesis. Activation of PPARγ has been shown to promote LD accumulation and lipid storage, whereas PPARα was found to promote lipid use. The role of PPARγ in the activation of lipogenic genes may contribute to the development of steatosis, and PPARγ is overexpressed in the fatty liver of obese human subjects [39]. Adiponectin has been shown to be increased by PPARγ, which also contributes to insulin sensitivity as well as upregulating PPARα expression.

6.2.8 LD Lipolysis

LD lipolysis has been investigated principally in adipocytes. Lipolysis generally proceeds via several steps. In the first step, adipose triglyceride lipase (ATGL) preferentially hydrolyzes TGs, with this rate-limiting reaction yielding DAGs and FAs. In the second step, hormone-sensitive lipase (HSL) hydrolyzes TGs, DAGs, monoacylglycerols (MAG), and cholesteryl esters. Finally, monoglyceride lipase (MGL) cleaves MAG, leading to the formation of glycerol and FA. In the basal state, HSL remains in the cytosol, while ATGL, perilipin, and the ATGL co-activator CGI-58 (comparative gene identification 58) are located at the LD surface. When stimulated by catecholamines, activated protein kinase A phosphorylates HSL and perilipin during lipolysis, resulting in an altered conformation that allows HSL and other lipases to function on the LD [40]. Perilipin phosphorylation is responsible for CGI-58 release and translocation to the ATGL [41], initiating TG breakdown [42–44]. Phosphorylated HSL migrates from the cytosol to the LD, where it is enzymatically active, and initiates lipolysis.

Less is known, however, about LD lipolysis in hepatocytes, cells that express very low levels of perilipin and in which adipophilin may be the primary PAT-family protein. Adipophilin localizes to the surface of the LD as well as the plasma membrane. Although perilipin and adipophilin may play a lipolysis-limiting role by forming a physical barrier between core TG and lipases, perilipin can also promote lipolysis when phosphorylated in adipocytes. CGI-58, which specifically enhances ATGL activity, can interact with adipophilin as well as perilipin [41, 45, 46]. Because adipophilin appears to be unphosphorylated [3], it may not be essential for lipolysis. In adipophilin-deficient mice, hepatic TG content was downregulated and the absence of adipophilin was not compensated for by other PAT-family proteins [3, 47], findings indicating the importance of adipophilin in maintaining hepatic TG homeostasis. Tip-47 as well as adipophilin is ubiquitously expressed in cells containing LDs. Liver cells expressing reduced levels of these PAT-family proteins show increased lipolysis, perhaps because of greater ATGL localization to the LD [48].

6.3 Cholesterol Metabolism

Hepatic cholesterol metabolism includes: (1) the cholesterol–LXRα–SREBP1c signaling pathway, leading to FA synthesis, (2) de novo cholesterol synthesis, (3) uptake of serum cholesterol through lipoproteins, (4) cholesterol absorption from bile, (5) cholesterol secretion into plasma as VLDL, (6) cholesterol secretion into bile, and (7) bile acid synthesis and secretion. Generally, most intracellular cholesterol is esterified with FAs by ACATs, which catalyze the formation of cholesteryl ester from cholesterol and fatty acyl-CoA [49]. Therefore, it is likely that an abundance of cholesterol promotes FA production for its esterification. In hepatocytes, LXRα regulates cholesterol and FA metabolism, and its endogenous agonistic ligands include the oxysterols, oxidized derivatives of cholesterol [50–53].

Plasma LDL-cholesterol is taken into hepatocytes via the LDLR. Hepatocyte uptake of dietary cholesterol in chylomicron remnants results in the suppression by exogenous cholesterol of the cholesterol-synthesizing system in the liver. Therefore, the cholesterol balance must be controlled in the body. The protein Niemann-Pick C1-like 1 (NPC1L1), located on the canalicular aspect of hepatocytes, is essential for the absorption/reabsorption of cholesterol from bile [54, 55].

SREBP1c and SREBP2 are expressed in the liver. SREBP1c preferentially affects the transcription of genes that regulate de novo FA synthesis, while SREBP2 is a key factor for cholesterol synthesis, and regulates genes involved in cholesterol biosynthesis and metabolism. SREBP2 synchronously activates the gene expression of LDLR and HMG-CoA reductase (HMGR), a key enzyme in cholesterol synthesis. Physiologically, accumulated cholesterol in hepatocytes and LXRα combine to downregulate SREBP2 activity, thus reducing cholesterol synthesis and uptake [56].

Cholesterol 7α-hydroxylase (CYP7A1) is a key enzyme involved in bile acid synthesis, the expression of which is negatively regulated by FXR. Bile acid is transported into bile by bile salt export pump (BSEP), the expression of which is positively regulated by FXR. For secretion to serum, cholesterol is packed into VLDL particles, together with TGs and apoB, by MTP. Cholesterol is also secreted into bile via the ATP-binding cassette (ABC) G5/ABCG8. A schematic showing cholesterol metabolism in the liver is presented in Fig. 6.2 [57, 58].

6.4 Phospholipid Metabolism

Bile is mainly composed of bile acids, cholesterol, and phospholipids, which are excreted at the canalicular membranes of hepatocytes by their specific transporters, BSEP, ABCG5/G8, and multidrug resistance 3 (MDR3/ABCB4), respectively [59, 60]. In humans, two hydrophobic primary bile acids, taurocholic acid and glycocholic acid, constitute approximately 80 % of total bile acids. When these hydrophobic bile acids reach levels higher than the critical micellar level, they form mixed micelles with phosphatidylcholine (PC), reducing their detergent activity [59, 60]. These mixed micelles can subsequently accept cholesterol to form secondary micelles. The primary function of biliary PC excretion is to protect the membranes of biliary epithelial cells from cytotoxic bile salts.

Hepatocytic phospholipid metabolism includes the pathways involved in choline uptake, PC synthesis, and PC excretion. Choline uptake at hepatocytic sinusoidal membranes in humans involves two choline transporters, low-affinity polyspecific organic cation transporter 1 (OCT1), which is primarily responsible for choline uptake, and choline transporter-like protein 1 (CTL1) [61, 62]. During PC synthesis, the enzyme CTP:phosphocholine cytidylyltransferase (Pcyt1) catalyzes the

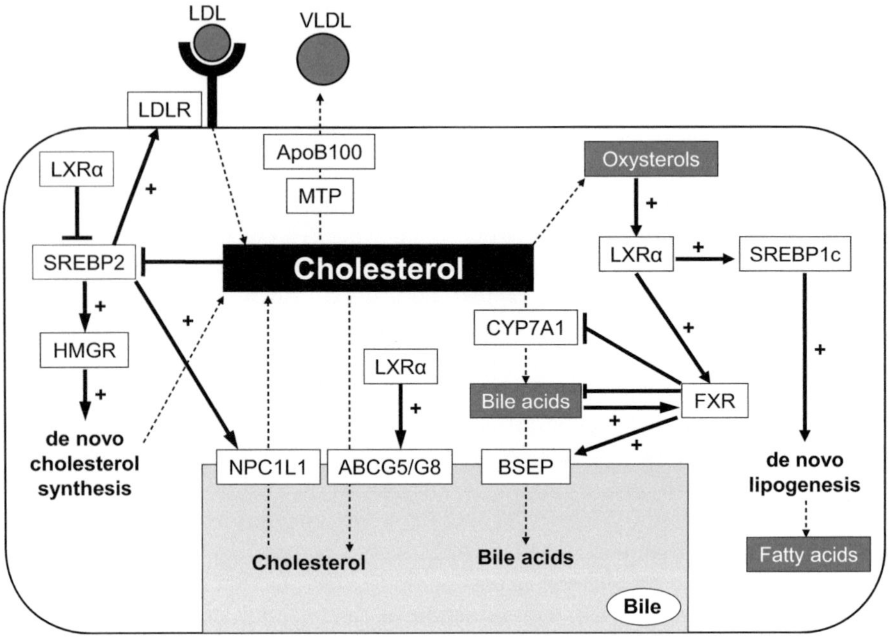

Fig. 6.2 Schematic of cholesterol metabolism in the liver. Abbreviations: *LDL* low-density lipoprotein, *VLDL* very low-density lipoprotein, *LDLR* LDL receptor, *LXR* liver X receptor, *SREBP* sterol regulatory element-binding protein, *MTP* microsomal triglyceride transfer protein, *ApoB* apolipoprotein B, *HMGR* HMG-CoA reductase, *NPC1L1* Niemann-Pick C1 like 1, *ABC* ATP-binding cassette, *CYP7A1* cholesterol 7α-hydroxylase, *FXR* farnesoid X receptor, *BSEP*, bile salt export pump

rate-limiting step of the CDP-choline pathway, whereas phosphatidylethanolamine N-methyltransferase (PEMT) and betaine-homocysteine methyltransferase (BHMT) are the key enzymes in the phosphatidylethanolamine methylation pathway [62]. During PC excretion, the expression and canalicular redistribution of MDR3 are enhanced by PPARα and FXR [63–65]. A schematic of phospholipid metabolism in the liver is presented in Fig. 6.3 [66, 67].

6.5 Lipid Metabolism in Diseased Liver

6.5.1 Nonalcoholic Fatty Liver Disease

The liver plays a major role in controlling systemic lipid metabolism by importing free FAs and manufacturing, storing, and exporting lipids. An imbalance between lipid acquisition (FA uptake and de novo lipogenesis) and removal (β-oxidation and

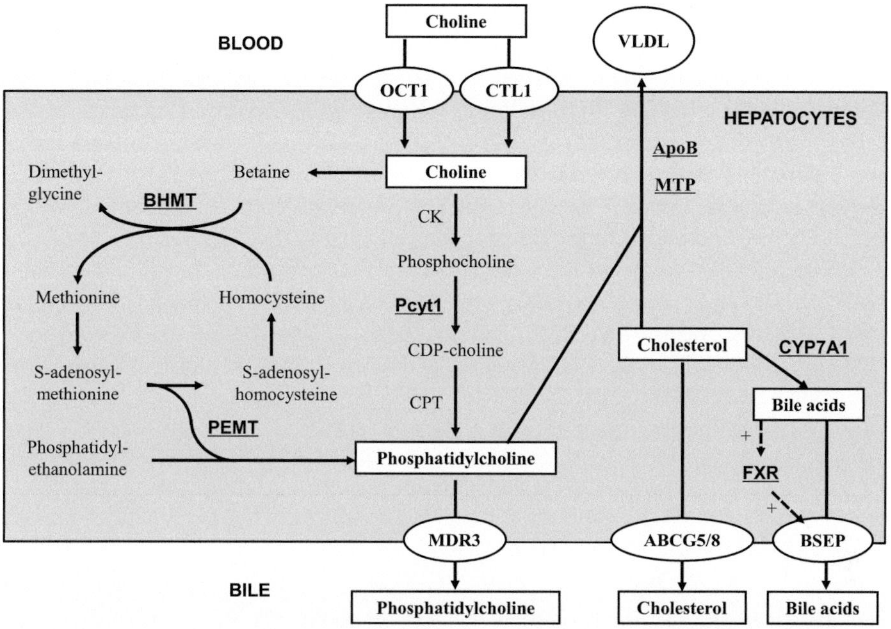

Fig. 6.3 Schematic of phospholipid metabolism in the liver. Abbreviations: *VLDL* very low-density lipoprotein, *OCT* organic cation transporter, *CTL* choline transporter-like protein, *Pcyt1* CTP:phosphocholine cytidylyltransferase, *BHMT* betaine-homocysteine methyltransferase, *PEMT* phosphatidylethanolamine-N-methyltransferase, *MTP* microsomal triglyceride transfer protein, *ApoB* apolipoprotein B, *ABC* ATP-binding cassette, *CYP7A1* cholesterol 7α-hydroxylase, *FXR* farnesoid X receptor, *BSEP* bile salt export pump, *MDR* multidrug resistance

VLDL secretion) can lead to the development of insulin resistance and its associated disorders, including nonalcoholic fatty liver disease (NAFLD).

Insulin resistance in peripheral adipose tissues enhances lipolysis, increasing plasma levels of free FAs and the delivery of adipose-derived free FAs to the liver. Elevated intrahepatic FAs result in increased DAG formation and TG synthesis, which have been observed in patients with NAFLD. Thus, hepatic fat accumulation has been strongly associated with insulin resistance [68, 69]. Although TG synthesis may protect against the damage caused by free FAs and lipid intermediates, accumulating DAG interferes with insulin signaling in hepatocytes by activating protein kinase C and reducing insulin-stimulated tyrosine phosphorylation of the IRS2, increasing insulin resistance [70–72]. NAFLD has been associated with increased hepatic expression of several genes involved in de novo lipogenesis [57, 58, 73–76]. Hyperinsulinemia leads to the activation of SREBP1c, a key transcription factor regulating de novo lipogenesis and TG synthesis. For example, PPARγ was found to be overexpressed in the fatty liver of obese human subjects [39]. PPARγ activation was found to reduce circulating free FA levels, improve insulin sensitivity, and increase adiponectin levels [77].

Hepatic FAs can enter the mitochondria to undergo β-oxidation, as well as be esterified into TGs, with reactive oxygen species (ROS) generated via the mitochondrial respiratory chain. Abundant FAs in NAFLD increase β-oxidation and lipotoxicity by inducing ROS release, which causes structural changes in the mitochondria and mitochondrial dysfunction, as well as increasing inflammation and apoptosis, and enhances the progression to nonalcoholic steatohepatitis (NASH) and fibrogenesis. Elevated FA levels can also lead to ER stress, which has also been implicated in the development of NAFLD/NASH.

Enhanced CB1-mediated EC tone, which also contributes to the pathogenesis of NAFLD/NASH, is characterized by upregulation of adipose tissue and hepatocyte CB1 receptors and by increased liver synthesis of anandamide in experimental NAFLD models [22, 78]. CB1 receptor activation results in upregulation of the lipogenic transcription factor, SREBP1c, and its target enzymes, ACC1 and FAS, as well as concurrent downregulation of CPT1 [20–22].

6.5.2 HCV Infection

Hepatic steatosis and insulin resistance are frequently present in patients with chronic hepatitis C. The lipid-producing machinery of hepatocytes is commandeered by HCV for its benefit. Thus, lipogenesis is elevated and cholesterol synthesis impaired during HCV infection and progression [79, 80]. Plasma cholesterol level and cholesterol synthesis were found to be lower in patients with than without HCV infection [81]. HCV appears to upregulate cholesterol synthetic genes [57, 82] but may interrupt cholesterol synthesis by diverting the intermediate geranyl pyrophosphate, which appears to be required for viral replication [83, 84]. Specifically, HCV may upregulate the process of cholesterogenesis, while the actual synthesis of cholesterol is impaired.

Expression of various HCV proteins may lead to alterations in lipid metabolism and transport, with the HCV core protein thought to contribute especially to hepatic steatosis and ROS production. The HCV core protein localizes at the surface of LDs within the cytoplasm [85] and interacts with the cell machinery involved in lipid metabolism, resulting in TG accumulation and storage in hepatocytes [86]. The HCV core protein also upregulates SREBP1c [87] and binds to the DNA-binding domain of retinoid X receptor α, a nuclear receptor that regulates several genes involved in cellular lipid synthesis, thus promoting de novo lipogenesis [88]. Furthermore, the HCV core protein interferes with the assembly of VLDL particles by reducing the level of MTP and with the insulin signaling pathway, which can induce accumulation of unsecreted TG, resulting in steatosis [89].

HCV core protein was also found to accumulate in mitochondria, impairing electron transport and increasing ROS production [90]. Oxidative stress results in the peroxidation of lipids and structural proteins, disturbing cellular trafficking and VLDL secretion [91]. Moreover, the HCV core protein was also found to reduce the expression of PPARα, which regulates the transcription of mitochondrial CPT1, one of the rate-limiting enzymes in β-oxidation, by mediating the entry of FAs into mitochondria [92].

6.5.3 *Primary Biliary Cholangitis*

Primary biliary cholangitis (PBC) represents a physiological response of the liver to intracellular cholesterol accumulation; specifically, cholesterol uptake and synthesis are suppressed, while secretion and excretion are enhanced [66]. The transcription levels of SREBP2, LDLR, HMGR, and NPC1L1, all of which are associated with cholesterol uptake and synthesis, were found to be downregulated. Conversely, the levels of MTP and apoB, which are involved in VLDL formation and excretion; ABCG5, a transporter of cholesterol excretion into bile; and CYP7A1, which is needed for bile acid synthesis from cholesterol, were markedly increased. Cholesterol levels and the cholesterol/TG ratio in plasma VLDL fraction were also markedly increased in patients with PBC. Based on the expression profiles of cholesterol metabolism-associated genes and the composition of plasma VLDL in PBC patients, PC synthesis should be activated in PBC liver because PC is required for VLDL formation and bile acid/cholesterol efflux into bile. These changes may lead to elevated plasma cholesterol levels, a symptom frequently observed in patients with PBC. In contrast, we observed no changes in the expression levels of genes associated with bile acid synthesis and excretion.

The expression of *PEMT* and *BHMT*, which encode key enzymes involved in PC synthesis, as well as MDR3, was enhanced in PBC liver. These expression profiles are physiologically reasonable because PC secretion into bile may be increased to deal with increased levels of cholesterol and bile acid. Increased PC consumption may be compensated for by a sufficient supply of choline; however, intracellular choline levels were much lower, while plasma choline levels were much higher, in PBC patients than in healthy individuals [67]. Differences in expression of hepatic OCT1, the main choline transporter in hepatocytes, have been associated with cholestasis [93], and single nucleotide polymorphisms in the OCT1 gene, such as the rs683369 (CG/GG) and rs622342 (CC) variants, were found to be closely associated with susceptibility to the progression of PBC [94].

6.6 Conclusion

This chapter provides an overview of lipid metabolism in the liver.

References

1. Hajri T, Abumrad NA. Fatty acid transport across membranes: relevance to nutrition and metabolic pathology. Ann Rev Nutr. 2002;22:383–415.
2. Robenek H, Robenek MJ, Buers I, Lorkowski S, Hofnagel O, Troyer D, Severs NJ. Lipid droplets gain PAT family proteins by interaction with specialized plasma membrane domains. J Biol Chem. 2005;280:26330–8.
3. Chang BH, Li L, Paul A, Taniguchi S, Nannegari V, Heird WC, Chan L. Protection against fatty liver but normal adipogenesis in mice lacking adipose differentiation-related protein. Mol Cell Biol. 2006;26:1063–76.
4. Berlanga A, Guiu-Jurado E, Porras JA, Auguet T. Molecular pathways in non-alcoholic fatty liver disease. Clin Exp Gastroenterol. 2014;7:221–39.
5. Ekstedt M, Franzén LE, Mathiesen UL, Thorelius L, Holmqvist M, Bodemar G, Kechagias S. Long-term follow-up of patients with NAFLD and elevated liver enzymes. Hepatology. 2006;44:865–73.
6. Kawano Y, Cohen DE. Mechanisms of hepatic triglyceride accumulation in non-alcoholic fatty liver disease. J Gastroenterol. 2013;48:434–41.
7. Nguyen P, Leray V, Diez M, Serisier S, Le Bloc'h J, Siliart B, Dumon H. Liver lipid metabolism. J Anim Physiol Anim Nutr. 2008;92:272–83.
8. Horton JD, Goldstein JL, Brown MS. SREBPs: activators of the complete program of cholesterol and fatty acid synthesis in the liver. J Clin Invest. 2002;109:1125–31.
9. Osborne TF. Sterol regulatory element-binding proteins (SREBPs): key regulators of nutritional homeostasis and insulin action. J Biol Chem. 2000;275:32379–82.
10. Matsuzaka T, Shimano H, Yahagi N, Amemiya-Kudo M, Okazaki H, Tamura Y, et al. Insulin-independent induction of sterol regulatory element-binding protein-1c expression in the livers of streptozotocin-treated mice. Diabetes. 2004;53:560–9.
11. Wolfrum C, Asilmaz E, Luca E, Friedman JM, Stoffel M. Foxa2 regulates lipid metabolism and ketogenesis in the liver during fasting and in diabetes. Nature. 2004;432:1027–32.
12. Shimano H, Shimomura I, Hammer RE, Herz J, Goldstein JL, Brown MS, Horton JD. Elevated levels of SREBP-2 and cholesterol synthesis in livers of mice homozygous for a targeted disruption of the SREBP-1 gene. J Clin Invest. 1997;100:2115–24.
13. Yahagi N, Shimano H, Hasty AH, Matsuzaka T, Ide T, Yoshikawa T, et al. Absence of sterol regulatory element-binding protein-1 (SREBP-1) ameliorates fatty livers but not obesity or insulin resistance in Lep(ob)/Lep(ob) mice. J Biol Chem. 2002;277:19353–7.
14. Zhou G, Myers R, Li Y, Chen Y, Shen X, Fenyk-Melody J, et al. Role of AMP-activated protein kinase in mechanism of metformin action. J Clin Invest. 2001;108:1167–74.
15. Woods A, Azzout-Marniche D, Foretz M, Stein SC, Lemarchand P, Ferré P, et al. Characterization of the role of AMP-activated protein kinase in the regulation of glucose-activated gene expression using constitutively active and dominant negative forms of the kinase. Mol Cell Biol. 2000;20:6704–11.
16. Fuchs M. Non-alcoholic fatty liver disease: the bile acid-activated farnesoid x receptor as an emerging treatment target. J Lipids. 2012;2012:934396.
17. Yang ZX, Shen W, Sun H. Effects of nuclear receptor FXR on the regulation of liver lipid metabolism in patients with non-alcoholic fatty liver disease. Hepatol Int. 2010;4:741–8.
18. Watanabe M, Houten SM, Wang L, Moschetta A, Mangelsdorf DJ, Heyman RA, et al. Bile acids lower triglyceride levels via a pathway involving FXR, SHP, and SREBP-1c. J Clin Invest. 2004;113:1408–18.
19. Zhang W, Patil S, Chauhan B, Guo S, Powell DR, Le J, et al. FoxO1 regulates multiple metabolic pathways in the liver: effects on gluconeogenic, glycolytic, and lipid metabolism. J Biol Chem. 2006;281:10105–17.
20. Kunos G, Osei-Hyiaman D. Endocannabinoids and liver disease. IV. Endocannabinoid involvement in obesity and hepatic steatosis. Am J Physiol Gastrointest Liver Physiol. 2008;294:G1101–4.

21. Osei-Hyiaman D, Depetrillo M, Pacher P, Liu J, Radaeva S, Bátkai S, et al. Endocannabinoid activation at hepatic CB(1) receptors stimulates fatty acid synthesis and contributes to diet-induced obesity. J Clin Invest. 2005;115:1298–305.
22. Osei-Hyiaman D, Liu J, Zhou L, Godlewski G, Harvey-White J, Jeong WI, et al. Hepatic CB1 receptor is required for development of diet-induced steatosis, dyslipidemia, and insulin and leptin resistance in mice. J Clin Invest. 2008;118:3160–9.
23. Toyoda M, Kitaoka A, Machida K, Nishinakagawa T, Yada R, Kohjima M, et al. Association between lipid accumulation and the cannabinoid system in Huh7 cells expressing HCV genes. Int J Mol Med. 2011;27:619–24.
24. Chumurzynska A. The multigene family of fatty acid-binding proteins (FABPs): function, structure and polymorphism. J Appl Genet. 2006;47:39–48.
25. Mandard S, Müller M, Kersten S. Peroxisome proliferator-activated receptor alpha target genes. Cell Mol Life Sci. 2004;61:393–416.
26. Harano Y, Yasui K, Toyama T, Nakajima T, Mitsuyoshi H, Mimani M, et al. Fenofibrate, a peroxisome proliferator-activated receptor alpha agonist, reduces hepatic steatosis and lipid peroxidation in fatty liver Shionogi mice with hereditary fatty liver. Liver Int. 2006;26:613–20.
27. Yamazaki T, Sasaki E, Kakinuma C, Yano T, Miura S, Ezaki O. Increased very low density lipoprotein secretion and gonadal fat mass in mice overexpressing liver DGAT1. J Biol Chem. 2005;280:21506–14.
28. Stone SJ, Myers HM, Watkins SM, Brown BE, Feingold KR, Elias PM, Farese Jr RV. Lipopenia and skin barrier abnormalities in DGAT2-deficient mice. J Biol Chem. 2004;279:11767–76.
29. Liang JJ, Oelkers P, Guo C, Chu PC, Dixon JL, Ginsberg HN, Sturley SL. Overexpression of human diacylglycerol acyltransferase 1, acyl-CoA:cholesterol acyltransferase 1, or acyl-CoA: cholesterol acyltransferase 2 stimulates secretion of apolipoprotein B-containing lipoproteins in McA-RH7777 cells. J Biol Chem. 2004;279:44938–44.
30. Gibbons GF, Wiggins D. Intracellular triacylglycerol lipase: its role in the assembly of hepatic very-low-density lipoprotein (VLDL). Adv Enzym Regul. 1995;35:179–98.
31. Innerarity TL, Boren J, Yamanaka S, Olofsson SO. Biosynthesis of apolipoprotein B48-containing lipoproteins. Regulation by novel post-transcriptional mechanisms. J Biol Chem. 1996;271:2353–6.
32. Zammit VA. Role of insulin in hepatic fatty acid partitioning: emerging concepts. Biochem J. 1996;314:1–14.
33. Shelness GS, Sellers JA. Very-low-density lipoprotein assembly and secretion. Curr Opin Lipidol. 2001;12:151–7.
34. Shi YC, Lau J, Lin Z, Zhang H, Zhai L, Sperk G, et al. Arcuate NPY controls sympathetic output and BAT function via a relay of tyrosine hydroxylase neurons in the PVN. Cell Metab. 2013;17:236–48.
35. Bruinstroop E, Fliers E, Kalsbeek A. Hypothalamic control of hepatic lipid metabolism via the autonomic nervous system. Best Prac Res Clin Endocrinol Matab. 2014;28:673–84.
36. Bruinstroop E, Pei L, Ackermans MT, Foppen E, Borgers AJ, Kwakkel J, et al. Hypothalamic neuropeptide Y controls hepatic VLDL-triglyceride secretion in rat via sympathetic nervous system. Diabetes. 2012;61:1043–50.
37. Straub BK, Gyoengyoesi B, Koenig M, Hashani M, Pawella LM, Herpel E, et al. Adipophilin/perilipin-2 as a lipid droplet-specific marker for metabolically active cells and diseases associated with metabolic dysregulation. Histopathology. 2013;62:617–31.
38. Robenek H, Hofnagel O, Buers I, Robenek MJ, Troyer D, Severs NJ. Adipophilin-enriched domains in the ER membrane are sites of lipid droplet biogenesis. J Cell Sci. 2006;119:4215–24.
39. Westerbacka J, Kolak M, Kiviuoto T, Arkkila P, Sirén J, Hamsten A, et al. Genes involved in fatty acid partitioning and binding, lipolysis, monocyte/macrophage recruitment, and

inflammation are overexpressed in the human fatty liver of insulin-resistant subjects. Diabetes. 2007;56:2759–65.
40. Marcinkiewicz A, Gauthier D, Garcia A, Brasaemle DL. The phosphorylation of serine 492 of perilipin a directs lipid droplet fragmentation and dispersion. J Biol Chem. 2006;281:11901–9.
41. Granneman JG, Moore HP, Krishnamoorthy R, Rathod M. Perilipin controls lipolysis by regulating the interactions of AB-hydrolase containing 5 (Abhd5) and adipose triglyceride lipase (Atgl). J Biol Chem. 2009;284:34538–44.
42. Bezaire V, Mairal A, Ribet C, Lefort C, Girousse A, Jocken J, et al. Contribution of adipose triglyceride lipase and hormone-sensitive lipase to lipolysis in hMADS adipocytes. J Biol Chem. 2009;284:18282–91.
43. Subramanian V, Rothenberg A, Gomez C, Cohen AW, Garcia A, Bhattacharyya S, et al. Perilipin A mediates the reversible binding of CGI-58 to lipid droplets in 3T3-L1 adipocytes. J Biol Chem. 2004;279:42062–71.
44. Yamaguchi T, Omatsu N, Matsushita S, Osumi T. CGI-58 interacts with perilipin and is localized to lipid droplets. Possible involvement of CGI-58 mislocalization in Chanarin-Dorfman syndrome. J Biol Chem. 2004;279:30490–7.
45. Lass A, Zimmermann R, Oberer M, Zechner R. Lipolysis—a highly regulated multi-enzyme complex mediates the catabolism of cellular fat stores. Prog Lipid Res. 2011;50:14–27.
46. Lass A, Zimmermann R, Haemmerle G, Riederer M, Schoiswohl G, Schweiger M, et al. Adipose triglyceride lipase-mediated lipolysis of cellular fat stores is activated by CGI-58 and defective in Chanarin-Dorfman syndrome. Cell Metab. 2006;3:309–19.
47. Girousse A, Langin D. Adipocyte lipases and lipid droplet-associated proteins: insight from transgenic mouse models. Int J Obes. 2012;36:581–94.
48. Bell M, Wang H, Chen H, McLenithan JC, Gong DW, Yang RZ, et al. Consequences of lipid droplet coat protein downregulation in liver cells: abnormal lipid droplet metabolism and induction of insulin resistance. Diabetes. 2008;57:2037–45.
49. Buhman KK, Chen HC, Farese Jr RV. The enzymes of neutral lipid synthesis. J Biol Chem. 2001;276:40369–72.
50. Chen G, Liang G, Ou J, Goldstein JL, Brown MS. Central role for liver x receptor in insulin-mediated activation of Srebp-1c transcription and stimulation of fatty acid synthesis in liver. Proc Natl Acad Sci U S A. 2004;101:11245–50.
51. Laffitte BA, Joseph SB, Walczak R, Pei L, Wilpitz DC, Collins JL, Tontonoz P. Autoregulation of the human liver x receptor α promoter. Mol Cell Biol. 2001;21:7558–68.
52. Tobin KA, Steineger HH, Alberti S, Spydevold O, Auwerx J, Gustafsson JA, Nebb HI. Cross-talk between fatty acid and cholesterol metabolism mediated by liver x receptor α. Mol Endocrinol. 2000;14:741–52.
53. Tobin KA, Ulven SM, Schuster GU, Steineger HH, Andresen SM, Gustafsson JA, Nebb HI. Liver x receptor α as insulin-mediating factors in fatty acid and cholesterol biosynthesis. J Biol Chem. 2002;277:10691–7.
54. Kidambi S, Patel SB. Cholesterol and non-cholesterol sterol transporters: ABCG5, ABCG8 and NPC1L1: a review. Xenobiotica. 2008;38:1119–39.
55. Enjoji M, Machida K, Kohjima M, Kato M, Kotoh K, Matsunaga K, et al. NPC1L1 inhibitor ezetimibe is a reliable therapeutic agent for non-obese patients with nonalcoholic fatty liver disease. Lipids Health Dis. 2010;9:29.
56. Wójcicka G, Jamroz-Wiśniewska A, Horoszewicz K, Bełtowski J. Liver X receptors (LXRs). Part I: structure, function, regulation of activity, and role in lipid metabolism. Postepy Hig Med Dosw. 2007;61:736–59.
57. Nakamuta M, Yada R, Fujino T, Yada M, Higuchi N, Tanaka M, et al. Changes in the expression of cholesterol metabolism-associated genes in HCV-infected liver: a novel target for therapy? Int J Mol Med. 2009;24:825–8.
58. Nakamuta M, Fujino T, Yada R, Yada M, Yasutake K, Yoshimoto T, et al. Impact of cholesterol metabolism and the LXRα–SREBP-1c pathway on nonalcoholic fatty liver disease. Int J Mol Med. 2009;23:603–8.

59. Van Erpecum KJ. Biliary lipids, water and cholesterol gallstones. Biol Cell. 2005;97:815–22.
60. Oude Elfrrink RPJ, Paulusma CC. Function and pathophysiological importance of ABCB4 (MDR3 P-glycoprotein). Eur J Physiol. 2007;453:601–10.
61. Sinclair CJ, Chi KD, Subramanian V, Ward KL, Green RM. Functional expression of a high affinity mammalian hepatic choline/organic cation transporter. J Lipid Res. 2000;41:1841–8.
62. Michel V, Yuan Z, Ramsubir S, Bakovic M. Choline transport for phospholipid synthesis. Exp Biol Med. 2006;231:490–504.
63. Shoda J, Inada Y, Tsuji A, Kusama H, Ueda T, Ikegami T, et al. Bezafibrate stimulates canalicular localization of NBD-labeled PC in HepG2 cells by PPARα-mediated redistribution of ABCB4. J Lipid Res. 2004;45:1813–25.
64. Chinale J, Vollrath V, Wielandt AM, Amigo L, Rigotti A, Nervi F, et al. Fibrate induce mdr2 gene expression and biliary phospholipids secretion in the mouse. Biochem J. 1996;314:781–6.
65. Shoda J, Okada K, Inada Y, Kusama H, Utsunomiya H, Oda K, et al. Bezafibrate induces multidrug-resistance P-glycoprotein 3 expression in cultured human hepatocytes and humanized livers of chimeric mice. Hepatol Res. 2007;37:548–56.
66. Enjoji M, Yada R, Fujino T, Yoshimoto T, Yada M, Harada N, et al. The state of cholesterol metabolism in the liver of patients with primary biliary cirrhosis: the role of MDR3 expression. Hepatol Int. 2009;3:490–6.
67. Kohjima M, Enjoji M, Yada R, Yoshimoto T, Nakamura T, Fukuizumi K, et al. Pathophysiological analysis of primary biliary cirrhosis focusing on choline/phospholipid metabolism. Liver Int. 2015;35:1095–102.
68. Petta S, Muratore C, Craxi A. Non-alcoholic fatty liver disease pathogenesis: the present and the future. Dig Liver Dis. 2009;41:615–25.
69. Magkos F, Su X, Bradley D, Fabbrini E, Conte C, Eagon JC, et al. Intrahepatic diacylglycerol content is associated with hepatic insulin resistance in obese subjects. Gastroenterology. 2012;142:1444–6.
70. Jornayvaz FR, Birkenfeld AL, Jurezak MJ, Kanda S, Guigni BA, Jiang DC, et al. Hepatic insulin resistance in mice with hepatic overexpression of diacylglycerol acyltransferase 2. Proc Natl Acad Sci U S A. 2011;108:5748–52.
71. Choi SS, Diehl AM. Hepatic triglyceride synthesis and nonalcoholic fatty liver disease. Curr Opin Lipidol. 2008;19:295–300.
72. Yamaguchi K, Yang L, McCall S, Huang J, Yu XX, Pandey SK, et al. Inhibiting triglyceride synthesis improves hepatic steatosis but exacerbate liver damage and fibrosis in obese mice with nonalcoholic steatohepatitis. Hepatology. 2007;45:1366–74.
73. Kohjima M, Enjoji M, Higuchi N, Kato M, Kotoh K, Yoshimoto T, et al. Re-evaluation of fatty acid metabolism-related gene expression in nonalcoholic fatty liver disease. Int J Mol Med. 2007;20:351–8.
74. Kohjima M, Higuchi N, Kato M, Kotoh K, Yoshimoto T, Fujino T, et al. SREBP-1c, regulated by the insulin and AMPK signaling pathways, plays a role in nonalcoholic fatty liver disease. Int J Mol Med. 2008;21:507–11.
75. Nakamuta M, Kohjima M, Higuchi N, Kato M, Kotoh K, Yoshimoto T, et al. The significance of differences in fatty acid metabolism between obese and non-obese patients with nonalcoholic fatty liver disease. Int J Mol Med. 2008;22:663–7.
76. Higuchi N, Kato M, Tanaka M, Miyazaki M, Takao S, Kohjima M, et al. Effects of insulin resistance and hepatic lipid accumulation on hepatic mRNA expression levels of apoB, MTP and L-FABP in non-alcoholic fatty liver disease. Exp Ther Med. 2011;2:1077–81.
77. Ahmadian M, Suh JM, Hah N, Liddle C, Atkins AR, Downes M, Evans RM. PPARgamma signaling and metabolism: the good, the bad and the future. Nat Med. 2013;19:557–66.
78. Tam J, Vemuri VK, Liu J, Bátkai S, Mukhopadhyay B, Godlewski G, et al. Peripheral CB1 cannabinoid receptor blockade improves cardiometabolic risk in mouse models of obesity. J Clin Invest. 2010;120:2953–66.

79. Negro F. Abnormalities of lipid metabolism in hepatitis C virus infection. Gut. 2010;59:1279–87.
80. Huang H, Sun F, Owen DM, Li W, Chen Y, Gale Jr M, Ye J. Hepatitis C virus production by human hepatocytes dependent on assembly and secretion of very low-density lipoproteins. Proc Natl Acad Sci U S A. 2007;104:5848–53.
81. Corey KE, Kane E, Munroe C, Barlow LL, Zheng H, Chung RT. Hepatitis C virus infection and its clearance alter circulating lipids: implications for long-term follow-up. Hepatology. 2009;50:1030–7.
82. Fujino T, Nakamuta M, Yada R, Aoyagi Y, Yasutake K, Kohjima M, et al. Expression profile of lipid metabolism-associated genes in hepatitis C virus-infected human liver. Hepatol Res. 2010;40:923–9.
83. Kapadia SB, Chisari FV. Hepatitis C virus RNA replication is regulated by host geranylgeranylation and fatty acids. Proc Natl Acad Sci U S A. 2005;102:2561–6.
84. Ye J, Wang C, Sumpter Jr R, Brown MS, Goldstein JL, Gale Jr M. Disruption of hepatitis C virus RNA replication through inhibition of host protein geranylgeranylation. Proc Natl Acad Sci U S A. 2003;100:15865–70.
85. Moradpour D, Englert C, Wakita T, Wands JR. Characterization of cell lines allowing tightly regulated expression of hepatitis c virus core protein. Virology. 1996;222:51–63.
86. Barba G, Harper F, Harada T, Kohara M, Goulinet S, Matsuura Y, et al. Hepatitis C virus core protein shows a cytoplasmic localization and associates to cellular lipid storage droplets. Proc Natl Acad Sci U S A. 1997;94:1200–5.
87. Kim KH, Hong SP, Kim K, Park MJ, Kim KJ, Cheong J. HCV core protein induces hepatic lipid accumulation by activating SREBP1 and PPARgamma. Biochem Biophys Res Commun. 2007;355:883–8.
88. Tsutsumi T, Suzuki T, Shimoike T, Suzuki R, Moriya K, Shintani Y, et al. Interaction of hepatitis C virus core protein with retinoid X receptor alpha modulates its transcriptional activity. Hepatology. 2002;35:937–46.
89. Perlemuter G, Sabile A, Letteron P, Vona G, Topilco A, Chrétien Y, et al. Hepatitis C virus core protein inhibits microsomal triglyceride transfer protein activity and very low density lipoprotein secretion: a model of viral-related steatosis. FASEB J. 2002;16:185–94.
90. Okuda M, Li K, Beard MR, Showalter LA, Scholle F, Lemon SM, Weinman SA. Mitochondrial injury, oxidative stress, and antioxidant gene expression are induced by hepatitis C virus core protein. Gastroenterology. 2002;122:366–75.
91. Negro F. Mechanism and significance of liver steatosis in hepatitis C virus infection. World J Gastroenterol. 2006;12:6756–65.
92. Dharancy S, Malapel M, Perlemuter G, Roskams T, Cheng Y, Dubuquoy L, et al. Impaired expression of the peroxisome proliferator-activated receptor alpha during hepatitis C virus infection. Gastroenterology. 2005;128:334–42.
93. Nies AT, Koepsell H, Winter S, Burk O, Klein K, Kerb R, et al. Expression of organic cation transporters OCT1 (SLC22A1) and OCT3 (SLC22A3) is affected by genetic factors and cholestasis in human liver. Hepatology. 2009;50:1227–40.
94. Ohishi Y, Nakamuta M, Ishikawa N, Saitoh O, Nakamura H, Aiba Y, et al. Genetic polymorphisms of OCT-1 confer susceptibility to severe progression of primary biliary cirrhosis in Japanese patients. J Gastroenterol. 2014;49:332–42.

Chapter 7
Metal Metabolism and Liver

Keisuke Hino and Masaru Harada

Abstract The liver is the central organ for the metabolism of iron and copper. Therefore, primary metabolic disorders of iron and copper give rise to liver diseases, and secondary iron and copper disorders induced by chronic liver diseases potentially modify or aggravate the clinical courses of the original liver diseases. This chapter will review and discuss (1) iron and copper metabolism, (2) hemochromatosis and Wilson disease as primary iron and copper metabolic disorders, and (3) mechanisms underlying secondary iron metabolic disorders induced by chronic liver diseases such as chronic hepatitis C and nonalcoholic fatty liver disease (NAFLD). The degree of hepatic iron accumulation in chronic hepatitis C and NAFLD is not as severe as that in hereditary hemochromatosis. However, mild to moderate hepatic iron accumulation potentially modifies the disease progression and induces the development of hepatocellular carcinoma (HCC) in chronic hepatitis C and NAFLD. Abnormal metabolism of copper in the liver is detected in patients with Wilson disease. This is a peculiar disease, because it is a rare genetic metabolic disorder that can be treated by pharmacological treatments. However, prompt recognition, diagnosis, and adequate treatment are essential, because inadequate management is fatal for the patients.

Keywords Hepcidin • Iron regulatory protein • Iron responsive element • Ceruloplasmin • Wilson disease

---

K. Hino (✉)
Department of Hepatology and Pancreatology, Kawasaki Medical School, 577 Matsushima, Kurashiki, Okayama 701-0192, Japan
e-mail: khino@med.kawasaki-m.ac.jp

M. Harada
Third Department of Internal Medicine, School of Medicine, University of Occupational and Environmental Health, 1-1 Iseigaoka, Yahatanishi-ku, Kitakyushu 807-8555, Japan

H. Ohira (ed.), *The Liver in Systemic Diseases*, DOI 10.1007/978-4-431-55790-6_7

7.1 Introduction

Essential trace elements such as iron, copper, and zinc are biologically indispensable for mitochondrial electron transport, signal transduction, redox reaction, oxygen transport, and/or physiological catalytic reactions such as hydrolysis. Because these elements are transition metals, they also function as active regions for various enzymes, cytokines, and hormones. Thus, metabolic disturbances of these elements result in critical disorders of biological functions, leading to the development of various diseases.

The liver is a crucial organ for metabolism of iron and copper. Therefore, primary metabolic disorders of iron and copper give rise to liver diseases, and secondary metabolic disorders of iron and copper induced by liver diseases potentially modify or aggravate the clinical courses of the original liver diseases. This chapter will review and discuss (1) iron and copper metabolism, (2) hemochromatosis and Wilson disease as primary iron and copper metabolic disorders, and (3) mechanisms underlying secondary iron metabolic disorder induced by chronic liver diseases such as chronic hepatitis C and nonalcoholic fatty liver disease (NAFLD).

7.2 Iron Metabolism

7.2.1 Iron Absorption

Iron can be absorbed from the diet in two forms in the proximal intestine as inorganic (nonheme) iron predominantly released from foods such as vegetables or cereals or as heme iron from the breakdown of hemoglobin and myoglobin contained in red meat [1]. Heme (ferrous protoporphyrin IX) is more efficiently absorbed than inorganic iron from the diet. The mechanism responsible for heme uptake is not yet well understood, but it is known to occur via receptor-mediated endocytosis. Heme-carrier protein 1 (HCP1) has been identified as the most probable receptor involved in this process [2]. However, it has low affinity to heme and is more involved in folate absorption [3]. Once in the enterocyte, heme is broken down by heme oxygenase 1 (HO1) and iron is released in its ferric state.

Nonheme iron exists primarily in the bio-unavailable, oxidized form (Fe^{3+}), which must first be reduced to Fe^{2+} for transport across the intestinal epithelium. At the apical membrane, there is a cytochrome b-like ferrireductase (Dcytb) [4]. Fe^{2+} enters the cell through divalent metal transporter 1 (Dmt1), an iron transporter. Dmt1 is responsible for the absorption of the ionic forms of iron, cobalt, zinc, cadmium, and other metals and takes advantage of the proton gradient existing between the gut lumen and the enterocyte cytoplasm to perform the transport of Fe^{2+} coupled with H^+ [5].

In the cytoplasm, iron is transferred to the basolateral membrane of the enterocyte or stored in ferritin, a multisubunit protein shell that can accommodate up to 4,500 atoms of iron. The export of iron from the enterocyte to the circulation is a critical step for the entrance of iron in the body. The mammalian iron transporter ferroportin-1 exists on the basolateral membrane of the enterocyte [6]. Ferroportin-1 transports Fe^{2+} to the extracellular side of the basolateral membrane, where it is oxidized by the ferroxidase, hephaestin, and ceruloplasmin in order to associate with the circulatory transferrin [7, 8].

7.2.2 Hepatocellular Iron Transport

Hepatocytes take up iron through at least two distinct pathways. They have a functional transferrin cycle and a transport system to take up non-transferrin-bound iron. The cellular uptake of transferrin-bound iron is mainly mediated by transferrin receptor 1 (TfR1). The molecules important for non-transferrin-bound iron transport have not yet been identified. Hepatocytes store iron in ferritin. When iron is needed elsewhere in the body, they can release it to transferrin. The mechanism of hepatocyte export is not well known, but it may involve ferroportin-1. Ceruloplasmin seems to aid in iron export from hepatocytes, but its precise function has not yet been defined.

7.2.3 Regulation of Iron Homeostasis

Systemic iron homeostasis, the control of iron balance throughout the body, requires controlled absorption, recycling, and storage because there is no efficient pathway for iron excretion in the human body. All the stages required for keeping iron homeostasis are strictly regulated at both the systemic and cellular levels.

7.2.3.1 Hepcidin

The major systemic regulator of iron homeostasis is hepcidin, which is a 25-amino acid peptide hormone exclusively synthesized in the liver and a soluble regulator that acts to attenuate both intestinal iron absorption and iron release from reticuloendothelial macrophages [9, 10]. Hepcidin acts by triggering internalization of ferroportin-1 and consequent degradation and traps iron in absorptive enterocytes, macrophages, and hepatocytes [11]. Thus, coupling the internalization of ferroportin-1 to hepcidin levels generates a homeostatic loop regulating the iron plasma level and the tissue distribution of iron. Hepcidin is expressed by the *hepcidin antimicrobial peptide* (*HAMP*) gene on the long arm of chromosome 19. Increase of iron levels and inflammation upregulates the transcription of the *HAMP* gene, whereas reactive oxygen species (ROS), hypoxia, and anemia/erythropoiesis repress its expression [12–16].

Hemojuvelin (Hjv), HFE, TfR1, and TfR2, which are located on the hepatocyte surface, are considered to be "iron sensors." The Hjv-hepcidin axis is the most important mechanism for the upregulation of *HAMP* expression during iron overload. Bone morphogenetic protein (BMP) binding to the Hjv and BMP receptor complexes induces the phosphorylation of cytosolic sons of mothers against decapentaplegic (SMADs) 1, 5, and 8 [12, 17]. The phosphorylated SMADs form complexes with SMAD4 that are translocated to the nucleus where they bind to the BMP-responsive elements present at the *HAMP* promoter, inducing its transcription [18]. Proinflammatory cytokine interleukin 6 (IL-6) activates *HAMP* gene transcription through a pathway that involves Janus kinase (JAK)-signal transducer and activator of transcription (STAT) signaling and a binding site for the transcription factor STAT3 [15, 19]. The transcription factor CCAAT/enhancer-binding protein α (C/EBPα) is also clearly involved in regulating hepcidin transcription [20].

7.2.3.2 Iron Regulatory Protein (IRP)/Iron Responsive Element (IRE) System

In addition to the systemic regulation of iron homeostasis by hepcidin, the IRP/IRE system controls both mRNA stability and translation of transcripts coding proteins involved in iron uptake (Dmt1 and TfR1), storage (ferritin), and export (ferroportin-1) [21, 22]. Proteins IRP1 and IRP2 are the main regulators of cellular iron in humans, but IPR2 is assumed to play a central role in the IRP/IRE system [23]. Under iron-deficient conditions, IRP binds to the IRE present at the 5′- or 3′-untranslated regions (UTRs) of mRNAs that code for iron regulatory proteins. Under iron-depleted condition in cells, IRPs bind to the IREs present at 5′-UTRs of *FTH*, *FHL* (genes coding ferritin heavy and light chains), and *SLC40A1* (the gene coding ferroportin-1), preventing ribosome assembly and further translation [24, 25], while they bind to the IREs present at 3′-UTR of TfR1 and *SLC11A2* (the gene coding Dmt1), increasing the stability of transcripts and subsequently their translation [26, 27]. Thus, cellular iron depletion downregulates iron storage and export and upregulates iron uptake. Alternatively, a cellular iron increase renders IRPs unable to bind to the IREs, resulting in suppression of iron acquisition. Cellular regulation other than via the IRP/IRE system for iron homeostasis will be discussed elsewhere.

7.3 Iron-Overload Disorders and Liver Diseases

Iron overload, especially excess divalent iron, can be highly toxic, mainly via the Fenton reaction producing hydroxyl radicals [28]. This is particularly relevant for iron-overload liver diseases such as hemochromatosis, chronic hepatitis C, and nonalcoholic steatohepatitis (NASH), in which oxidative stress has been proposed as a major mechanism of liver injury. Oxidative stress and increased iron levels strongly favor DNA damage, genetic instability, and tumorigenesis. Indeed, a significant correlation between 8-hydroxy-2′-deoxyguanosine (8-OHdG), a marker of oxidatively generated DNA damage [29], and hepatic iron excess has been shown in iron-overload liver diseases.

7.3.1 Primary Iron-Overload Disorder and Liver

Hereditary hemochromatosis is a heterogeneous group of inherited iron-overload conditions that is characterized by increased intestinal absorption and deposition of iron in vital organs, including the liver, heart, and pancreas. To date, mutations in five genes (*HFE*, *HAMP*, *Hjv*, *TFR2*, and *SLC40A1*) and four types of hemochromatosis have been found: (1) *HFE*-associated hemochromatosis, (2) juvenile hemochromatosis, (3) *TFR2*-associated hemochromatosis, and (4) ferroportin disease. The hemochromatosis group shows common features with respect to increased transferrin saturation and parenchymal iron deposition in organs, resulting in the development of liver cirrhosis, hepatocellular carcinoma (HCC), heart failure, diabetes, and hypogonadism, even though the severity of the different forms of hemochromatosis varies. The molecular mechanism common to all types of hereditary hemochromatosis is failure to regulate hepcidin expression in response to cellular iron levels.

Type I hereditary hemochromatosis, also known as classic hemochromatosis, is affected by *HFE* mutations and accounts for approximately 90 % of all cases of hereditary hemochromatosis. It is characterized by mild disease progression with a gradual iron deposition in organs [30, 31]. *HFE* encodes an atypical histocompatibility class I protein that heterodimerizes with β-2 microglobulin [31]. Most affected patients are homozygous for a missense mutation (C282Y) that partially disrupts HFE function [31]. Therefore, mutated HFE protein cannot bind to β-2 microglobulin and be transferred to the cell surface, which presumably results in failure to regulate hepcidin expression.

Type II hereditary hemochromatosis, which is affected by *Hjv* or *HAMP* mutations, is also known as juvenile hemochromatosis and is a rare but more progressive disease. Juvenile hemochromatosis is further classified into two types: (i) - Hjv-associated hemochromatosis [32] and (ii) HAMP-associated hemochromatosis [33]. Type III hemochromatosis is affected by *TFR2* mutations on chromosome 7 [34]. This type of hemochromatosis affects middle-aged adults but also adolescents and young adults and resembles type I hemochromatosis. Type IV hemochromatosis, which is affected by *SLC40A1* mutations, is also known as ferroportin disease and is less rare than type II or III [30]. This disease is phenotypically heterogeneous with two forms (A and B). In form A, the loss of function mutants of ferroportin is unable to export iron from cells, resulting in cellular (especially macrophage) iron accumulation and decreased availability of iron for transferrin

[30]. In form B, ferroportin mutations are responsible for a gain of function with full iron export capability but insensitivity to downregulation by hepcidin, leading to a phenotype similar to other hepcidin deficiency-based types of hemochromatosis [30, 35]. Thus, ferroportin disease form B shows elevated transferrin saturation-associated tissue iron accumulation, preferentially within hepatocytes.

7.3.2 Iron-Overload Disorder in Chronic Liver Diseases

The liver is the major iron storage organ in the body, and therefore, iron metabolic disorders are sometimes involved in chronic liver diseases. Mild to moderate degrees of hepatic iron accumulation are common in chronic hepatitis C and NASH [36–39]. This section highlights the current concept of the hepatic iron-overload status in chronic hepatitis C and nonalcoholic steatohepatitis (NASH) and discusses how iron metabolic disorders develop in both chronic liver diseases and the impact of hepatic iron overload on disease progression and its relevance to hepatocarcinogenesis.

7.3.2.1 Chronic Hepatitis C

Hepatic Iron Content

Based on the assumption that one-third of iron stores are normally in the liver, this would translate to a normal median hepatic iron content of 0.27 g for men and 0.13 g for women [40]. Extensive studies have reported median hepatic iron concentrations of 396 [range, 0–2,105] and 458 [range, 114–2,190] μg/g dry-weight liver tissue in patients with chronic hepatitis C [41, 42]. These results suggest that the hepatic iron content in patients with chronic hepatitis C is approximately 0.50–0.69 g, equivalent to two to five times the normal hepatic iron content if the liver weight is estimated to be 1,500 g. In contrast, a hepatic iron index (μmol Fe/g liver tissue/patients age) of 1.9 or more has been reported to be typical of patients with hereditary hemochromatosis [43]. If the hepatic iron index of a patient aged 60 with hereditary hemochromatosis is 1.9, the hepatic iron concentration of this patient is assumed to be 6,384 μg/g liver tissue. Thus, we should understand that hepatic iron content is much less in chronic hepatitis C than in hereditary hemochromatosis, even though chronic hepatitis C is recognized to be one of the liver diseases that show hepatic iron accumulation. There also remains uncertainty as to whether iron predominantly accumulates in hepatocytes or the reticuloendothelial system, mainly Kupffer cells, in patients with chronic hepatitis C. Some clinical studies showed that iron was mainly localized in the reticuloendothelial system [44], whereas others reported its localization in hepatocytes [45]. Interestingly, Fiel et al. documented that even ribavirin-associated hemolysis deposited iron preferentially in hepatocytes in patients with chronic hepatitis C [46].

Mechanisms Underlying Hepatic Iron Overload

The role of *HFE* mutations in chronic hepatitis C has been well reviewed [47]. In general, patients with chronic hepatitis C seem to have no difference in the prevalence of heterozygosity for *HFE* mutations as compared with a control population. It is still controversial as to whether *HFE* mutations are associated with hepatic iron overload in chronic hepatitis C, probably because of the different methodologies used to measure hepatic iron and/or confounding variables such as demographic parameters, environmental factors, hepatic inflammatory activity, and the duration of hepatitis C virus (HCV) infection among the reported studies.

The levels of hepatic hepcidin mRNA and serum hepcidin, which is a 25-amino acid bioactive hepcidin, are reported to be lower in patients with chronic hepatitis C than in those with chronic hepatitis B or controls despite a significant correlation between hepcidin and serum ferritin and the histological iron scores in both groups [48, 49]. Thus, the relatively decreased synthesis of hepcidin in chronic hepatitis C contrasts with the absolute deficit or lack of hepcidin synthesis observed in hereditary hemochromatosis and may account for the mild to moderate hepatic iron overload observed in some patients with chronic hepatitis C.

HCV core protein induces the production of ROS through inhibition of mitochondrial electron transport [50]. Alcohol metabolism-mediated ROS have been shown to suppress hepcidin transcription via C/EBPα [16]. The mechanisms underlying HCV-related hepatic iron overload appear to have some similarities to alcohol-induced iron overload in terms of disrupted hepcidin transcription through suppressed activity of C/EBPα. The activity of the hepcidin promoter and the DNA-binding activity of C/EBPα are downregulated concomitant with an increase in C/EBP homology protein (CHOP), an inhibitor of C/EBP DNA-binding activity, and increased levels of ROS in transgenic mice expressing the HCV polyprotein [51]. It is also reported that HCV-induced ROS inhibit the binding activity of C/EBPα to the hepcidin promoter through increased histone deacetylase activity in hepatoma cell lines [52].

Hepcidin is potentially regulated through the BMP/SMAD cascade by both circulating transferrin-bound iron and intracellular iron stores in chronic hepatitis C. Taking into account the significant correlation between hepcidin expression and serum ferritin or the histological iron score [48, 49], hepcidin transcription seems to be properly regulated in response to the iron concentration in chronic hepatitis C. Thus, the opposing effects of HCV-induced hepcidin-suppressive factors and iron load-induced hepcidin-stimulation factors potentially regulate hepcidin transcription in chronic hepatitis C.

Inflammation also regulates hepcidin transcription. Proinflammatory cytokines such as IL-6 mediate this response by inducing transcription of hepcidin mRNA via STAT3, which binds to a STAT-responsive element within the hepcidin promoter [15]. A possible pitfall in transgenic mouse models is the absence of hepatic inflammation, which is different from what is observed in patients with chronic hepatitis C. Serum levels of IL-6 have been shown to be elevated in patients with HCV-related chronic liver disease [53], which raises the possibility that IL-6 acts to

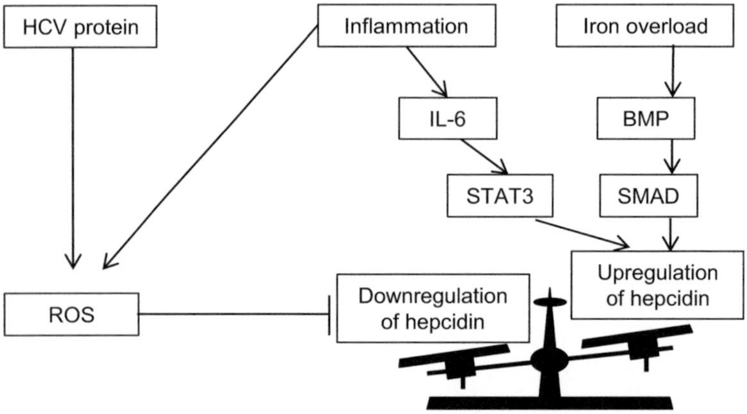

Fig. 7.1 Schematic diagram depicting the assumed mechanisms underlying the hepatic iron accumulation in patients with chronic hepatitis C. Hepcidin transcription in chronic hepatitis C may be potentially regulated by the opposing effects of HCV-related ROS-induced hepcidin suppression and iron load-induced hepcidin stimulation. Inflammation may also have the opposing effects of stimulation and suppression of hepcidin transcription through the IL-6/STAT pathway and ROS pathway, respectively. Consequent relative suppression of hepcidin expression is potentially one of the mechanisms underlying the hepatic iron accumulation in patients with chronic hepatitis C. *HCV* hepatitis C virus, *ROS* reactive oxygen species, *IL-6* interleukin 6, *STAT* signal transducer and activator of transcription, *BMP* bone morphogenetic protein, *SMAD* sons of mothers against decapentaplegic

stimulate hepcidin expression through the STAT3 pathway. This would be expected to counteract the decrease in hepcidin transcription caused by HCV-induced ROS. However, no significant relationship has been found between serum IL-6 and hepcidin in patients with chronic hepatitis C [49, 54], even though a paracrine effect of local IL-6 release on hepcidin transcription in the liver cannot be excluded. On the other hand, chronic inflammation with production of proinflammatory cytokines has the potential to deliver an additional burden of ROS, which would be expected to reinforce the decrease in hepcidin transcription. Most likely, during chronic inflammation states in vivo like chronic hepatitis C, the regulation of hepcidin is more complex and may depend on many variables, including the particular stage of systemic and/or hepatic inflammatory disease. This might explain the variations in hepatic iron concentrations reported among patients with HCV-related chronic liver diseases. The schematic outline in Fig. 7.1 depicts the assumed mechanisms underlying the hepatic iron accumulation in chronic hepatitis C.

Relevance of Hepatic Iron Overload to Hepatocarcinogenesis

Studies of HCV-infected and uninfected chimpanzees have demonstrated that iron loading does exacerbate liver injury in the infected chimpanzees and that infection increases the susceptibility of the liver to injury following iron loading

[55]. In addition, it has been prospectively shown that stainable iron in hepatocytes and portal tract cells predicts progression and outcomes (Child Pugh Score >7, ascites, encephalopathy, variceal bleeding, spontaneous bacterial peritonitis, HCC, and death) in advanced chronic hepatitis C [56]. Thus, iron is a cofactor that influences the severity and progression of chronic hepatitis C.

There also are several lines of evidence that suggest the association of hepatic iron overload with hepatocarcinogenesis in chronic hepatitis C. Hepatic iron storage is strongly correlated with hepatic 8-OHdG levels, and subsequent oxidative DNA damage in the liver is associated with an increased risk of HCC development [57]. The decrease in hepatic 8-OHdG content caused by phlebotomy lowers the risk of progression to HCC, which indeed shows the critical role of the iron-overload state in the development of HCC in patients with chronic hepatitis C [58]. Transgenic mice expressing the HCV polyprotein also reproduce the synergistic effect of iron loading on the development of HCC [59]. In these mice, the hepatic iron content is increased even in the absence of exogenous iron loading, and because the levels of hepcidin mRNA in the liver are simultaneously reduced, a defect in iron regulation caused by the HCV polyprotein is indicated [59]. Thus, there is a close relationship between the development of HCC and oxidative DNA damage synergistically induced by hepatic iron accumulation and HCV proteins.

7.3.2.2 NAFLD

Relevance of Hepatic Iron Overload to Pathogenesis, Disease Progression, and Hepatocarcinogenesis

NAFLD is present in 10–30 % of the world's population. A relative minority of subjects with NAFLD develop liver injury histologically characterized as NASH. A recent large cohort study showed that 35 % of subjects enrolled in the NASH Clinical Research Network had stainable hepatic iron [60]. In animal models of fatty liver, iron loading is associated with the development of hepatic inflammation and fibrosis [61]. Early reports on the association of hepatic iron with NAFLD and NASH were controversial. However, more recent studies have strongly suggested a causative role for iron, with several studies demonstrating that increased hepatic iron contributes to progression of NAFLD [36, 62]. In addition to the induction of oxidative stress, iron has been implicated as a cofactor in the pathogenesis of insulin resistance, which is universal among individuals with NAFLD and is implicated in the progression of liver injury [63]. Iron also appears to be a risk factor for the development of HCC in patients with NASH. Iron overload in patients with NASH-related cirrhosis is reported to be potentially associated with HCC development [64].

Mechanisms Underlying Hepatic Iron Overload

The precise mechanisms by which some patients with NASH are prone to hepatic iron accumulation remain elusive. However, several mechanisms have been proposed (Table 7.1). Aigner et al. suggested impaired release of iron from liver cells as an underlying mechanism for iron accumulation in NAFLD [65]. They found downregulation of ferroportin-1 and the *Hjv* gene, probably due to an increase in tumor necrosis-alpha (TFN-α). This also explains the characteristic pattern of iron deposition in NAFLD, which is different from the pattern seen in hereditary hemochromatosis, i.e., hepatic and sinusoidal deposition without a zonal gradient. Transgenic mice expressing the retinoic acid receptor alpha-dominant negative form in hepatocytes develop steatohepatitis and liver tumors [66]. Hepatic iron accumulates in these mice, and retinoid treatment decreases hepatic iron content through suppression of Hjv expression [67]. These results suggest that impaired retinoic acid function is responsible for hepatic iron accumulation in NASH. Otogawa et al. indicated that the engulfment of phosphatidylserine-externalized, apoptotic signal-positive erythrocytes by hepatic macrophages might lead to the accumulation of iron derived from hemoglobin in the NASH liver [68]. Interestingly, a recent study has demonstrated that duodenal iron absorption increases through upregulation of Dmt1 regardless of elevation of serum hepcidin in patients with NASH [69]. Undetermined humoral factor(s) contained in sera of NASH

Table 7.1 Proposed mechanisms by which hepatic iron accumulates in NAFLD/NASH

Factor(s) related to iron metabolic disorders	Intermediary molecules	Molecules responsible for iron accumulation	Affected pathway in iron transport	References
Increased TNF-α[a] production	Hemojuvelin	Ferroportin-1	Iron release from hepatocytes and Kupffer cells	[65]
Impaired retinoic acid signaling	Hemojuvelin, TfR2[c]	Ferroportin-1	Iron release from hepatocytes and Kupffer cells	[66, 67]
Erythrocytes		Phosphatidylserine	Erythrocyte phagocytosis by Kupffer cells	[68]
Undetermined humoral factor(s)	IRP1	Dmt1[d]	Duodenal iron absorption	[69]
Copper deficiency	Ceruloplasmin	Ferroportin-1	Iron release from hepatocytes and Kupffer cells	[70]
ROS[b] production	Ceruloplasmin	Ferroportin-1	Iron release from hepatocytes and Kupffer cells	[71]

[a]Tumor necrosis factor alpha
[b]Reactive oxygen species
[c]Transferrin receptor 2
[d]Divalent metal transporter

patients activate IRP1, which subsequently upregulates Dmt1 expression through the IRP/IRE system [69].

Iron accumulation may be linked to copper homeostasis. One study reported that copper status was linked to iron homeostasis in NAFLD, suggesting that low copper bioavailability causes increased hepatic iron stores via decreased ferroportin-1 expression and ceruloplasmin ferroxidase activity, thus blocking liver iron export in copper-deficient subjects [70]. In addition, oxidative stress/ROS in hepatic cells has been demonstrated to downregulate ceruloplasmin via a novel mRNA decay mechanism that may contribute to hepatic iron accumulation by decreasing hepatic iron release [71].

7.4 Copper Metabolism

Copper is an essential trace element that plays roles in many important cellular processes. These biological processes include mitochondrial energy generation (cytochrome c oxidase), iron metabolism regulation (ceruloplasmin), melanin formation (tyrosinase), oxygen-radical scavenging (superoxide dismutase), and collage cross-linking (lysyl oxidase) [72–74]. However, excess copper is toxic because it can induce ROS via the Fenton reaction. Thus, both a shortage and an excess of copper can induce serious problems as illustrated by Menkes disease and Wilson disease [75]. Therefore, accurate regulation of copper uptake, utilization, storage, and excretion are necessary for health. In this section, we describe the copper metabolism in normal and abnormal conditions.

7.4.1 Copper Absorption

The average diet of an adult human contains from 0.6 to 1.6 mg of copper per day. Shellfish are rich in copper, as are organ meats such as the liver. Freshwater contains very little copper. Seawater is rich in copper and the concentrations rise with the increase of depth. Therefore, fish and shellfish from the ocean flower contain much copper. In mammals, copper absorption mainly occurs in the small intestine. From 12 to 56 % of copper in food is absorbed by adult humans depending on the copper content of the diet [76–78]. The requirement for copper is rather low; therefore, we need a way to excrete copper from the body. Most dietary copper is Cu^{2+}. This is reduced before uptake at the apical membrane of the enterocyte, because copper is absorbed as Cu^{+} [79]. Copper transporter 1 (CTR1) transports copper across the membrane [80]. Some copper may be transported by divalent metal transporter 1 (DMT1), which is important for iron metabolism [79]. The copper in the cytoplasm of enterocytes is delivered to Atox1, a copper chaperone [81], which then delivers copper to ATP7A [81]. In copper-depleted conditions, ATP7A localizes in the trans-Golgi network (TGN) and localizes in the peripheral vesicles in copper-rich conditions [82]. Copper-containing vesicles release copper from the basolateral membrane to the interstitial space of the small intestine via exocytosis.

7.4.2 Copper Transport to the Liver

Copper absorbed from the gastrointestinal tract enters the portal circulation. It binds to albumin, transcuprein, or histidine [72, 83]. About 15 % of absorbed copper is transported to various tissues, and the rest is excreted from the body from hepatocytes via bile [84]. The liver is the central organ of copper metabolism and takes up copper from the portal circulation [72, 84]. CTR1 transports copper across the plasma membrane [85]. CTR1-mediated copper uptake into the cells is regulated by its degradation as it is endocytosed and degraded in lysosomes when cells are exposed to a high concentration of copper [86].

7.4.3 Copper Metabolism in Hepatocytes

Copper in the cytoplasm binds to the copper chaperones ATOX1, the copper chaperone for superoxide dismutase 1 (CCS1), and cytochrome C oxidase assembly factor 17 (COX17) or to the copper ligands glutathione and metallothionein because free copper may be toxic to the cells [83, 84, 87]. The mechanisms of copper metabolism were deduced by phenotypes of Wilson disease. Wilson disease is an autosomal recessive inherited disorder of copper metabolism. It is characterized by the accumulation of copper in the body because of decreased biliary copper excretion from hepatocytes to the bile canaliculi. The Wilson disease gene has been cloned and shown to encode a homology to the cation-transporting P-type ATPase [88–91]. It is clear that ATP7B functions in both incorporation of copper into apoceruloplasmin to form stable (mature) holoceruloplasmin and biliary copper excretion [92, 93]. The Long-Evans Cinnamon (LEC) rat is an animal model of Wilson disease, and it has a mutated *Atp7b* gene, the rat gene homologous to *ATP7B* [94]. Introduction of ATP7B protein to hepatocytes of the LEC rat restores the normal ceruloplasmin secretion and biliary copper excretion [92, 93]. The proper intracellular localization is very important for the protein function. First, the gene product, ATP7B (Wilson disease protein), was detected in the trans-Golgi network (TGN) by two different institutes [95, 96]; however, the localization is still controversial [97–103]. We examined the intracellular localization of green fluorescent protein ATP7B (GFP-ATP7B), ATP7B-DsRed, transfected ATP7B, and endogenous ATP7B in primary isolated rat hepatocytes, OUMS29 (a human hepatocyte cell line), Huh7 and Hep3B (human hepatoma cell lines), and HEK293 and MDCK cells [97–103]. Our examinations demonstrated that ATP7B colocalized with lysosome-associated protein (lamp) 1 (a late

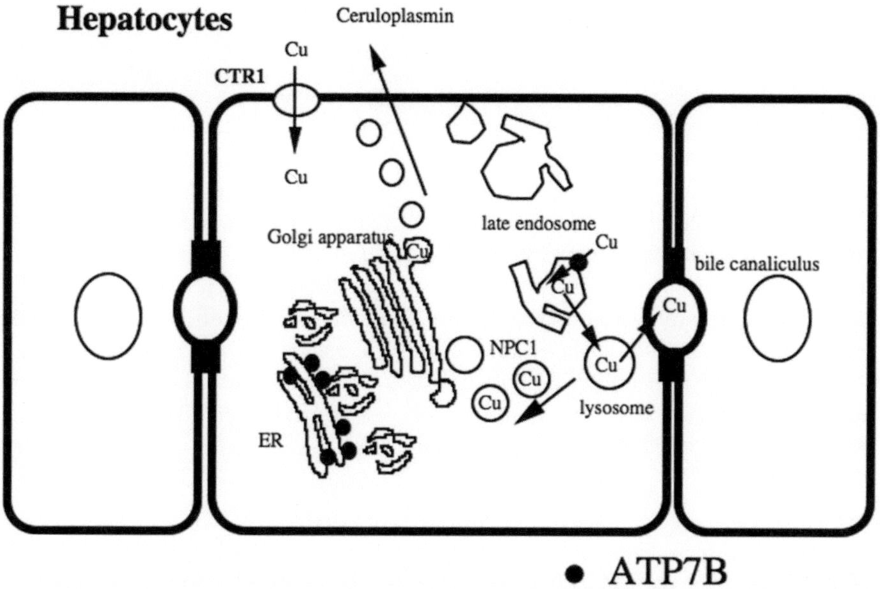

Fig. 7.2 Copper transporter 1 (CTR 1) in the sinusoidal membrane of hepatocytes transports copper from the bloodstream to the cytoplasm of hepatocytes. ATP7B translocates copper from the cytoplasm into the late endosomal lumen. Copper in the late endosome is transported to the lysosomes and is excreted to the bile canaliculus via biliary lysosomal excretion. Copper is also transported to the *trans*-Golgi network (TGN) via Niemann-Pick C1 protein (NPC1), incorporated into ceruloplasmin and secreted into the bloodstream. Abbreviation: *ER* endoplasmic reticulum

endosome/lysosome-localized protein), lamp 2 (a late endosome/lysosome-localized protein), Rab7 (a late endosome-localized protein), Niemann-Pick C1 protein (NPC1, a late endosome-localized protein), and incubated rhodamine dextran (localized in all endocytic structures), but not with galactosyltransferase (a - TGN-localized protein), γ-adaptin (a TGN-localized protein), 58-kd Golgi protein (a TGN-localized protein), cathepsin D (a lysosome-localized protein), or lysosomal glycoprotein 85 (a lysosome-localized protein) [97–103]. Therefore, we consider that ATP7B localizes in late endosomes. ATP7B translocates copper from the cytoplasm into the late endosomes. Lysosomes are important for biliary copper excretion [104–106]. Therefore, copper in the late endosomes is transported to the lysosomes and excreted to the bile canaliculi (Fig. 7.2). For the copper incorporation into ceruloplasmin, we demonstrated the importance of Niemann-Pick C1 protein (NPC1) in experiments with NPC1 knockdown and NPC1 transfection using cultured hepatocytes and hepatoma cells [102, 103]. Recent studies of cultured cells, mice, and humans support our hypothesis that NPC1 plays an important role in copper metabolism in hepatocytes [107, 108].

7.5 Hepatic Disorder of Copper Metabolism

The most important hepatic disorder of copper metabolism is Wilson disease, although copper metabolism is disturbed in various chronic cholestatic conditions. Wilson disease is an autosomal recessive disorder characterized by the accumulation of copper in the body [73, 74, 109]. Samuel Alexander Kinnier Wilson was the first to describe strange familial cases with nervous system disorders and liver cirrhosis as progressive lenticular degeneration in 1912 [110]. Copper accumulation in the liver and central nervous system is associated with this disease [111]. The serum ceruloplasmin concentration was found to be low in patients with this disease [112]. Wilson disease was a fatal disorder until treatments were established a half century ago. It was one of the first genetic metabolic disorders for which effective pharmacological treatment was established [73, 74, 109, 113]. The prevalence of Wilson disease is estimated to be 1 in 35,000–45,000 individuals [73, 74, 109].

7.5.1 Clinical Manifestations of Wilson Disease

Clinical manifestations of patients with Wilson disease vary greatly and the onset of the manifestations is also variable [114], as is the age of the onset. Typical symptoms are hepatic disorders, neuropsychiatric disorders, Kayser-Fleischer rings, and hemolysis in association with acute liver failure. Various other abnormalities of other organs such as the kidney, heart, bone, muscle, and endocrine organs are possible.

Hepatic manifestations range from asymptomatic mild liver function abnormality to cirrhosis. Some patients may present with acute liver failure. HCC is also possible, although the prevalence of HCC is not so high. We have little experience with aged Wilson disease patients because this disease was fatal before the introduction of chelating therapy with D-penicillamine. Therefore, we must be careful to screen for HCC, especially in aged cirrhotic patients [74, 83, 115].

Some patients manifest a broad spectrum of neurological, behavioral, and psychiatric symptoms. These include changes in behavior, deterioration of school life, difficulty in writing, tremors, abnormal speech, Parkinson disease-like symptoms, dysarthria, dystonia, slavering, depression, anxiety, and psychosis. Most, probably all, patients with neurological manifestations have some degree of liver abnormality.

There are some eye presentations in patients with Wilson disease. Kayser-Fleischer rings represent deposition of copper in Descemet's membrane of the cornea. Sunflower cataract represents copper deposition in the lens. These findings in the eyes represent copper deposition in the extrahepatic tissues including the central nervous system [73, 74, 83].

Other manifestations include renal dysfunction, cardiac abnormalities, hemolysis, gall bladder stones, myopathy, osteoarthritis, and infertility or repeated spontaneous abortions [73, 74, 83].

Although uncontrolled Wilson disease patients cannot become pregnant, patients with successful treatment can [116, 117]. Treatment must be continued throughout the duration of pregnancy. D-Penicillamine, trientine, and zinc have been demonstrated to be safe for pregnant patients with Wilson disease and the fetus [73, 74, 118, 119]. Interruption of the treatment during pregnancy may induce acute liver failure [73, 74, 109]. The dose of chelating agents should be reduced in the late period of pregnancy to avoid insufficient copper supply to the fetus and insufficient wound healing of the mother [73, 74, 109].

7.5.2 *Diagnosis of Wilson Disease*

There is no single test to diagnose Wilson disease. Therefore, combined evaluation of clinical and biochemical findings is important. The Wilson disease scoring system is useful for diagnosis (Table 7.2) [109, 120]. If the cumulative score

Table 7.2 Scoring system for the diagnosis of Wilson disease proposed at the 8th international meeting on Wilson disease

Symptoms and tests	Points
Kayser-Fleisher ring	2
Neurologic symptoms or MRI findings	2
Coombs-negative hemolytic anemia	1
Urinary copper 1–2 × ULN	1
>2×	2
Normal, but >5× after D-penicillamine	2
Liver copper content	
1–5 × ULN	1
>5×	2
Normal	−1
Rhodanine staining	
Positive[a]	1
Serum ceruloplasmin (mg/dL)	
10–20	1
<10	2
Mutation analysis	
Disease causing mutations on both chromosomes	4
Disease causing mutations on one chromosome	1

Total score

4 or more: diagnosis of Wilson disease highly likely

2–3: diagnosis of Wilson disease probable, do more investigation

0–1: diagnosis of Wilson disease unlikely

ULN upper limit of normal, urinary copper <40 μg/day, liver copper content <50 μg/g

Serum ceruloplasmin < 20 mg/dL

[a]If measurement of liver copper content is not available

obtained using this system is four or more, the diagnosis of Wilson disease is very likely.

7.5.3 Treatment for Wilson Disease

Wilson disease was fatal until a treatment was introduced. Now, it is a rare genetic metabolic disorder that can be treated with some drugs. The treatments are based on the use of copper chelators to remove accumulated copper from the body and zinc to reduce absorption of copper in the small intestine [73, 74, 109]. Since chocolate, nuts, mushrooms, shellfish, and organ meats contain high concentrations of copper, patients should avoid these foods.

D-Penicillamine promotes urinary excretion of copper from the body. Side effects appear in approximately 30 % of patients treated with this drug. The side effects include fever, eruptions, lymphadenopathy, neutropenia, thrombocytopenia, proteinuria, nephrotoxicity, lupus-like symptoms, lichen planus, myasthenia gravis, polymyositis, and hepatotoxicity [73, 74, 109]. Usually, the initial dose is 200–400 mg/day. The maintenance dose is usually 800–1,500 mg/day. D-Penicillamine should be taken 1 h before or 2 h after meals, because food in the gastrointestinal tract inhibits absorption of the drug. The long-term prognosis of most patients treated with D-penicillamine is favorable, although some patients need to change the treatment due to adverse events [121].

Trientine, introduced in 1969, is another copper chelator that promotes urinary excretion of copper from the body [122, 123]. When patients suffer from severe adverse effects due to the use of D-penicillamine, trientine should be administrated [73, 74, 109]. Because trientine has few adverse effects, it is an effective treatment for Wilson disease [73, 124]. The therapeutic effect of trientine is sufficient after the change from D-penicillamine [123]. In general, the adverse effects due to D-penicillamine resolve when trientine replaces it. Typical dosages are 750–1,500 mg/day and maintenance dosages are usually 750–1,000 mg/day. A recent long-term observation demonstrated that trientine produced outcomes comparable to those for D-penicillamine with fewer adverse events [121].

Zinc is also used for the treatment of Wilson disease. It induces the expression of metallothionein, a metal binding protein, in various cells, including epithelial cells of the small intestine (enterocytes) [125, 126]. Metallothionein has greater affinity with copper than zinc. Copper binds with metallothionein in the cytoplasm of enterocytes. Therefore, copper is not absorbed but is lost into the intestinal lumen with enterocytes. Foods interfere with the absorption of zinc; therefore, it should be administrated 1 h before or 2 h after meals. Zinc has very few side effects [124]. However, we must be careful, because long-term excessive intake of zinc can produce toxic effects [127]. Zinc is used for presymptomatic patients or for maintenance of those who have already received chelation therapy because zinc monotherapy is not as effective as chelating agents according to a long-term observation of symptomatic patients [128].

Combination therapy using trientine and zinc for hepatic decompensated patients with Wilson disease was successful [129]. Combination of D-penicillamine and zinc can also be used for treatment for patients with Wilson disease [130].

Patients with acute liver failure or decompensated liver failure who do not respond to standard therapy may require liver transplantation [73, 74, 109]. Living donor liver transplantation from a family member who has heterozygote mutation is also successful [131]. However, liver transplantation does not always improve the neurological manifestations [73]. Therefore, we should carefully consider the indication for transplantation in such cases. It is not recommended for patients with neurological manifestations with stable liver function. For consideration of the indication for liver transplantation for patients with Wilson disease, the revised King's College score is very useful [132].

7.5.4 Prognosis of Wilson Disease

Patients with Wilson disease who receive adequate care usually have a favorable prognosis. However, there are problems in some patients. The prognosis is poor in patients diagnosed after the development of cirrhosis or with advanced neurological symptoms [124, 133]. When patients with Wilson disease are not promptly diagnosed or adequately treated, the hepatic and neurological abnormalities progress. Even experienced hepatologists may misdiagnose patients with Wilson disease [134]. Discontinuance of treatment induces intractable hepatic failure even in patients who had been well treated effectively [135–137]. Suicide is one of the problems of patients with Wilson disease [136, 137]. Education of patients and careful attention to their situation are important to prevent these serious problems.

7.6 Conclusions

The liver is the central organ for the metabolism of iron and copper. Iron metabolic disorders occur not only in primary (genetic) diseases such as hereditary hemochromatosis but also in chronic liver diseases such as chronic hepatitis C and NAFLD/NASH. The degree of hepatic iron accumulation in chronic hepatitis C and NAFLD/NASH is not as severe as that in hereditary hemochromatosis. However, mild to moderate hepatic iron accumulation potentially modifies the disease progression and induces the development of HCC in chronic hepatitis C and NAFLD/NASH. Thus, iron metabolic disorders are a critical pathologic feature in chronic hepatitis C and NAFLD/NASH.

Abnormal metabolism of copper in the liver is detected in patients with Wilson disease. It is an unusual disease because it is a rare genetic metabolic disorder that can be treated by pharmacological treatments. Therefore, recognition, prompt diagnosis, and adequate treatment are essential for these patients because inadequate management is fatal for them.

References

1. Silva B, Faustino R. An overview of molecular basis of iron metabolism regulation and the associated pathologies. Biochim Biophys Acta. 1852;2015:1347–59.
2. Shayeghi M, Latunde-Dada GO, Oakhill JS, Laftah AH, Takeuchi K, Halliday N, et al. Identification of an intestinal heme transporter. Cell. 2005;122:789–801.
3. Laftah AH, Latunde-Dada GO, Fakih S, Hider RC, Simpson RJ, McKie AT. Haem and folate transport by proton-coupled folate transporter/haem carrier protein 1 (SLC46A1). Br J Nutr. 2009;101:1150–6.
4. McKie AT, Barrow D, Latunde-Dada GO, Rolfs A, Sager G, Mudaly E, et al. An iron-regulated ferric reductase associated with the absorption of dietary iron. Science. 2001;291: 1755–9.
5. Gunshin H, Mackenzie B, Berger UV, Gunshin Y, Romero MF, Boron WF, et al. Cloning and characterization of a mammalian proton-coupled metal-ion transporter. Nature. 1997;388: 482–8.
6. Donovan A, Brownlie A, Zhou Y, Shepard J, Pratt SJ, Moynihan J, et al. Positional cloning of zebrafish ferroportin1 identifies a conserved vertebrate iron exporter. Nature. 2000;403: 776–81.
7. Yeh KY, Yeh M, Mims L, Glass J. Iron feeding induces ferroportin 1 and hephaestin migration and interaction in rat duodenal epithelium. Am J Physiol Gastrointest Liver Physiol. 2009;296:G55–65.
8. Brittin GM, Chee QT. Relation of ferroxidase (ceruloplasmin) to iron absorption. J Lab Clin Med. 1969;74:53–9.
9. Park CH, Valore EV, Waring AJ, Ganz T. Hepcidin, a urinary antimicrobial peptide synthesized in the liver. J Biol Chem. 2001;276:7806–10.
10. Ganz T. Hepcidin, a key regulator of iron metabolism and mediator of anemia of inflammation. Blood. 2003;102:783–8.
11. Nemeth E, Tuttle MS, Powelson J, Vaughn MB, Donovan A, Ward DM, et al. Hepcidin regulates cellular iron efflux by binding to ferroportin and inducing its internalization. Science. 2004;306:2090–3.
12. Zhang AS, Gao J, Koeberl DD, Enns CA. The role of hepatocyte hemojuvelin in the regulation of bone morphogenic protein-6 and hepcidin expression in vivo. J Biol Chem. 2010;285:16416–23.
13. Schmidt PJ, Toran PT, Giannetti AM, Bjorkman PJ, Andrews NC. The transferrin receptor modulates Hfe-dependent regulation of hepcidin expression. Cell Metab. 2008;7:205–14.
14. Gao J, Chen J, Kramer M, Tsukamoto H, Zhang AS, Enns CA. Interaction of the hereditary hemochromatosis protein HFE with transferrin receptor 2 is required for transferrin-induced hepcidin expression. Cell Metab. 2009;9:217–27.
15. Pietrangelo A, Dierssen U, Valli L, Garuti C, Rump A, Corradini E, et al. STAT3 is required for IL-6-gp130-dependent activation of hepcidin in vivo. Gastroenterology. 2007;132: 294–300.
16. Harrison-Findik DD, Schafer D, Klein E, Timchenko NA, Kulaksiz H, Clemens D, et al. Alcohol metabolism-mediated oxidative stress down-regulates hepcidin transcription and leads to increased duodenal iron transporter expression. J Biol Chem. 2006;281: 22974–82.
17. Babitt JL, Huang FW, Wrighting DM, Xia Y, Sidis Y, Samad TA, et al. Bone morphogenetic protein signaling by hemojuvelin regulates hepcidin expression. Nat Genet. 2006;38:531–9.

18. Truksa J, Lee P, Beutler E. Two BMP responsive elements, STAT, and bZIP/HNF4/COUP motifs of the hepcidin promoter are critical for BMP, SMAD1, and HJV responsiveness. Blood. 2009;113:688–95.
19. Wrighting DM, Andrews NC. Interleukin-6 induces hepcidin expression through STAT3. Blood. 2006;108:3204–9.
20. Courselaud B, Pigeon C, Inoue Y, Inoue J, Gonzalez FJ, Leroyer P, et al. C/EBPalpha regulates hepatic transcription of hepcidin, an antimicrobial peptide and regulator of iron metabolism. Cross-talk between C/EBP pathway and iron metabolism. J Biol Chem. 2002; 277:41163–70.
21. Anderson CP, Shen M, Eisenstein RS, Leibold EA. Mammalian iron metabolism and its control by iron regulatory proteins. Biochim Biophys Acta. 2012;1823:1468–83.
22. Hentze MW, Muckenthaler MU, Andrews NC. Balancing acts: molecular control of mammalian iron metabolism. Cell. 2004;117:285–97.
23. Meyron-Holtz EG, Ghosh MC, Iwai K, LaVaute T, Brazzolotto X, Berger UV, et al. Genetic ablations of iron regulatory proteins 1 and 2 reveal why iron regulatory protein 2 dominates iron homeostasis. EMBO J. 2004;23:386–95.
24. Sammarco MC, Ditch S, Banerjee A, Grabczyk E. Ferritin L and H subunits are differentially regulated on a post-transcriptional level. J Biol Chem. 2008;283:4578–87.
25. Lymboussaki A, Pignatti E, Montosi G, Garuti C, Haile DJ, Pietrangelo A. The role of the iron responsive element in the control of ferroportin1/IREG1/MTP1 gene expression. J Hepatol. 2003;39:710–5.
26. Casey JL, Koeller DM, Ramin VC, Klausner RD, Harford JB. Iron regulation of transferrin receptor mRNA levels requires iron-responsive elements and a rapid turnover determinant in the 3′ untranslated region of the mRNA. EMBO J. 1989;8:3693–9.
27. Gunshin H, Allerson CR, Polycarpou-Schwarz M, Rofts A, Rogers JT, Kishi F, et al. Iron-dependent regulation of the divalent metal ion transporter. FEBS Lett. 2001;509:309–16.
28. Fenton HJH. Oxidation of tartaric acid in presence of iron. J Chem Soc. 1894;65:899–910.
29. Shibutani S, Takeshita M, Grollman AP. Insertion of specific bases during DNA synthesis past the oxidation-damaged base 8-oxodG. Nature. 1991;349:431–4.
30. Pietrangelo A. Hereditary hemochromatosis: pathogenesis, diagnosis, and treatment. Gastroenterology. 2010;139:393–408. 408 e1–2.
31. Feder JN, Gnirke A, Thomas W, Tsuchihashi Z, Ruddy DA, Basava A, et al. A novel MHC class I-like gene is mutated in patients with hereditary haemochromatosis. Nat Genet. 1996;13:399–408.
32. Papanikolaou G, Samuels ME, Ludwig EH, MacDonald ML, Franchini PL, Dube MP, et al. Mutations in HFE2 cause iron overload in chromosome 1q-linked juvenile hemochromatosis. Nat Genet. 2004;36:77–82.
33. Roetto A, Papanikolaou G, Politou M, Alberti F, Girelli D, Christakis J, et al. Mutant antimicrobial peptide hepcidin is associated with severe juvenile hemochromatosis. Nat Genet. 2003;33:21–2.
34. Camaschella C, Roetto A, Cali A, De Gobbi M, Garozzo G, Carella M, et al. The gene TFR2 is mutated in a new type of haemochromatosis mapping to 7q22. Nat Genet. 2000;25:14–5.
35. Sham RL, Phatak PD, West C, Lee P, Andrews C, Beutler E. Autosomal dominant hereditary hemochromatosis associated with a novel ferroportin mutation and unique clinical features. Blood Cells Mol Dis. 2005;34:157–61.
36. George DK, Goldwurm S, MacDonald GA, Cowley LL, Walker NI, Ward PJ, et al. Increased hepatic iron concentration in nonalcoholic steatohepatitis is associated with increased fibrosis. Gastroenterology. 1998;114:311–8.
37. Sumida Y, Nakashima T, Yoh T, Furutani M, Hirohama A, Kakisaka Y, et al. Serum thioredoxin levels as a predictor of steatohepatitis in patients with nonalcoholic fatty liver disease. J Hepatol. 2003;38:32–8.

38. Farinati F, Cardin R, De Maria N, Della Libera G, Marafin C, Lecis E, et al. Iron storage, lipid peroxidation and glutathione turnover in chronic anti-HCV positive hepatitis. J Hepatol. 1995;22:449–56.
39. Di Bisceglie AM, Axiotis CA, Hoofnagle JH, Bacon BR. Measurements of iron status in patients with chronic hepatitis. Gastroenterology. 1992;102:2108–13.
40. Rouault TA, Gordeuk V, Anderson G. The central role of the liver in iron storage and regulation of systemic iron homeostasis. In: Arias IM et al., editors. The liver: biology and pathobiology. 5th ed. Hoboken: Weiley-Blackwell; 2009. p. 235–50.
41. Hofer H, Osterreicher C, Jessner W, Penz M, Steindl-Munda P, Wrba F, et al. Hepatic iron concentration does not predict response to standard and pegylated-IFN/ribavirin therapy in patients with chronic hepatitis C. J Hepatol. 2004;40:1018–22.
42. Rulyak SJ, Eng SC, Patel K, McHutchison JG, Gordon SC, Kowdley KV. Relationships between hepatic iron content and virologic response in chronic hepatitis C patients treated with interferon and ribavirin. Am J Gastroenterol. 2005;100:332–7.
43. Bassett ML, Halliday JW, Powell LW. Value of hepatic iron measurements in early hemochromatosis and determination of the critical iron level associated with fibrosis. Hepatology. 1986;6:24–9.
44. Bonkovsky HL, Banner BF, Rothman AL. Iron and chronic viral hepatitis. Hepatology. 1997; 25:759–68.
45. Brunt EM. Pathology of hepatic iron overload. Semin Liver Dis. 2005;25:392–401.
46. Fiel MI, Schiano TD, Guido M, Thung SN, Lindsay KL, Davis GL, et al. Increased hepatic iron deposition resulting from treatment of chronic hepatitis C with ribavirin. Am J Clin Pathol. 2000;113:35–9.
47. Pietrangelo A. Hemochromatosis gene modifies course of hepatitis C viral infection. Gastroenterology. 2003;124:1509–23.
48. Fujita N, Sugimoto R, Takeo M, Urawa N, Mifuji R, Tanaka H, et al. Hepcidin expression in the liver: relatively low level in patients with chronic hepatitis C. Mol Med. 2007;13:97–104.
49. Girelli D, Pasino M, Goodnough JB, Nemeth E, Guido M, Castagna A, et al. Reduced serum hepcidin levels in patients with chronic hepatitis C. J Hepatol. 2009;51:845–52.
50. Korenaga M, Wang T, Li Y, Showalter LA, Chan T, Sun J, et al. Hepatitis C virus core protein inhibits mitochondrial electron transport and increases reactive oxygen species (ROS) production. J Biol Chem. 2005;280:37481–8.
51. Nishina S, Hino K, Korenaga M, Vecchi C, Pietrangelo A, Mizukami Y, et al. Hepatitis C virus-induced reactive oxygen species raise hepatic iron level in mice by reducing hepcidin transcription. Gastroenterology. 2008;134:226–38.
52. Miura K, Taura K, Kodama Y, Schnabl B, Brenner DA. Hepatitis C virus-induced oxidative stress suppresses hepcidin expression through increased histone deacetylase activity. Hepatology. 2008;48:1420–9.
53. Migita K, Abiru S, Maeda Y, Daikoku M, Ohata K, Nakamura M, et al. Serum levels of interleukin-6 and its soluble receptors in patients with hepatitis C virus infection. Hum Immunol. 2006;67:27–32.
54. Aoki CA, Rossaro L, Ramsamooj R, Brandhagen D, Burritt MF, Bowlus CL. Liver hepcidin mRNA correlates with iron stores, but not inflammation, in patients with chronic hepatitis C. J Clin Gastroenterol. 2005;39:71–4.
55. Bassett SE, Di Bisceglie AM, Bacon BR, Sharp RM, Govindarajan S, Hubbard GB, et al. Effects of iron loading on pathogenicity in hepatitis C virus-infected chimpanzees. Hepatology. 1999;29:1884–92.
56. Lambrecht RW, Sterling RK, Naishadham D, Stoddard AM, Rogers T, Morishima C, et al. Iron levels in hepatocytes and portal tract cells predict progression and outcomes of patients with advanced chronic hepatitis C. Gastroenterology. 2011;140:1490–500. e3.
57. Tanaka H, Fujita N, Sugimoto R, Urawa N, Horiike S, Kobayashi Y, et al. Hepatic oxidative DNA damage is associated with increased risk for hepatocellular carcinoma in chronic hepatitis C. Br J Cancer. 2008;98:580–6.

58. Kato J, Kobune M, Nakamura T, Kuroiwa G, Takada K, Takimoto R, et al. Normalization of elevated hepatic 8-hydroxy-2′-deoxyguanosine levels in chronic hepatitis C patients by phlebotomy and low iron diet. Cancer Res. 2001;61:8697–702.
59. Furutani T, Hino K, Okuda M, Gondo T, Nishina S, Kitase A, et al. Hepatic iron overload induces hepatocellular carcinoma in transgenic mice expressing the hepatitis C virus polyprotein. Gastroenterology. 2006;130:2087–98.
60. Nelson JE, Wilson L, Brunt EM, Yeh MM, Kleiner DE, Unalp-Arida A, et al. Relationship between the pattern of hepatic iron deposition and histological severity in nonalcoholic fatty liver disease. Hepatology. 2011;53:448–57.
61. Imeryuz N, Tahan V, Sonsuz A, Eren F, Uraz S, Yuksel M, et al. Iron preloading aggravates nutritional steatohepatitis in rats by increasing apoptotic cell death. J Hepatol. 2007;47:851–9.
62. Nelson JE, Bhattacharya R, Lindor KD, Chalasani N, Raaka S, Heathcote EJ, et al. HFE C282Y mutations are associated with advanced hepatic fibrosis in Caucasians with nonalcoholic steatohepatitis. Hepatology. 2007;46:723–9.
63. Smith BW, Adams LA. Nonalcoholic fatty liver disease and diabetes mellitus: pathogenesis and treatment. Nat Rev Endocrinol. 2011;7:456–65.
64. Sorrentino P, D'Angelo S, Ferbo U, Micheli P, Bracigliano A, Vecchione R. Liver iron excess in patients with hepatocellular carcinoma developed on non-alcoholic steato-hepatitis. J Hepatol. 2009;50:351–7.
65. Aigner E, Theurl I, Theurl M, Lederer D, Haufe H, Dietze O, et al. Pathways underlying iron accumulation in human nonalcoholic fatty liver disease. Am J Clin Nutr. 2008;87:1374–83.
66. Yanagitani A, Yamada S, Yasui S, Shimomura T, Murai R, Murawaki Y, et al. Retinoic acid receptor alpha dominant negative form causes steatohepatitis and liver tumors in transgenic mice. Hepatology. 2004;40:366–75.
67. Tsuchiya H, Akechi Y, Ikeda R, Nishio R, Sakabe T, Terabayashi K, et al. Suppressive effects of retinoids on iron-induced oxidative stress in the liver. Gastroenterology. 2009;136:341–50. e8.
68. Otogawa K, Kinoshita K, Fujii H, Sakabe M, Shiga R, Nakatani K, et al. Erythrophagocytosis by liver macrophages (Kupffer cells) promotes oxidative stress, inflammation, and fibrosis in a rabbit model of steatohepatitis: implications for the pathogenesis of human nonalcoholic steatohepatitis. Am J Pathol. 2007;170:967–80.
69. Hoki T, Miyanishi K, Tanaka S, Takada K, Kawano Y, Sakurada A, et al. Increased duodenal iron absorption through up-regulation of divalent metal transporter 1 from enhancement of iron regulatory protein 1 activity in patients with nonalcoholic steatohepatitis. Hepatology. 2015. doi:10.1002/hep.27774.
70. Aigner E, Theurl I, Haufe H, Seifert M, Hohla F, Scharinger L, et al. Copper availability contributes to iron perturbations in human nonalcoholic fatty liver disease. Gastroenterology. 2008;135:680–8.
71. Tapryal N, Mukhopadhyay C, Das D, Fox PL, Mukhopadhyay CK. Reactive oxygen species regulate ceruloplasmin by a novel mRNA decay mechanism involving its 3′-untranslated region: implications in neurodegenerative diseases. J Biol Chem. 2009;284:1873–83.
72. Linder MC, Hazegh-Azam M. Copper biochemistry and molecular biology. Am J Clin Nutr. 1996;63:797S–811.
73. Roberts EA, Schilsky ML. Diagnosis and treatment of Wilson disease: an update. Hepatology. 2008;47:2089–111.
74. Harada M. Pathogenesis and management of Wilson disease. Hepatol Res. 2014;44:395–402.
75. de Bie P, Muller P, Wijmenga C, Klomp LW. Molecular pathogenesis of Wilson and Menkes disease: correlation of mutations with molecular defects and disease phenotypes. J Med Genet. 2007;44:673–88.
76. Turnlund JR, Keyes WR, Anderson HL, Acord LL. Copper absorption and retention in young men at three levels of dietary copper by use of the stable isotope 65Cu. Am J Clin Nutr. 1989;49:870–8.

77. Turnlund JR, Keyes WR, Peiffer GL, Scott KC. Copper absorption, excretion, and retention by young men consuming low dietary copper determined by using the stable isotope 65Cu. Am J Clin Nutr. 1998;67:1219–25.
78. Peña MM, Lee J, Thiele DJ. A delicate balance: homeostatic control of copper uptake and distribution. J Nutr. 1999;129:1251–60.
79. Lönnerdal B. Intestinal regulation of copper homeostasis: a developmental perspective. Am J Clin Nutr. 2008;88:846S–50.
80. Nose Y, Rees EM, Thiele DJ. Structure of the Ctr1 copper trans'PORE'ter reveals novel architecture. Trends Biochem Sci. 2006;31:604–7.
81. Lutsenko S, Barnes NL, Bartee MY, Dmitriev OY. Function and regulation of human copper-transporting ATPases. Physiol Rev. 2007;87:1011–46.
82. Nyasae L, Bustos R, Braiterman L, Eipper B, Hubbard A. Dynamics of endogenous ATP7A (Menkes protein) in intestinal epithelial cells: copper-dependent redistribution between two intracellular sites. Am J Physiol Gastrointest Liver Physiol. 2007;292:G1181–94.
83. Harada M. Wilson disease. Med Electron Microsc. 2002;35:61–6.
84. Wijmenga C, Klomp LW. Molecular regulation of copper excretion in the liver. Proc Nutr Soc. 2004;63:31–9.
85. Zhou B, Gitschier J. hCTR1: a human gene for copper uptake identified by complementation in yeast. Proc Natl Acad Sci U S A. 1997;94:7481–6.
86. Petris MJ, Smith K, Lee J, Thiele DJ. Copper-stimulated endocytosis and degradation of the human copper transporter, hCtr1. J Biol Chem. 2003;278:9639–46.
87. Rae TD, Schmidt PJ, Pufahl RA, Culotta VC, O'Halloran TV. Undetectable intracellular free copper: the requirement of a copper chaperone for superoxide dismutase. Science. 1999;284: 805–8.
88. Bull PC, Thomas GR, Rommens JM, Forbes JR, Cox DW. The Wilson disease gene is a putative copper transporting P-type ATPase similar to the Menkes gene. Nat Genet. 1993;5: 327–37.
89. Petrukhin K, Fischer SG, Pirastu M, Tanzi RE, Chernov I, Devoto M, et al. Mapping, cloning and genetic characterization of the region containing the Wilson disease gene. Nat Genet. 1993;5:338–43.
90. Tanzi RE, Petrukhin K, Chernov I, Pellequer JL, Wasco W, Ross B, et al. The Wilson disease gene is a copper transporting ATPase with homology to the Menkes disease gene. Nat Genet. 1993;5:344–50.
91. Yamaguchi Y, Heiny ME, Gitlin JD. Isolation and characterization of a human liver cDNA as a candidate gene for Wilson disease. Biochem Biophys Res Commun. 1993;197:271–7.
92. Terada K, Nakako T, Yang XL, Iida M, Aiba N, Minamiya Y, et al. Restoration of holoceruloplasmin synthesis in LEC rat after infusion of recombinant adenovirus bearing WND cDNA. J Biol Chem. 1998;273:1815–20.
93. Terada K, Aiba N, Yang XL, Iida M, Nakai M, Miura N, et al. Biliary excretion of copper in LEC rat after introduction of copper transporting P-type ATPase, ATP7B. FEBS Lett. 1999;448:53–6.
94. Yamaguchi Y, Heiny ME, Shimizu N, Aoki T, Gitlin JD. Expression of the Wilson disease gene is deficient in the Long-Evans Cinnamon rat. Biochem J. 1994;301:1–4.
95. Hung IH, Suzuki M, Yamaguchi Y, Yuan DS, Klausner RD, Gitlin JD. Biochemical characterization of the Wilson disease protein and functional expression in the yeast Saccharomyces cerevisiae. J Biol Chem. 1997;272:21461–6.
96. Yang XL, Miura N, Kawarada Y, Terada K, Petrukhin K, Gilliam T, et al. Two forms of Wilson disease protein produced by alternative splicing are localized in distinct cellular compartments. Biochem J. 1997;326:897–902.
97. Harada M, Sakisaka S, Terada K, Kimura R, Kawaguchi T, Koga H, et al. Role of ATP7B in biliary copper excretion in a human hepatoma cell line and normal rat hepatocytes. Gastroenterology. 2000;118:921–8.

98. Harada M, Sakisaka S, Kawaguchi T, Kimura R, Taniguchi E, Koga H, et al. Copper does not alter the intracellular distribution of ATP7B, a copper-transporting ATPase. Biochem Biophys Res Commun. 2000;275:871–6.
99. Harada M, Sakisaka S, Terada K, Kimura R, Kawaguchi T, Koga H, et al. A mutation of the Wilson disease protein, ATP7B, is degraded in the proteasomes and forms protein aggregates. Gastroenterology. 2001;120:967–74.
100. Harada M, Kumemura H, Sakisaka S, Shishido S, Taniguchi E, Kawaguchi T, et al. Wilson disease protein ATP7B is localized in the late endosomes in a polarized human hepatocyte cell line. Int J Mol Med. 2003;11:293–8.
101. Harada M, Kawaguchi T, Kumemura H, Terada K, Ninomiya H, Taniguchi E, et al. The Wilson disease protein ATP7B resides in the late endosomes with Rab7 and the Niemann-Pick C1 protein. Am J Pathol. 2005;166:499–510.
102. Yanagimoto C, Harada M, Kumemura H, Koga H, Kawaguchi T, Terada K, et al. Niemann-Pick C1 protein transports copper to the secretory compartment from late endosomes where ATP7B resides. Exp Cell Res. 2009;315:119–26.
103. Yanagimoto C, Harada M, Kumemura H, Abe M, Koga H, Sakata M, et al. Copper incorporation into ceruloplasmin is regulated by Niemann-Pick C1 protein. Hepatol Res. 2011;41:484–91.
104. Gross Jr JB, Myers BM, Kost LJ, Kuntz SM, LaRusso NF. Biliary copper excretion by hepatocyte lysosomes in the rat. Major excretory pathway in experimental copper overload. J Clin Invest. 1989;83:30–9.
105. Harada M, Sakisaka S, Yoshitake M, Shakadoh S, Gondoh K, Sata M, et al. Biliary copper excretion in acutely and chronically copper-loaded rats. Hepatology. 1993;17:111–7.
106. Polishchuk EV, Concilli M, Iacobacci S, Chesi G, Pastore N, Piccolo P, et al. Wilson disease protein ATP7B utilizes lysosomal exocytosis to maintain copper homeostasis. Dev Cell. 2014;29:686–700.
107. Connemann BJ, Gahr M, Schmid M, Runz H, Freudenmann RW. Low ceruloplasmin in a patient with Niemann-Pick type C disease. J Clin Neurosci. 2012;19:620–1.
108. Vázquez MC, Martínez P, Alvarez AR, González M, Zanlungo S. Increased copper levels in in vitro and in vivo models of Niemann-Pick C disease. Biometals. 2012;25:777–86.
109. European Association for the Study of the Liver. EASL clinical practice guidelines: Wilson's disease. J Hepatol. 2012;56:671–85.
110. Wilson SAK. Progressive lenticular degeneration: a familial nervous disease associated with cirrhosis of the liver. Brain. 1912;34:295–507.
111. Cumings JN. The copper and iron content of brain and liver in the normal and in hepatolenticular degeneration. Brain. 1948;71:410–5.
112. Scheinberg IH, Gitlin D. Deficiency of ceruloplasmin in patients with hepatolenticular degeneration (Wilson's disease). Science. 1952;116:484–5.
113. Walshe JM. Wilson's disease. New oral therapy. Lancet. 1956;i:25–6.
114. Ferenci P, Członkowska A, Merle U, et al. Late-onset Wilson's disease. Gastroenterology. 2007;132:1294–8.
115. Harada M. Wilson disease and hepatocellular carcinoma. Intern Med. 2004;43:1012–3.
116. Scheinberg IH, Sternlieb I. Pregnancy in penicillamine-treated patients with Wilson's disease. N Engl J Med. 1975;293:1300–2.
117. Sinha S, Taly AB, Prashanth LK, Arunodaya GR, Swamy HS. Successful pregnancies and abortions in symptomatic and asymptomatic Wilson's disease. J Neurol Sci. 2004;217:37–40.
118. Brewer GJ, Johnson VD, Dick RD, Hedera P, Fink JK, Kluin KJ. Treatment of Wilson's disease with zinc. XVII: treatment during pregnancy. Hepatology. 2000;31:364–70.
119. Sternlieb I. Wilson's disease and pregnancy. Hepatology. 2000;31:531–2.
120. Ferenci P, Caca K, Loudianos G, Mieli-Vergani G, Tanner S, Sternlieb I, et al. Diagnosis and phenotypic classification of Wilson disease. Liver Int. 2003;23:139–42.

121. Weiss KH, Thurik F, Gotthardt DN, Schäfer M, Teufel U, Wiegand F, et al. Efficacy and safety of oral chelators in treatment of patients with Wilson disease. Clin Gastroenterol Hepatol. 2013;11:1028–35.
122. Walshe JM. Management of penicillamine nephropathy in Wilson's disease: a new chelating agent. Lancet. 1969;2:1401–2.
123. Walshe JM. Treatment of Wilson's disease with trientine dihydrochloride. Lancet. 1982;1: 643–7.
124. Merle U, Schaefer M, Ferenci P, Stremmel W. Clinical presentation, diagnosis and long-term outcome of Wilson's disease: a cohort study. Gut. 2007;56:115–20.
125. Shimizu N, Fujiwara J, Ohnishi S, Sato M, Kodama H, Kohsaka T, et al. Effects of long-term zinc treatment in Japanese patients with Wilson disease: efficacy, stability, and copper metabolism. Transl Res. 2010;156:350–7.
126. Brewer GJ, Terry CA, Aisen AM, Hill GM. Treatment of Wilson's disease. Semin Neurol. 1987;7:209–20.
127. Plum LM, Rink L, Haase H. The essential toxin: impact of zinc on human health. Int J Environ Res Public Health. 2010;7:1342–65.
128. Weiss KH, Gotthardt DN, Klemm D, Merle U, Ferenci-Foerster D, Schaefer M, et al. Zinc monotherapy is not as effective as chelating agents in treatment of Wilson disease. Gastroenterology. 2011;140:1189–98.
129. Askari FK, Greenson J, Dick RD, Johnson VD, Brewer GJ. Treatment of Wilson's disease with zinc. XVIII. Initial treatment of the hepatic decompensation presentation with trientine and zinc. J Lab Clin Med. 2003;142:385–90.
130. Sini M, Sorbello O, Sanna F, Battolu F, Civolani A, Fanni D, et al. Histologic evolution and long-term outcome of Wilson's disease: results of a single-center experience. Eur J Gastroenterol Hepatol. 2013;25:111–7.
131. Yoshitoshi EY, Takada Y, Oike F, Sakamoto S, Ogawa K, Kanazawa H, et al. Long-term outcomes for 32 cases of Wilson's disease after living-donor liver transplantation. Transplantation. 2009;87:261–7.
132. Petrasek J, Jirsa M, Sperl J, Kozak L, Taimr P, Spicak J, et al. Revised King's College score for liver transplantation in adult patients with Wilson's disease. Liver Transpl. 2007;13: 55–61.
133. Beinhardt S, Leiss W, Stättermayer AF, Graziadei I, Zoller H, Stauber R, et al. Long-term outcomes of patients with Wilson disease in a large Austrian cohort. Clin Gastroenterol Hepatol. 2014;12:683–9.
134. Honma Y, Harada M, Sato M, Katsuki Y, Hiura M, Shibata M, et al. Late diagnosed Wilson disease with hepatic and neurological manifestations. Hepatol Res. 2011;41:270–6.
135. Walshe JM, Dixon AK. Dangers of non-compliance in Wilson's disease. Lancet. 1986;327: 845–7.
136. Tatsumi Y, Hattori A, Hayashi H, Ikoma J, Kaito M, Imoto M, et al. Current state of Wilson disease patients in central Japan. Intern Med. 2010;49:809–15.
137. Harada M. Wilson disease and its current problems. Intern Med. 2010;49:807–8.

Part II
Clinical Research

Chapter 8
Metabolic Syndrome and the Liver

Hitoshi Yoshiji

Abstract Metabolic syndrome (MS) is characterized by metabolic disturbance, which leads to many types of organ disorders including the liver. MS is frequently associated with nonalcoholic fatty liver disease (NAFLD). NAFLD ranges from simple steatosis to cirrhosis. Nonalcoholic fatty liver (NAFL) has been recognized as a benign and nonprogressive condition. However, nonalcoholic steatohepatitis (NASH) is now widely known as a potent liver disease, which may progress to liver cirrhosis and finally hepatocellular carcinoma (HCC). Several metabolic factors exert close relation to NAFLD. Almost half of patients with NAFLD possess type 2 diabetes mellitus (DM), hypertension, and dyslipidemia. Clinical approaches to NAFLD are mostly common to the principles of management of MS. Several clinical agents for type 2 DM, hypertension, and dyslipidemia have shown to be some clinical beneficial effects on NASH. In this chapter, the possible interactions between MS and the liver, especially in conjunction with NASH, will be reviewed.

Keyword Metabolic syndrome • NASH • Hepatocellular carcinoma

8.1 Nonalcoholic Steatohepatitis

Nonalcoholic fatty liver disease (NAFLD) is one of the major consequences of the current obesity epidemic [1–3]. NAFLD is now widely spread on approximately one-third of the population worldwide, and its incidence continues to increase with the increasing prevalence of metabolic diseases such as diabetes mellitus (DM) and hypertension (Fig. 8.1). NAFLD ranges from simple steatosis to cirrhosis. Fatty liver (FL) has been recognized as a benign and nonprogressive condition. However, nonalcoholic steatohepatitis (NASH) is now widely known as a potent liver disease which may progress to liver cirrhosis and finally hepatocellular carcinoma (HCC). Cirrhosis could occur about one-fourth of NASH. Although weight loss based on diet and exercise therapies is very effective and improves steatosis and

H. Yoshiji (✉)
Third Department of Internal Medicine, Nara Medical University, 840 Shijo-cho, Kashihara, Nara 634-0813, Japan
e-mail: yoshijih@naramed-u.ac.jp

H. Ohira (ed.), *The Liver in Systemic Diseases*, DOI 10.1007/978-4-431-55790-6_8

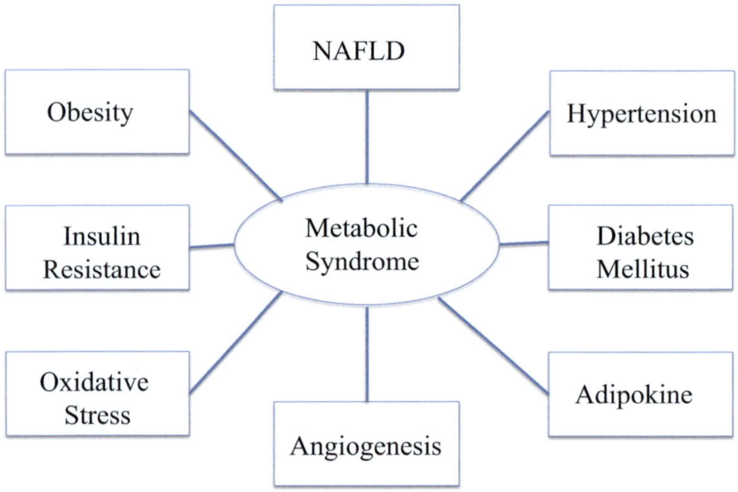

Fig. 8.1 Metabolic syndrome interacts many biological phenomenon and several diseases

inflammation in the liver, many NAFLD patients cannot change their lifestyle, and it is then necessary to employ additional therapy [4–6]. Accordingly, efforts are currently directed worldwide at overcoming NAFLD, especially NASH. However, no widely accepted therapeutic modalities have been established in the clinical practice yet.

8.1.1 Pathogenesis

8.1.1.1 Insulin Resistance

The accumulation of fat in the liver is a result of increased free fatty acid (FFA) along with reduced beta-oxidation. Patients with NAFLD usually have insulin resistance (IR). Cross-sectional human studies showed that insulin resistance (IR), i.e., coexistence of high glucose and insulin, is a consistent finding in patients with type 2 DM [7]. Experimental evidence for the contribution of hepatitis C virus (HCV) in the development of IR and DM has been found in the HCV-transgenic mouse model [8]. Moreover, several human studies demonstrated that IR is a risk factor of advanced fibrosis in patients with chronic hepatitis C (CHC), and IR itself may contribute to the liver fibrosis progression in CHC [9–11]. Moreover, a similar close interaction could be observed in patients with other morbidities, such as NASH [12]. Either high glucose or insulin increased the production and expression of collagen genes in the activated hepatic stellate cells (HSCs), which play a pivotal role in the liver fibrosis development in vitro [13, 14]. DM is associated with a two- to threefold increase in the risk of HCC regardless of the etiology of chronic liver diseases [15, 16]. Several reports have shown that IR increased the risk for the development and recurrence of HCC [15–18]. NASH is well known as a liver disease that frequently complicates IR status [19]. Current evidences point to IR and subsequent hyperinsulinemia as the key pathogenic factors in NAFLD and progression from simple FL to NASH [19]. It has been reported that the IR status accelerated the progression in the NASH animal model and that the insulin-sensitizing agent could reverse the underlying pathogenesis involved through improvement of IR [20]. We also have demonstrated that IR itself significantly promoted the liver fibrosis development in diabetic rats [3]. Several studies have shown that the insulin-sensitizing agents improved the metabolic and histologic parameters, most notably liver injury and fibrosis, not only in the experimental model but also in patients with NASH [21, 22].

8.1.1.2 Oxidative Stress and Angiogenesis

The pathogenesis of NASH is reportedly a multifactorial process [23].

Recently, reactive oxidative stress (ROS) has been focused upon as a common pathogenic mechanism in various liver diseases, including NASH [24, 25]. It has been found that hepatic 4-hydroxy-2-noneal (4-HNE) and 8-hydroxydeoxyguanosine (8-OHdG), as reliable ROS markers of lipid peroxidation and oxidative DNA-damage, respectively, significantly increased in the animal models and human samples of NASH [26, 27]. However, it has not been elucidated yet whether ROS is a crucial factor for progression of NASH, since, as in DM, NASH is almost certainly a polygenic disease affected by several factors related to "multiple hits" (Fig. 8.2) [23]. Animal models of hepatic steatosis and steatohepatitis have improved the understanding of the pathogenesis of NASH. The different animal models of NASH have been extensively reviewed [28]. Among them, we and other groups employed a choline-deficient, amino acid-defined (CDAA) diet model. This model induces histological processes similar to those of the human NASH, namely, hepatic steatosis, steatohepatitis, liver fibrosis, cirrhosis, and finally HCC development associated with elevation of several markers of ROS, such as TBARS and 8-OHdG [29]. A downside of the CDAA model is lack of the first-hit status, i.e., obesity, insulin resistance, and hyperglycemia [28]. Zucker rats, which lack functional leptin receptor (Ob-R) due to a missense mutation, have these first-hit conditions [30]. Several studies have shown impaired liver fibrogenesis in Zucker rats and *ob/ob* mice, which are leptin deficient [31–33. Similarly, leptin signal impairment did not develop either liver fibrosis or HCC, indicating that leptin-mediated signaling cascade plays a pivotal role in the pathogenesis of NASH.

Angiogenesis, i.e., the formation of new vessels by sprouting from the preexisting vasculature, is of central importance for the embryonic development and organogenesis. In adults, physiological angiogenesis occurs during the female reproductive cycle and in wound healing [34]. Abnormally pathological angiogenesis is observed in rheumatoid arthritis, psoriasis, diabetic retinopathy, tumor growth, and even fibrogenesis [34]. Although previous studies conducted to

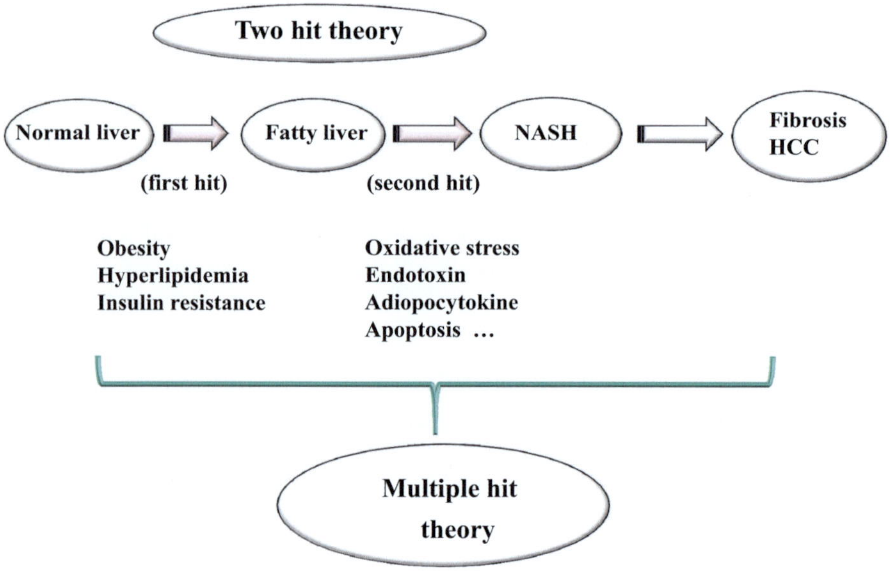

Fig. 8.2 Pathogenesis pathway of NASH. Although the two-hit theory has been widely accepted, recent studies suggest that several factors are involved simultaneously – multiple-hit theory

determine the molecular process associated with fibrosis and angiogenesis were performed independently, recent studies have revealed that both biological phenomena emerged synergistically [35]. It was shown that neovascularization significantly increased during the development of liver fibrosis both in human and animal experimental studies [36, 37]. Among the identified angiogenic factors to date, the vascular endothelial growth factor (VEGF) is one of the most potent and central factors in many physiological and pathological processes [38]. In liver fibrosis, the VEGF expression increased both in the human chronic liver diseases and in the experimental fibrogenesis [37, 39, 40]. The VEGF expression reportedly correlates with the chronic liver disease-associated angiogenesis and sinusoidal capillarization [39, 41]. These results suggest that VEGF-mediated angiogenesis also plays an important role in the development of liver fibrosis. In the NASH experimental model, we previously demonstrated that angiogenesis, which coordinates with VEGF, plays an important role in the progression of NASH [42]. A reported study has shown that ROS significantly increased in the liver with FL as well as NASH [43], indicating that FL and NASH are both affected by ROS despite the different clinical outcomes. It has been reported that the increased production of ROS occurs very early in the histological spectrum of NAFLD [27]. It has also been demonstrated that, even at the earliest stage of NAFLD, a considerable oxidative stress already exists [44]. Taken together, it is feasible that the onset and progression of NASH can be initiated by introducing an additional factor based on augmentation of ROS. It has been reported that leptin-mediated angiogenesis plays an important role of the pathogenesis of NASH [42].

8.1.1.3 Adipokine

Because NAFLD is a common manifestation of MS, various adipocytokines are involved in the progression of NASH [45, 46]. Among them, adiponectin and leptin are well known to be involved in the pathogenesis of NASH [31, 45, 47]. Adiponectin administration alleviates NAFLD progression in mice, and liver fibrosis is accelerated in adiponectin knockout mice, indicating the protective effect of adiponectin against liver fibrosis development in NASH [48]. In the NASH patients, the circulating adiponectin reportedly decreases [47], and we also observed that the serum level of adiponectin in NASH significantly decreased more than in FL. On the other hand, recent reports have revealed that leptin exerts a profibrogenic activity. Hepatic fibrogenesis is impaired in the leptin- and leptin receptor-deficient animals [31, 32]. Leptin also enhances proliferation of the activated HSC, which plays a central role in the liver fibrosis development [49]. In addition to these direct effects on HSC, recent studies have revealed that leptin possesses an angiogenic activity [42, 50]. We previously reported that leptin exerted a potent angiogenic activity and that leptin-mediated neovascularization plays an important role in the development of liver fibrosis in the rat NASH model [42]. The serum leptin level was significantly higher in NASH than in FL. Although the original findings of leptin indicated that leptin plays a crucial role in the regulation of appetite and the size of body fat mass, some recent studies have revealed that leptin elicits the multiplicity of biological effects [51]. Recently, it has been shown that leptin exerted a potent pro-angiogenic activity both in vitro and in vivo [50, 52]. It has been shown that Ob-R was expressed on EC and that leptin induced the proliferation of EC in a dose-dependent manner [50]. Leptin induced the neovascularization in the corneas of normal rats but not in Zucker rats [50]. Synergistic stimulation of angiogenesis by leptin with VEGF and impairment of VEGF production in the leptin receptor-deficient (*db/db*) mice have been also reported [53, 54]. We previously showed that, even in the absence of the leptin signaling cascade, steatohepatitis and augmentation of oxidative stress could be observed in the rat NASH experimental model. However, without leptin signaling, neither fibrosis nor HCC developed, suggesting that leptin played a pivotal role in the progression of fibrogenesis and carcinogenesis in NASH. Leptin-mediated neovascularization, which coordinated with VEGF, significantly increased almost in parallel with the progression of liver fibrogenesis and carcinogenesis.

8.1.1.4 Gut-Liver Axis

Recent studies have revealed that the innate immunity is activated in chronic liver diseases [55]. The liver is constantly exposed to some intestine-derived bacterial products such as lipopolysaccharide (LPS) through the portal vein. Toll-like receptors (TLRs) are family of pattern recognition receptors that recognize pathogen-derived molecules called pathogen-associated molecular patterns (PAMPs), which are structural components unique to bacteria, fungi, and viruses. To date, 13 TLRs have been found in mice and 11 in humans. Within this family of TLR proteins, TLR4 was discovered first and is the most important Toll homolog. TLR4 recognizes LPS, a Gram-negative bacterial cell component that is enriched within the intestinal lumen and its associated portal circulation. The breakdown of liver homeostasis and intestinal barrier functions in chronic liver disorders may activate the innate immunity system through LPS-TLR4 signaling cascade. In the liver, Kupffer cells (KCs) and HSCs, which are known to exert a pivotal role in liver fibrogenesis, express high levels of TLR4 [56]. The relative effects of TLR4 on KCs and HSCs in liver fibrosis have been studied recently [57]. Although the KCs are regarded as the main targets of TLR ligands in the liver, the HSCs were found to play a more important role in liver fibrosis development than the KC through activation of the myeloid differentiation factor (MyD88) and nuclear factor-κB (NF-κB). The HSCs are the cells responsible for TLR4 signaling in liver fibrosis, and several mechanisms mediated by TLR4 in the HSC promote liver fibrogenesis. Recent clinical studies reported that endotoxin/TLR4 signaling played an important role in the activation of inflammatory pathways associated with NASH. TLR4 is a pattern recognition receptor which recognizes endotoxin and signals through adaptor molecules termed MyD88 and Toll/interleukin 1 receptor domain-containing adaptor-inducing interferon-β (TRIF) to activate transcription factors that initiate innate immunity. TLR4 is expressed on multiple liver cell types including liver vascular endothelial cells (LVECs), KCs, and HSCs. Indeed, TLR4 on HSC plays a dominant role in fibrosis development through effects on transforming growth factor-β (TGF-β)-dependent collagen production [57]. The liver is the main target of intestinally derived bacterial products, and the rate of bacterial translocation increases in various models of hepatic disease, rendering LPS, a likely candidate mediator of TLR4-dependent profibrogenic effects. Polymyxins are antibiotics with a general structure consisting of a cyclic peptide with a long hydrophobic tail and are selectively toxic to Gram-negative bacteria such as *E. coli*, *Pseudomonas aeruginosa*, *Enterobacteriaceae*, and *Pneumobacillus* due to their specificity for the LPS molecule that exists within many Gram-negative outer membranes. They are produced by nonribosomal peptide synthetase systems in Gram-positive bacteria such as *Paenibacillus polymyxa* and disrupt the structure of the bacterial cell membrane by interacting with its phospholipids. They are not absorbed through gastrointestinal tract. In clinical settings, they are used for patients with Gram-negative bacterial infections and column of endotoxin apheresis against endotoxemia. Translocated LPS derived from the gut microflora mediates TLR4 activation in the liver. But this translocation might be independent of intestinal TLR4. Guo et al. reported that LPS caused an increase in intestinal permeability via an intracellular mechanism involving TLR4-dependent upregulation of CD14 membrane expression [58]. The relationship between LPS and TLR4 on intestinal permeability has been still controversial. NAFLD is associated with increased intestinal permeability and small intestinal bacteria overgrowth. The increased intestinal permeability might be the condition for the hypothesis of the contribution of gut-liver axis to the development of NAFLD. The intestinal barrier defect might be caused by disruption, imbalance of proliferation and apoptosis, intestinal mucosal atrophy and edema associated with portal hypertension or absence of bile acids, and systemic increases in inflammatory cytokines and oxidative stress produced from the liver. LPS causes an increase in intestinal permeability via an intracellular mechanism involving TLR4-dependent upregulation of CD14 membrane expression. Caco-2 cells grown in zinc-deficient media have reduced transepithelial electrical resistance (TEER) and altered expression of ZO-1 and occludin compared with Caco-2 cells grown in zinc-replete media [59]. In clinical practice, zinc deficiency is likely to occur in patients with liver cirrhosis. Zinc deficiency in patients with liver cirrhosis may reduce tight junction proteins in the intestine and increase the permeability. In the NASH model, CDAA-induced hepatic fibrosis, endogenous LPS, and systemic increases in inflammatory cytokines might disrupt intestinal-tight junction proteins. From this point of view, the recruitment of tight junction proteins by using probiotics and zinc preparation, for example, would be a new strategy for NASH treatment. Intestinal microflora is involved in liver fibrosis. In this in vivo model, dietary habits through increasing the percentage of intestinal endotoxin producers, such as Gram-negative bacteria, might accelerate liver fibrogenesis, introducing dysbiosis as a cofactor contributing to chronic liver injury in NAFLD. Endo et al. also showed butyrate-producing probiotics reduced NAFLD progression in rats [60]. These data indicated that intestinal microflora could be a new target for NASH treatment. Taken together, inhibition of LPS-**TLR4** signaling with poorly absorbable antibiotics attenuated the liver fibrosis development of NASH via inhibition of HSC activation indicating that reduction of LPS and restoration of the intestinal tight junction protein might be a new therapeutic strategy for the treatment of the liver fibrosis development in NASH.

8.2 Diagnosis

Although liver biopsy is currently the gold standard for diagnosing progressive NASH, it has many weak points, such as sampling error and risk of complications. Furthermore, it is not realistic to perform liver biopsies on all NAFLD patients. Furthermore, pathologists differ in their diagnosis and recognition of liver biopsy results, and there is no established treatment method for NASH even when it is diagnosed by liver biopsy. In the guidelines recently published by the AASLD, liver biopsy is suggested for complications of metabolic syndrome and a high serum ferritin level in patients with NASH, as well as in those suspected of having advanced fibrosis [61]. Nevertheless, NASH can only be diagnosed by liver biopsy. However, noninvasive techniques have been developed to identify whether it is NASH or not. Diagnosis of NASH using various biomarkers, scoring systems, and imaging methods, such as elastography, has recently been attempted. Shimada et al. reported that early NASH and simple steatosis could be differentiated by a combination of three values: adiponectin ($\leq$4.0 μg/mL), homeostasis model assessment of insulin resistance (HOMA-IR) ($\geq$3.0), and type 4 collagen 7S

(≥5.0 ng/mL) [62]. However, adiponectin cannot be measured at general practice sites and is not covered by health insurance. Sumida proposed the NAFIC score, which comprises three items – ferritin, fasting insulin, and type 4 collagen 7S – for the screening of NASH. These three variables were extracted as factors independently contributing to NASH in an analysis of 177 NAFLD patients. The NAFIC system assigns one point for 200 (female) or 300 (male) ng/mL or higher ferritin, one point for 10 μU/mL or higher fasting insulin, and two points for 5.0 ng/mL or higher type 4 collagen 7S. The total of these points is regarded as the NAFIC score, and the possibility of NASH is high when the NAFIC score is 2 or higher. The usefulness of this scoring system has been verified in a validation study involving 442 patients. The three variables constituting the NAFIC score are parameters associated with the pathology of NASH, such as oxidative stress, IR, and fibrosis. Sumida proposed that based on the results of the multicenter study performed by JSG-NAFLD, it can be concluded that the FIB-4 index is useful for excluding advanced fibrosis patients, whereas the NAFIC score is useful for detecting NASH [63].

Recent evidences have suggested that increased hepatocyte apoptosis has an important role in progression from simple NAFL to NASH and correlates with disease severity and hepatic fibrosis [64, 65]. During apoptosis, some intracellular proteins are cleaved by caspase. A neoepitope in cytokeratin 18 (CK18), the major intermediate filament protein in the liver, becomes available at an early caspase cleavage event during apoptosis and is not detectable in the viable or necrotic cells [66]. It has been reported that CK18 fragments were markedly elevated in the NAFLD patients as compared with the healthy control and that the plasma levels of CK18 correlated with the expression levels in the liver. A significant increase of CK18 expression could be observed in patients with NASH as compared with the simple FL patients, and the expression level of CK18 correlated with the presence of fibrosis [65]. The same group recently conducted a multicenter validation study that yielded similar results, and CK18 was an independent predictor of NASH [67].

Genome-wide association studies (GWASs) offer a powerful technique for discovering novel associations between single nucleotide polymorphisms (SNPs) and disease phenotypes. Romeo et al. [70] first reported that an SNP in patatin-like phospholipase domain-containing protein 3 (PNPLA3) (rs738409 [G], encoding I148M), also termed adiponutrin, on chromosome 22 was strongly associated with increased hepatic fat levels, as well as with hepatic inflammation. This allele was most commonly observed in Hispanics, the group most susceptible to NAFLD among the 2111 subjects that comprised a mixed study population of Hispanics, African Americans, and European Americans. PNPLA3 is highly expressed in adipose tissue as well as in the liver, and the overexpression of PNPA3 promotes lipogenesis in mouse primary hepatocytes. In humans, hepatic PNPLA3 messenger RNA expression appears to be correlated with hepatic triglyceride content. Association studies [71–75], including one meta-analysis [75], confirm that the I148M polymorphism is also a strong modifier of NASH and progressive hepatic injury in various populations throughout the world. However, not only in NASH, it has been reported that PNPLA3 SNP possesses the interaction with the pathogenesis of CHC and alcoholic liver injury. Further studies are required whether this SNP is specific factor for NASH or not. In addition to PNPLA3, other SNPs associated with NAFLD include neurocan, lysophospholipase-like 1, glucokinase regulatory protein, protein phosphatase 1 regulatory subunit 3b, and apolipoprotein C3 [76–78]. However, it is unknown whether screening for these SNPs can facilitate the diagnosis of NASH or advanced fibrosis.

8.3 Treatment

Although weight loss based on diet and exercise therapies is very effective and improves steatosis and inflammation in the liver, many NAFLD patients cannot change their lifestyle, and it is then necessary to employ additional therapy [4–6]. There are several focused areas about the therapeutic strategy against NASH as well as lifestyle modification. Targeting the component of metabolic syndrome would be one of the promising approaches in the clinical practice. Many efforts are currently directed toward overcoming NASH; however, the optimal treatment for NASH has not been established in the clinical practice.

8.3.1 Antihypertension

8.3.1.1 Hepatocellular Carcinoma

The renin-angiotensin system (RAS) is a key mediator in the regulation of the arterial blood pressure and body fluid homeostasis [68–70]. Recent studies have revealed that RAS has been postulated as an accelerator of injury and wound-healing responses. It has further been postulated that unrestrained angiotensin 1 (AT1) activation is the cause of fibrosis in chronic inflammation [71]. RAS also plays an important role in the regulation of the local hemodynamics in several organs. In the liver, it has been shown that RAS is frequently activated in the patients with chronic liver disease, such as cirrhosis [72–74]. Angiotensin II (AT-II), an octapeptide produced mainly through proteolytic cleavage of its precursor (AT-I) by angiotensin I-converting enzyme (ACE), is considered a potential mediator of portal hypertension because its plasma level is significantly increased in patients with liver cirrhosis, and its administration induces elevation of the portal pressure [75, 76]. AT-II reportedly stimulates neovascularization [77–80] and is also involved in several biological activities [81–85]. AT-II has been shown to induce VEGF in a dose-dependent manner both in vitro and in vivo [86–89]. A retrospective cohort study on 5207 patients receiving ACE-I or other antihypertensive drugs with a 10-year follow-up showed that ACE-I decreased the incident cancer and fetal cancer (Glasgow study) [90]. The other antihypertensive drugs, e.g., calcium channel blockers, diuretics, and β-blockers, had no apparent effects on the risk of cancer development. On the contrary, another study did not disclose such an inhibitory effect for ACE-I [91]. However, in this report, the standardized cancer incidence ratio (SIR) was quite variable according to the type of cancer. SIR of the liver cancer was low (0.5), whereas that of the renal cancer was high (1.6). A cohort study on 1051 patients has demonstrated that users of ACE-I or ARB had a lower incidence of cancer than nonusers [92]. It has been reported that addition of ACE-I or ARB to platinum-based chemotherapy may prolong the survival of patients with advanced lung cancer [93]. Also, several clinical studies have been reported such as a pilot study of ARB in advanced hormone-refractory prostate cancer [94, 95]. It has been reported that the serum ACE activity was a marker in the HCC patients [96]. ACE-I significantly suppressed the tumor growth in the murine HCC experimental model even after the tumor was fully established [87–89]. To date, several other clinically available agents have also been shown to inhibit the tumor development and angiogenesis in animal experiments [97, 98], but most of these drugs have been tested at very high doses as compared to the clinical dose range. Therefore, the clinical use of these agents does not appear feasible now.

Several studies demonstrated that neovascularization in the tumor was markedly suppressed by ACE-I and ARB [99, 100]. ACE-I significantly suppressed the VEGF mRNA expression in the tumor cells and EC in vitro and also significantly decreased the VEGF mRNA expression in the tumor. However, it has been reported that the use of anti-angiogenic agents as monotherapy in treating the patients with advanced cancer did not prove significantly effective [97]. Nevertheless, monotherapy with ACE-I would not exert a sufficient effect on the advanced tumor. It has been demonstrated that the combination treatment of anti-angiogenic agents exerted a synergistic inhibitory effect on the tumor development and angiogenesis [97, 101, 102]. The combination of ACE-I and interferon (IFN) had a greater suppressive effect on the HCC growth than ACE-I alone [103]. Other agents, such as 5-fluorouracil, also exerted a synergistic effect with ACE-I [104]. Moreover, ARB enhances the effects of radiation or gemcitabine on tumor growth and tumor-associated angiogenesis by reducing VEGF expression [105, 106]. In the future clinical applications of ACE-I, it is preferable to employ these combination therapies to improve their effectiveness. It has been suggested that angiogenesis is also involved in the early carcinogenesis step as well as tumor growth and metastasis [107–110]. Suppression of RAS significantly suppressed rat hepatocarcinogenesis at a clinically comparable low dose along with suppression of neovascularization [111]. Similar to the HCC growth, the combination treatment of ACE-I and vitamin K (VK) exerted a more potent inhibitory effect on rat hepatocarcinogenesis via angiogenesis suppression as compared with either single agent [112]. Not only in the experimental studies but also in the clinical practice this combination regimen could ameliorate hepatocarcinogenesis [113, 114]. A 48-month follow-up study revealed that the combination treatment with VK and ACE-I markedly inhibited the cumulative recurrence of HCC along with the suppression of the serum level of VEGF. The serum level of lectin-reactive alpha-fetoprotein was also suppressed almost in parallel with VEGF. These beneficial effects were not observed with single treatment using VK or ACE-I. The combination treatment of VK and ACE-I may suppress the cumulative recurrence of HCC after the curative therapy, at least partly through suppression of the VEGF-mediated neovascularization. Accordingly, this combination regimen may represent a new strategy for chemoprevention against HCC [115]. In morbidities other than cancer, angiogenesis has been shown to play an important role in several pathological processes, such as ocular neovascularization, arterial plaque formation, psoriasis, gastrointestinal ulcers, and rheumatoid arthritis [116–118]. The results of the EUCID study have highlighted the importance of RAS in the pathogenesis of diabetic retinopathy [119]. This study suggested that, lisinopril, an ACE-I, may slow the progression of diabetic retinopathy in the type 2 diabetes patients. Several clinical and experimental studies have suggested a strong correlation between RAS and diabetic retinopathy. The VEGF concentrations in the vitreous body were high in the patients with diabetic retinopathy, and the expression level of the retinal VEGF mRNA was increased in the streptozotocin-induced diabetic rats [120, 121]. Treatment with ACE-I significantly reduced the diabetes-associated changes in the VEGF gene expression and vascular permeability. Furthermore, recent studies have revealed the preventive effect of ARB against progression of diabetic retinopathy both in types 1 and 2 DM in randomized controlled trials [119, 122]. Nevertheless, new findings regarding the cancer are still accumulating, such as the association of ACE polymorphism and the cancer [123, 124].

Aldosterone (Ald), which is positioned in the downstream of AT-II in RAS, is a mineralocorticoid hormone that acts classically in blood pressure regulation and electrolyte balance via the mineralocorticoid receptors (MRs) [125, 126]. Recent data have suggested that Ald participates in endothelial dysfunction, vascular fibrosis, and inflammation in the vasculature and that it is involved in the pathogenesis of hypertension [127, 128]. Similar to AT-II, Ald was reportedly suggested to play an important role in angiogenesis (Fig. 8.1) [129–131]. Possible involvement of Ald and mineral corticoid receptor (MR) system in the ocular pathological neovascularization has been reported. Ald stimulated proliferation and tubulogenesis of EC and exacerbated angiogenesis in oxygen-induced retinopathy, and these events could be attenuated by spironolactone. Eplerenone, a selective Ald blocker (SAB), is clinically used for treatment of hypertension and heart failure in many countries including Japan. SAB is a selective MR antagonist with minimal binding to the progesterone and androgen receptors, of which selectivity is 100 times more than spironolactone. Treatment with SAB exerted a marked inhibitory effect on the HCC development along with suppression of VEGF-mediated angiogenesis [130]. Furthermore, a combination treatment of SAB and ACE-I exerted a remarkably more potent inhibitory effect than either single-agent treatment [132]. Since these agents are currently used widely in the clinical practice, the combination regimen using ACE-I, VK, BCAA, and SAB may represent a potential new therapeutic strategy against HCC in the future.

Renin is a rate-limiting enzyme of RAS, and several reports have shown that renin plays an important role in several pathological processes. A direct renin inhibitor (DRI), aliskiren, has shown to inhibit liver fibrosis development and glutathione-S-transferase placental form (GST-P)-positive preneoplastic lesions along with suppression of the Ac-HSCs and neovascularization in a dose-dependent manner. DRI also inhibited the hepatic expressions of transforming growth factor-beta 1 (TGF-beta 1), AT-II, and VEGF in a rat NASH model [133]. These data suggest that renin plays a pivotal role in the liver fibrosis development and hepatocarcinogenesis of NASH. Since DRI is already widely used in the clinical practice with safety, this drug may also represent a potential new strategy against the progression of NASH in the future.

8.3.1.2 Liver Fibrosis

It has been reported that the risk of HCC increases along with the progression of hepatic fibrosis [134]. Furthermore, the existence of fibrosis itself accelerates the experimental hepatocarcinogenesis [135, 136]. Taken together, an effective therapeutic strategy for suppressing liver fibrosis should improve the overall prognosis of the patients with HCC. Although emerging efforts are conducted to develop new drugs against liver fibrosis, there are no approved such anti-fibrotic agents to date. As in HCC, an alternative approach may be to find a clinically used orally available compound that also has inhibitory effects on liver fibrogenesis until new drugs become widely available. In addition to the transformed cells, extracellular matrix (ECM) remodeling has been shown to play an important role in the cancer development [137]. Recent studies have suggested that AT-II also plays an important role in the ECM remodeling. It has been demonstrated that the ECM remodeling is not a simple structural component, but it is an active process in the tumor development. For example, ECM provides the vascular supply that any tumor requires for satisfactory gas exchange, obtaining nutrients, and removal of waste products. In the human HCC, it has been recently shown that the increased ECM remodeling was associated with tumor progression [138]. Although the previous studies conducted to determine the molecular process associated with the ECM remodeling, such as liver fibrosis and angiogenesis, were performed independently, the recent studies have revealed that both biological phenomena emerged synergistically [35]. AT-II has also been shown to induce the contractility and proliferation of the HSC [139–143]. The gross remodeling of ECM in the fibrotic liver is likely to be regulated by synthesis and enzymatic degradation of ECM [139, 140, 144]. Matrix degradation is catalyzed by the activity of matrix metalloproteinases (MMPs). The activities of MMPs are inhibited by the tissue inhibitors of metalloproteinases (TIMPs) via formation of non-covalent 1:1 complexes with MMPs [145]. Four members of the TIMP family have been characterized so far. In the liver, TIMP-1 and TIMP-2 were identified, and TIMP-1 was suggested to play a more important role in the pathological processes in the liver than TIMP-2 [143, 146–151]. During liver fibrosis development, the TIMP-1 expression in the liver and the serum TIMP-1 level were markedly up-regulated in the murine liver fibrosis models and man [147, 148, 151–153]. In the cultured activated HSC, AT-II also increased TIMP-1 in dose- and time-dependent manners. ARB and LY 333531, an inhibitor of protein kinase C (PKC), blocked this augmentation in a dose-dependent manner. These results suggest that AT-II induces TIMP-1 via type-1 receptor and PKC as an intracellular signaling pathway in the Ac-HSC [154]. It has been reported that ACE-I and ARB had significant inhibitory effects on the experimental pig serum-induced liver fibrosis development, along with suppression of the HSC activation via AT1-R [155]. Similar suppressive effects have been noticed with AT-II blocking agents in several hepatic fibrosis experimental models [88, 156–162]. Not only the experimental studies but also several investigations in the clinical practice have shown beneficial effects of these agents. Several researchers showed that ARB markedly improved the liver fibrosis scores in the patients with HCV-related chronic hepatitis and NASH [163–167]. In the NASH experimental model, we previously demonstrated that angiogenesis plays an important role in the progression of NASH [42]. We also reported that neovascularization developed in patients with NASH, whereas no marked augmentation was observed in the FL or the healthy liver [168]. It has been reported that the IR status accelerated the progression in the NASH animal model and that the insulin-sensitizing agent could reverse the underlying pathogenesis involved through improvement of IR [20]. We also have demonstrated that IR itself significantly promoted the liver fibrosis development in diabetic rats [3].

It has been reported that IR plays a critical role in the pathogenesis of NASH [42]. Recent studies have revealed that the development of IR closely correlated with AT-II [169]. The suppressive effect of ARB may be linked with inhibition of IR. Moreover, a 10-year retrospective study on liver-transplanted patients with reinfection by HCV has revealed that the patients treated with RAS inhibitory agents – as an antihypertensive therapy – exerted protective effect against progression to liver cirrhosis as compared with those receiving other types of drugs [170]. This result is relevant since the aggressive fibrosis progression in the liver-transplanted patients with reinfection by HCV is one of the serious problems in the field of liver transplantation. A combination therapy against liver fibrosis may exert a synergistic rather than an additive effect. In some experimental studies, combination treatment of ACE-I with IFN or imatinib mesylate, a platelet-derived growth factor receptor tyrosine kinase inhibitor, significantly attenuated the liver fibrosis development as compared with either single-agent treatment [171, 172]. In a pilot study, the combination therapy of ACE-I and IFN significantly decreased the serum fibrosis markers in the patients with HCV-related chronic hepatitis refractory to IFN monotherapy. The inhibitory effect of this combination regimen was much more potent than that of either single agent [173]. Some recent studies have shown that Ald – in addition to AT-II – also stimulates the proliferation and the collagen synthesis of HSC [99, 155, 162, 174]. In addition to these above effects, several biological activities are involved in. It has been reported that AT-II induced the epithelial-mesenchymal transition (EMT) or chronic inflammation. Opinion is growing that the true nature of ARBs is actually anti-fibrotic and that the blood pressure effects are secondary. And the ECM remodeling is another manifestation of injury responses induced by RAS. The coordinated injury response-promoting angiogenesis, EMT, tissue destructive macrophage activity, and adaptive immune system are suppressed by the RAS inhibitors [175].

8.3.2 Branched-Chain Amino Acid

The branched-chain amino acids (BCAAs) are comprised of three essential amino acids, namely, leucine, isoleucine, and valine. Recent studies have shown that BCAA granules improved the nutritional status (e.g., hypoalbuminemia) and event-free survival in the patients with liver cirrhosis [176, 177]. Furthermore, BCAA suppressed the incidence of hepatocarcinogenesis in the patients with HCV-related cirrhosis and obesity that is often associated with IR [178]. BCAAs are also known to modulate insulin signaling. They induce glucose uptake and improve glucose metabolism in the rats with liver cirrhosis [179, 180]. They also improve IR in the patients with HCV-related liver diseases [181, 182]. Previously, we reported that the IR itself significantly augmented the VEGF-mediated hepatic neovascularization [3]. It has been reported that BCAA exerted a chemopreventive effect against HCC along with suppression of VEGF expression and hepatic neovascularization in the obese diabetic rats with IR [183]. In contrast to the animal studies, single BCAA treatment failed to suppress the first and second recurrence of HCC after the curative therapy in the clinical practice [184]. It has been reported that BCAA markedly inhibited the cumulative HCC recurrence after the curative therapy under the condition of high HOMA-IR along with suppression of several indices. It is well-known that the IR status in the patients with chronic liver diseases is usually associated with both high insulin and glucose levels [175]. We previously reported that the IR status itself significantly augmented the hepatocarcinogenesis [3], and BCAA could suppress the development of preneoplastic lesions under the IR condition in rats [183]. BCAA suppressed the recurrence of HCC in the patients with high IRI while glucose level did not influence the effect of BCAA. A recent report has shown that BCAA suppressed insulin-induced hepatic tumor cell proliferation [185]. We observed that IR was significantly improved by the BCAA treatment. This effect is also likely to play a clinically beneficial role since insulin is now recognized as a multifunctional protein involved in the tumor cell proliferation and antiapoptotic activity [3]. These results indicated that the suppressive effect of BCAA was, at least partly, mediated by the inhibition of insulin-induced HCC progression rather than the glucose-induced effects. It has been reported that the combination treatment of BCAA and the ACE-I significantly inhibited hepatocarcinogenesis along with suppression of VEGF-mediated angiogenesis than that of either single agent in a rat NASH model [80]. Noteworthy was the finding that these inhibitory effects were achieved at clinically comparable low doses. Since both agents are currently used widely in the clinical practice, this combination regimen may represent a potential new strategy for chemoprevention against IR-based HCC in the future.

It has been reported that the use of anti-angiogenic agents as monotherapy in treating the patients with advanced cancer has not yet shown a significant efficacy [97]. Nevertheless, monotherapy with ACE-I would not exert a sufficient effect on the advanced tumors. It has been clarified that a combination of anti-angiogenic therapy with cytotoxic therapy, such as chemotherapy or radiotherapy, increased the therapeutic curative effect in the tumor-bearing animals, for which either agent alone showed only an inhibitory effect. The limitations of the anti-angiogenic monotherapy in this setting were in fact predicted by preclinical studies using the angiogenesis inhibitors endostatin and angiostatin. It has been reported that the combination treatment of anti-angiogenic agents, such as endostatin and angiostatin, exerted a synergistic inhibitory effect on the tumor development and angiogenesis [97, 101, 102]. It has been also reported that the combination of TNP-470, which is one of the anti-angiogenic agents under clinical trials, and IFN inhibited angiogenesis synergistically [186]. We also observed that the combination of ACE-I and IFN-β showed a greater suppressive effect on the tumor growth than ACE-I alone [103]. Other agents, such as 5-fluorouracil, also exerted a synergistic effect with ACE [104]. For the future clinical applications of ACE-I, it will be preferable to employ these combination therapies to improve their effectiveness.

8.3.3 Anti-diabetes Mellitus and Others

The patients in NASH are frequently associated with type 2 DM. It has been reported that the IR plays a pivotal role in the pathogenesis of NASH. Recent studies have revealed a close relationship between IR and the progression of liver diseases, including liver cirrhosis and HCC [3, 187, 188]. Cross-sectional human studies showed that IR is a consistent finding in patients with type 2 DM, and more than 90 % of patients with liver cirrhosis may be glucose intolerant, and 30 % may be in clinically diabetic state [189]. In the presence of liver disease, the metabolic homeostasis of glucose is impaired as a result of disorders such as IR, glucose intolerance, and DM [190]. Previous report has demonstrated that serum insulin levels are higher in diabetic patients with chronic liver disease than those in patients with lifestyle-related DM [191]. Several reports suggested the possible involvement of a combination of increased FFA and decreased lipid peroxidation in the liver as a result of IR [192, 193]. Recently, it has also been reported that the IR status accelerated the progression of steatohepatitis and fibrosis in the NASH experimental model [20]. This study showed a close relationship between steatohepatitis and fibrosis through upregulation of lipogenesis-related genes. In addition to the liver fibrogenesis, a close interaction between DM and HCC has been documented. DM is associated with a two- to threefold increase in the risk of HCC regardless of the etiology of chronic liver diseases, including CHC and NASH [15, 16]. In a large longitudinal study in the United States, the incidence of HCC increased more than twofold among diabetic patients with higher increase in those with longer duration of follow-up [194]. The risk of HCC with DM remained elevated even after excluding patients who were subsequently diagnosed with HCV, HBV, alcohol use, and/or fatty liver disease at any time during the follow-up [16]. Furthermore, IR itself may directly contribute to the liver fibrosis progression and hepatocarcinogenesis [3]. In obese diabetic rats, experimental liver fibrosis was significantly developed compared to the control rats together with the proliferation of the activated HSC. It has also been revealed that either high glucose or insulin stimulated the proliferation of HSC and increased the production and expression of collagen genes in the activated HSC [3, 13, 14]. Similar to liver fibrosis, it has been demonstrated that the IR status itself directly accelerated hepatocarcinogenesis [3]. Recent evidence has suggested that hyperinsulinemia can promote the synthesis and biological activity of insulin-like growth factor 1 (IGF-1), which is a peptide hormone that regulates energy-dependent growth processes [195]. IGF-1 stimulates cell proliferation and inhibits apoptosis and has been shown to have strong mitogenic effects on a wide variety of cancer cell lines. Changes in the expression pattern of IGF system components have been observed in HCC patients, human HCC cell lines and their conditioned culture medium, as well as rodent models of hepatocarcinogenesis [196].

Moreover, it has been reported that both insulin and glucose can accelerate angiogenesis via induction of the VEGF expression [197]. We have reported that IR status may facilitate hepatocarcinogenesis via stimulation of hepatic neovascularization and VEGF expression in the rat carcinogenesis model [3]. An additive effect of high insulin and glucose on the EC tubular formation via phosphorylation of ERK1/ERK2 has been shown, and this promoting effect was markedly canceled by treatment with VEGF monoclonal antibody. The initial treatment of patients with mild hyperglycemia and compensated liver disease may be a lifestyle change. However, these therapeutic measures may be compromised by restrictive diets since they might aggravate malnutrition in some patients. On the other hand, physical exercise, which improves IR may not be an appropriate measure in the patients with active liver disease. To treat diabetic patients in advanced stage of liver disease, the administration of oral hypoglycemic drugs, especially exerting insulin-sensitizing effects such as metformin and pioglitazone, may be required [198, 199]. Moreover, recent reports have suggested that statins, a class of drugs used to lower cholesterol levels by inhibiting HMG-CoA reductase, significantly reduced the risk of HCC among patents with DM [200]. However, the use of only insulin sensitizer or statins could not sufficiently prevent the liver fibrosis development and hepatocarcinogenesis.

Dipeptidyl peptidase-4 inhibitor (DPP4-I) is clinically used as a new oral antidiabetic agent. DPP4-I can exert an antidiabetic action due to the enhancement of the function of incretin, including glucagon-like peptide 1 (GLP-1). GLP-1, a prominent active compound of the incretin family, is a gut-derived peptide secreted in a nutrient-dependent manner from the small intestine and stimulates glucose-dependent insulin production and secretion via specific receptors expressed on the islet β cells [201–204]. It potentiates insulin synthesis and secretion, inhibits glucagon secretion, increases islet cell proliferation, and decreases cell apoptosis. Although GLP-1 contributes to improve hyperglycemia, its functions are rapidly inactivated in serum because of the degradation of GLP-1 by DPP4. Therefore, continuous inhibition of DPP4 by DPP4-I can enhance the effects of GLP-1 and consequently may lower the serum glucose [201, 205]. Besides its key role in the regulation of incretin, DPP4 has multiple the functions in various organs

[206, 207]. In the liver, DPP4 also plays a role in fibronectin-mediated interaction of hepatocytes with ECM [206, 208, 209]. Moreover, it has been noted that DPP4 is possibly involved in several liver diseases, such as CHC, primary biliary cholangitis (PBC), chronic cholestasis, and HCC [210–214]. Previous reports revealed that DPP4 is expressed on the surface of reactive fibroblasts including Ac-HSCs [215–217]. We have reported that DPP4-I markedly inhibits liver fibrosis development in rats via suppression of HSCs proliferation and collagen synthesis. These suppressive effects are associated with dephosphorylation of ERK1/2, p38, and Smad2/3 in the HSCs. Since DPP4-I is widely used in clinical practice, this drug may represent a potential new therapeutic strategy against liver fibrosis in the near future [218].

8.3.4 Anti-endogenous Endotoxin

In both human and animal studies, it has been reported that NASH is associated with portal LPS levels through mechanisms involving bacterial translocation, and gut microbiota is thought to generate products like LPS, a cell-wall component of Gram-negative bacteria, which are delivered into liver via portal vein. Endotoxin production by gut microbiota could cause an inflammation in patients with obesity, diabetes, metabolic disorder, NAFLD, and NASH [219]. Plasma LPS levels are associated with small intestinal bacteria overgrowth, the change of composition of microbiota, and increased intestinal permeability [60]. Polymyxins are antibiotics with a general structure consisting of a cyclic peptide with a long hydrophobic tail and are selectively toxic to Gram-negative bacteria such as *E. coli*. In clinical settings, they are used for patients with Gram-negative bacterial infections and column of endotoxin apheresis against endotoxemia. Neomycins are aminoglycoside antibiotics and effective against both Gram-negative and Gram-positive bacteria. They are produced by Gram-positive bacteria such as *Streptomyces fradiae*. They inhibit protein synthesis of bacteria via binding to 30S ribosome. They are also hardly absorbed through gastrointestinal tract and are useful for Gram-negative bacterial infections in clinical settings. NAFLD is associated with increased intestinal permeability and small intestinal bacteria overgrowth. These findings have been thought to be associated with the severity of hepatic steatosis. Inhibition of LPS-TLR4 signaling with poorly absorbable antibiotics attenuated the liver fibrosis development associated with NASH via inhibition of HSC activation, indicating that hat reduction of LPS and restoration of the intestinal tight junction protein might be a new therapeutic strategy for treatment of the liver fibrosis development in NASH [220].

AT-II reportedly upregulated TLR4 by activating NF-κB of the mesangial cells. In the smooth muscle cells, the AT-II-induced inflammatory response was partly mediated via TLR4. In addition to these cells, the possible interaction between AT-II and TLR4 in the liver especially in conjunction with the HSC has been reported recently [221]. AT-II directly stimulated TLR4 mRNA expression in the Ac-HSC. The degree of NF-κB activation was reflected by detecting the

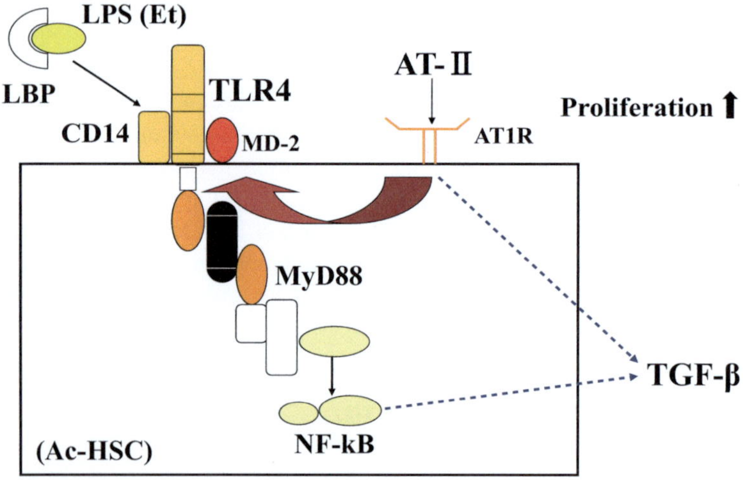

Fig. 8.3 AT-II and LPS-TLR4 interaction in the activated hepatic stellate cells (Ac-HSC). AT-II upregulates TLR4 and downstream signal such as MyD88, NF-κB, and TGF-β expressions

phosphorylation level of p65 NF-κB. LPS with AT-II significantly increased LPS-induced activation. And ARB significantly inhibited this augmentation. This effect was functional consequence of TLR4 upregulation by AT-II. TLR4 is not the downstream receptor of AT-II. AT-II just augmented the LPS-TLR4 signaling cascade via upregulation of TLR4. The AT-II-TGF-β signaling is independent cascade from TLR4-mediated signaling. AT-II has shown to induce the proliferation of the Ac-HSC through AT1-R, which is independent from TLR4-mediated cascade. This could explain why AT-II markedly augmented the LPS-induced MyD88 and NF-κB expressions, whereas AT-II could stimulate neither MyD88 nor NF-κB without LPS, and LPS only had little effect on TGF-β and no effect on Ac-HSC proliferation. In the rat peritoneal mesothelial cells and in the mouse mesangial cells, AT-II upregulated TLR4 through activation of TLR4 promoter which was dependent on the presence of functional AP-1 transcriptional sites. AT-II increased the AP-1-binding activity in the Ac-HSC. This effect was significantly inhibited by ARB. A similar mechanism may be involved in the Ac-HSC, at least partly, through activation of AP-1. Collectively, AT-II and LPS-TLR4 interaction plays a pivotal role in liver fibrosis development in NASH, at least partly, via activation of MyD88, NF-κB, and TGF-β expressions. ARB significantly attenuated the liver fibrosis development along with suppression of the Ac-HSC and TLR4 signaling cascade in the liver. ARB could represent a potential new therapeutic strategy against NASH from the aspect of LPS suppression (Fig. 8.3).

8.4 Conclusions and Future Perspectives

Obesity is keeping increase in all over the world, especially in advanced countries. Obesity is frequently associated with metabolic syndrome, cardiovascular disease, IR, and type 2 DM resulting in an increase of NAFLD. NAFLD is very common in the obese people. While simple steatosis seems benign and nonprogressive, NASH is recognized as a potentially progressive disease that may cause cirrhosis, an end-stage liver disease, and HCC. Furthermore, while a low-calorie diet has been recommended to treat obese NAFLD patients, it is sometimes difficult for many patients to change their lifestyle. Several mechanisms have shown to be involved in the pathogenesis of NASH, such as IR, angiogenesis, and innate immunity. Combination treatment with clinically available respective targeted agent would improve the prognosis in patients with NASH along with improvement of metabolic syndrome. Further studies are required to improve the prognosis of NASH from many points of view.

References

1. Angulo P. Nonalcoholic fatty liver disease. N Engl J Med. 2002;346:1221–31.
2. Yasui K, Hashimoto E, Tokushige K, et al. Clinical and pathological progression of non-alcoholic steatohepatitis to hepatocellular carcinoma. Hepatol Res. 2012;42:767–73.
3. Kaji K, Yoshiji H, Kitade M, et al. Impact of insulin resistance on the progression of chronic liver diseases. Int J Mol Med. 2008;22:801–8.
4. Kato J, Koda M, Kishina M, et al. Therapeutic effects of angiotensin II type 1 receptor blocker, irbesartan, on non-alcoholic steatohepatitis using FLS-ob/ob male mice. Int J Mol Med. 2012;30:107–13.
5. Kawai D, Takaki A, Nakatsuka A, et al. Hydrogen-rich water prevents progression of non-alcoholic steatohepatitis and accompanying hepatocarcinogenesis in mice. Hepatology. 2012;56:912–21.
6. Imarisio C, Alchera E, Sutti S, et al. Adenosine A2a receptor stimulation prevents hepatocyte lipotoxicity and nonalcoholic steatohepatitis (NASH) in rats. Clin Sci (Lond). 2012;123: 323–32.
7. Kahn CR. Insulin resistance, insulin insensitivity, and insulin unresponsiveness: a necessary distinction. Metabolism. 1978;27:1893–902.
8. Shintani Y, Fujie H, Miyoshi H, et al. Hepatitis C virus infection and diabetes: direct involvement of the virus in the development of insulin resistance. Gastroenterology. 2004;126:840–8.
9. Hui JM, Sud A, Farrell GC, et al. Insulin resistance is associated with chronic hepatitis C virus infection and fibrosis progression [corrected]. Gastroenterology. 2003;125:1695–704.
10. Petrides AS, Vogt C, Schulze-Berge D, et al. Pathogenesis of glucose intolerance and diabetes mellitus in cirrhosis. Hepatology. 1994;19:616–27.
11. Petit JM, Bour JB, Galland-Jos C, et al. Risk factors for diabetes mellitus and early insulin resistance in chronic hepatitis C. J Hepatol. 2001;35:279–83.
12. Bugianesi E, McCullough AJ, Marchesini G. Insulin resistance: a metabolic pathway to chronic liver disease. Hepatology. 2005;42:987–1000.
13. Sugimoto R, Enjoji M, Kohjima M, et al. High glucose stimulates hepatic stellate cells to proliferate and to produce collagen through free radical production and activation of mitogen-activated protein kinase. Liver Int. 2005;25:1018–26.

14. Svegliati-Baroni G, Ridolfi F, Di Sario A, et al. Insulin and insulin-like growth factor-1 stimulate proliferation and type I collagen accumulation by human hepatic stellate cells: differential effects on signal transduction pathways. Hepatology. 1999;29:1743–51.
15. Davila JA, Morgan RO, Shaib Y, et al. Diabetes increases the risk of hepatocellular carcinoma in the United States: a population based case control study. Gut. 2005;54:533–9.
16. El-Serag HB, Tran T, Everhart JE. Diabetes increases the risk of chronic liver disease and hepatocellular carcinoma. Gastroenterology. 2004;126:460–8.
17. El-Serag HB. Epidemiology of hepatocellular carcinoma in USA. Hepatol Res. 2007;37 Suppl 2:S88–94.
18. Imai K, Takai K, Nishigaki Y, et al. Insulin resistance raises the risk for recurrence of stage I hepatocellular carcinoma after curative radiofrequency ablation in hepatitis C virus-positive patients: a prospective, case series study. Hepatol Res. 2010;40:376–82.
19. Polyzos SA, Kountouras J, Zavos C. Nonalcoholic fatty liver disease: the pathogenetic roles of insulin resistance and adipocytokines. Curr Mol Med. 2009;9:299–314.
20. Ota T, Takamura T, Kurita S, et al. Insulin resistance accelerates a dietary rat model of nonalcoholic steatohepatitis. Gastroenterology. 2007;132:282–93.
21. Aithal GP, Thomas JA, Kaye PV, et al. Randomized, placebo-controlled trial of pioglitazone in nondiabetic subjects with nonalcoholic steatohepatitis. Gastroenterology. 2008;135:1176–84.
22. Ratziu V, Giral P, Jacqueminet S, et al. Rosiglitazone for nonalcoholic steatohepatitis: one-year results of the randomized placebo-controlled Fatty Liver Improvement with Rosiglitazone Therapy (FLIRT) Trial. Gastroenterology. 2008;135:100–10.
23. Reid AE. Nonalcoholic steatohepatitis. Gastroenterology. 2001;121:710–23.
24. Jaeschke H. Reactive oxygen and mechanisms of inflammatory liver injury. J Gastroenterol Hepatol. 2000;15:718–24.
25. Sato N. Central role of mitochondria in metabolic regulation of liver pathophysiology. J Gastroenterol Hepatol. 2007;22 Suppl 1:S1–6.
26. Seki S, Kitada T, Yamada T, et al. In situ detection of lipid peroxidation and oxidative DNA damage in non-alcoholic fatty liver diseases. J Hepatol. 2002;37:56–62.
27. Gao D, Wei C, Chen L, et al. Oxidative DNA damage and DNA repair enzyme expression are inversely related in murine models of fatty liver disease. Am J Physiol Gastrointest Liver Physiol. 2004;287:G1070–7.
28. Nanji AA. Animal models of nonalcoholic fatty liver disease and steatohepatitis. Clin Liver Dis. 2004;8:559–74, ix.
29. Nakae D, Yoshiji H, Mizumoto Y, et al. High incidence of hepatocellular carcinomas induced by a choline deficient L-amino acid defined diet in rats. Cancer Res. 1992;52:5042–5.
30. Carmiel-Haggai M, Cederbaum AI, Nieto N. A high-fat diet leads to the progression of non-alcoholic fatty liver disease in obese rats. FASEB J. 2005;19:136–8.
31. Leclercq IA, Farrell GC, Schriemer R, et al. Leptin is essential for the hepatic fibrogenic response to chronic liver injury. J Hepatol. 2002;37:206–13.
32. Honda H, Ikejima K, Hirose M, et al. Leptin is required for fibrogenic responses induced by thioacetamide in the murine liver. Hepatology. 2002;36:12–21.
33. Ikejima K, Takei Y, Honda H, et al. Leptin receptor-mediated signaling regulates hepatic fibrogenesis and remodeling of extracellular matrix in the rat. Gastroenterology. 2002;122:1399–410.
34. Carmeliet P. Angiogenesis in life, disease and medicine. Nature. 2005;438:932–6.
35. Kalluri R, Sukhatme VP. Fibrosis and angiogenesis. Curr Opin Nephrol Hypertens. 2000;9:413–18.
36. Yoshiji H, Kuriyama S, Yoshii J, et al. Vascular endothelial growth factor and receptor interaction is a prerequisite for murine hepatic fibrogenesis. Gut. 2003;52:1347–54.
37. Medina J, Caveda L, Sanz-Cameno P, et al. Hepatocyte growth factor activates endothelial proangiogenic mechanisms relevant in chronic hepatitis C-associated neoangiogenesis. J Hepatol. 2003;38:660–7.

38. Shibuya M. Structure and function of VEGF/VEGF-receptor system involved in angiogenesis. Cell Struct Funct. 2001;26:25–35.
39. Corpechot C, Barbu V, Wendum D, et al. Hypoxia-induced VEGF and collagen I expressions are associated with angiogenesis and fibrogenesis in experimental cirrhosis. Hepatology. 2002;35:1010–21.
40. Salcedo X, Medina J, Sanz-Cameno P, et al. The potential of angiogenesis soluble markers in chronic hepatitis C. Hepatology. 2005;42:696–701.
41. Nakamura K, Zen Y, Sato Y, et al. Vascular endothelial growth factor, its receptor Flk-1, and hypoxia inducible factor-1alpha are involved in malignant transformation in dysplastic nodules of the liver. Hum Pathol. 2007;38:1532–46.
42. Kitade M, Yoshiji H, Kojima H, et al. Leptin-mediated neovascularization is a prerequisite for progression of nonalcoholic steatohepatitis in rats. Hepatology. 2006;44:983–91.
43. Kojima H, Sakurai S, Uemura M, et al. Mitochondrial abnormality and oxidative stress in nonalcoholic steatohepatitis. Alcohol Clin Exp Res. 2007;31:S61–6.
44. Yang S, Zhu H, Li Y, et al. Mitochondrial adaptations to obesity-related oxidant stress. Arch Biochem Biophys. 2000;378:259–68.
45. Marra F, Aleffi S, Bertolani C, et al. Adipokines and liver fibrosis. Eur Rev Med Pharmacol Sci. 2005;9:279–84.
46. Larter CZ, Farrell GC. Insulin resistance, adiponectin, cytokines in NASH: which is the best target to treat? J Hepatol. 2006;44:253–61.
47. Musso G, Gambino R, Biroli G, et al. Hypoadiponectinemia predicts the severity of hepatic fibrosis and pancreatic Beta-cell dysfunction in nondiabetic nonobese patients with nonalcoholic steatohepatitis. Am J Gastroenterol. 2005;100:2438–46.
48. Kamada Y, Tamura S, Kiso S, et al. Enhanced carbon tetrachloride-induced liver fibrosis in mice lacking adiponectin. Gastroenterology. 2003;125:1796–807.
49. Saxena NK, Ikeda K, Rockey DC, et al. Leptin in hepatic fibrosis: evidence for increased collagen production in stellate cells and lean littermates of ob/ob mice. Hepatology. 2002;35:762–71.
50. Sierra-Honigmann MR, Nath AK, Murakami C, et al. Biological action of leptin as an angiogenic factor. Science. 1998;281:1683–6.
51. Huang L, Li C. Leptin: a multifunctional hormone. Cell Res. 2000;10:81–92.
52. Jin X, Fukuda N, Su J, et al. Effects of leptin on endothelial function with OB-Rb gene transfer in Zucker fatty rats. Atherosclerosis. 2003;169:225–33.
53. Lerman OZ, Galiano RD, Armour M, et al. Cellular dysfunction in the diabetic fibroblast: impairment in migration, vascular endothelial growth factor production, and response to hypoxia. Am J Pathol. 2003;162:303–12.
54. Cao R, Brakenhielm E, Wahlestedt C, et al. Leptin induces vascular permeability and synergistically stimulates angiogenesis with FGF-2 and VEGF. Proc Natl Acad Sci U S A. 2001;98:6390–5.
55. Soares JB, Pimentel-Nunes P, Roncon-Albuquerque R, et al. The role of lipopolysaccharide/toll-like receptor 4 signaling in chronic liver diseases. Hepatol Int. 2010;4:659–72.
56. Su GL, Klein RD, Aminlari A, et al. Kupffer cell activation by lipopolysaccharide in rats: role for lipopolysaccharide binding protein and toll-like receptor 4. Hepatology. 2000;31:932–6.
57. Seki E, De Minicis S, Osterreicher CH, et al. TLR4 enhances TGF-beta signaling and hepatic fibrosis. Nat Med. 2007;13:1324–32.
58. Guo H, Chen Y, Hu X, et al. The regulation of Toll-like receptor 2 by miR-143 suppresses the invasion and migration of a subset of human colorectal carcinoma cells. Mol Cancer. 2013;12:77.
59. Szabo G, Bala S, Petrasek J, et al. Gut-liver axis and sensing microbes. Dig Dis. 2010;28:737–44.
60. Endo H, Niioka M, Kobayashi N, et al. Butyrate-producing probiotics reduce nonalcoholic fatty liver disease progression in rats: new insight into the probiotics for the gut-liver axis. PLoS One. 2013;8:e63388.

61. Chalasani N, Younossi Z, Lavine JE, et al. The diagnosis and management of non-alcoholic fatty liver disease: practice guideline by the American Association for the Study of Liver Diseases, American College of Gastroenterology, and the American Gastroenterological Association. Am J Gastroenterol. 2012;107:811–26.
62. Shimada M, Kawahara H, Ozaki K, et al. Usefulness of a combined evaluation of the serum adiponectin level, HOMA-IR, and serum type IV collagen 7S level to predict the early stage of nonalcoholic steatohepatitis. Am J Gastroenterol. 2007;102:1931–8.
63. Sumida Y, Yoneda M, Hyogo H, et al. A simple clinical scoring system using ferritin, fasting insulin, and type IV collagen 7S for predicting steatohepatitis in nonalcoholic fatty liver disease. J Gastroenterol. 2011;46:257–68.
64. Canbay A, Friedman S, Gores GJ. Apoptosis: the nexus of liver injury and fibrosis. Hepatology. 2004;39:273–8.
65. Wieckowska A, Zein NN, Yerian LM, et al. In vivo assessment of liver cell apoptosis as a novel biomarker of disease severity in nonalcoholic fatty liver disease. Hepatology. 2006;44:27–33.
66. Ueno T, Toi M, Linder S. Detection of epithelial cell death in the body by cytokeratin 18 measurement. Biomed Pharmacother. 2005;59 Suppl 2:S359–62.
67. Feldstein AE, Wieckowska A, Lopez AR, et al. Cytokeratin-18 fragment levels as noninvasive biomarkers for nonalcoholic steatohepatitis: a multicenter validation study. Hepatology. 2009;50:1072–78.
68. Dzau VJ, Gibbons GH, Pratt RE. Molecular mechanisms of vascular renin-angiotensin system in myointimal hyperplasia. Hypertension. 1991;18:II100–5.
69. Ardaillou R. Angiotensin II receptors. J Am Soc Nephrol. 1999;10 Suppl 11:S30–9.
70. Matsusaka T, Ichikawa I. Biological functions of angiotensin and its receptors. Annu Rev Physiol. 1997;59:395–412.
71. Yoshiji H, Noguchi R, Ikenaka Y, Kitade M, Kaji K, Tsujimoto T, Uemura M, Fukui H. Renin-angiotensin system inhibitors as therapeutic alternatives in the treatment of chronic liver diseases. Curr Med Chem. 2007;14(26):2749–54.
72. Rockey DC, Weisiger RA. Endothelin induced contractility of stellate cells from normal and cirrhotic rat liver: implications for regulation of portal pressure and resistance. Hepatology. 1996;24:233–40.
73. Helmy A, Jalan R, Newby DE, et al. Role of angiotensin II in regulation of basal and sympathetically stimulated vascular tone in early and advanced cirrhosis. Gastroenterology. 2000;118:565–72.
74. Arroyo V, Bosch J, Mauri M, et al. Effect of angiotensin-II blockade on systemic and hepatic haemodynamics and on the renin-angiotensin-aldosterone system in cirrhosis with ascites. Eur J Clin Invest. 1981;11:221–9.
75. Ballet F, Chretien Y, Rey C, et al. Differential response of normal and cirrhotic liver to vasoactive agents. A study in the isolated perfused rat liver. J Pharmacol Exp Ther. 1988;244:283–9.
76. Garcia-Pagan JC, Bosch J, Rodes J. The role of vasoactive mediators in portal hypertension. Semin Gastrointest Dis. 1995;6:140–7.
77. Fernandez LA, Twickler J, Mead A. Neovascularization produced by angiotensin II. J Lab Clin Med. 1985;105:141–5.
78. Le Noble FA, Hekking JW, Van Straaten HW, et al. Angiotensin II stimulates angiogenesis in the chorio-allantoic membrane of the chick embryo. Eur J Pharmacol. 1991;195:305–6.
79. Heffelfinger SC. The renin angiotensin system in the regulation of angiogenesis. Curr Pharm Des. 2007;13:1215–29.
80. Yoshiji H, Noguchi R, Kaji K, et al. Attenuation of insulin-resistance-based hepatocarcinogenesis and angiogenesis by combined treatment with branched-chain amino acids and angiotensin-converting enzyme inhibitor in obese diabetic rats. J Gastroenterol. 2010;45:443–50.

81. Debernardi-Venon W, Martini S, Biasi F, et al. AT1 receptor antagonist Candesartan in selected cirrhotic patients: effect on portal pressure and liver fibrosis markers. J Hepatol. 2007;46:1026–33.
82. Ikura Y, Ohsawa M, Shirai N, et al. Expression of angiotensin II type 1 receptor in human cirrhotic livers: its relation to fibrosis and portal hypertension. Hepatol Res. 2005;32:107–16.
83. Iwata K, Sohda T, Irie M, et al. Angiotensin II type 1 receptor antagonist improves the prognosis in rats displaying liver cirrhosis induced by a choline-deficient diet. J Gastrointestin Liver Dis. 2008;17:21–5.
84. Oakley F, Teoh V, Ching ASG, et al. Angiotensin II activates I kappaB kinase phosphorylation of RelA at Ser 536 to promote myofibroblast survival and liver fibrosis. Gastroenterology. 2009;136:2334–2344 e1.
85. Toblli JE, Munoz MC, Cao G, et al. ACE inhibition and AT1 receptor blockade prevent fatty liver and fibrosis in obese Zucker rats. Obesity (Silver Spring). 2008;16:770–6.
86. Krishna P, Nakata M, Nakajima T, et al. Increased production of vascular endothelial growth factor (VEGF) by angiotensin II. Neurosci Res Commun. 1999;25:79–88.
87. Yoshiji H, Kuriyama S, Kawata M, et al. The angiotensin-I-converting enzyme inhibitor perindopril suppresses tumor growth and angiogenesis: possible role of the vascular endothelial growth factor. Clin Cancer Res. 2001;7:1073–8.
88. Yoshiji H, Kuriyama S, Fukui H. Angiotensin-I-converting enzyme inhibitors may be an alternative anti-angiogenic strategy in the treatment of liver fibrosis and hepatocellular carcinoma. Possible role of vascular endothelial growth factor. Tumour Biol. 2002;23:348–56.
89. Yoshiji H, Kuriyama S, Fukui H. Perindopril: possible use in cancer therapy. Anticancer Drugs. 2002;13:221–8.
90. Lever AF, Hole DJ, Gillis CR, et al. Do inhibitors of angiotensin-I-converting enzyme protect against risk of cancer? Lancet. 1998;352:179–84.
91. Friis S, Sorensen HT, Mellemkjaer L, et al. Angiotensin-converting enzyme inhibitors and the risk of cancer: a population-based cohort study in Denmark. Cancer. 2001;92:2462–70.
92. Christian JB, Lapane KL, Hume AL, et al. Association of ACE inhibitors and angiotensin receptor blockers with keratinocyte cancer prevention in the randomized VATTC trial. J Natl Cancer Inst. 2008;100:1223–32.
93. Wilop S, von Hobe S, Crysandt M, et al. Impact of angiotensin I converting enzyme inhibitors and angiotensin II type 1 receptor blockers on survival in patients with advanced non-small-cell lung cancer undergoing first-line platinum-based chemotherapy. J Cancer Res Clin Oncol. 2009;135:1429–35.
94. Brown M, Mackenzie I, Ashby M, et al. AT2 receptor stimulation may halt progression of pheochromocytoma. Ann N Y Acad Sci. 2006;1073:436–43.
95. Uemura H, Hasumi H, Kawahara T, et al. Pilot study of angiotensin II receptor blocker in advanced hormone-refractory prostate cancer. Int J Clin Oncol. 2005;10:405–10.
96. Kardum D, Huskic J, Fabijanic D, et al. Activity of serum angiotensin-converting enzyme as a tumour marker of hepatocellular carcinoma. Eur J Gastroenterol Hepatol. 1999;11:1209–13.
97. Kerbel RS. Clinical trials of antiangiogenic drugs: opportunities, problems, and assessment of initial results. J Clin Oncol. 2001;19:45S–51.
98. Kerbel RS, Viloria-Petit A, Klement G, et al. 'Accidental' anti-angiogenic drugs. anti-oncogene directed signal transduction inhibitors and conventional chemotherapeutic agents as examples. Eur J Cancer. 2000;36:1248–57.
99. Yoshiji H, Noguchi R, Ikenaka Y, et al. Renin-angiotensin system inhibitors as therapeutic alternatives in the treatment of chronic liver diseases. Curr Med Chem. 2007;14:2749–54.
100. Yoshiji H, Kuriyama S, Noguchi R, et al. Angiotensin-I converting enzyme inhibitors as potential anti-angiogenic agents for cancer therapy. Curr Cancer Drug Targets. 2004;4:555–67.

101. Scappaticci FA, Smith R, Pathak A, et al. Combination angiostatin and endostatin gene transfer induces synergistic antiangiogenic activity in vitro and antitumor efficacy in leukemia and solid tumors in mice. Mol Ther. 2001;3:186–96.
102. Scappaticci FA. Mechanisms and future directions for angiogenesis-based cancer therapies. J Clin Oncol. 2002;20:3906–27.
103. Noguchi R, Yoshiji H, Kuriyama S, et al. Combination of interferon-beta and the angiotensin-converting enzyme inhibitor, perindopril, attenuates murine hepatocellular carcinoma development and angiogenesis. Clin Cancer Res. 2003;9:6038–45.
104. Yanase K, Yoshiji H, Ikenaka Y, et al. Synergistic inhibition of hepatocellular carcinoma growth and hepatocarcinogenesis by combination of 5-fluorouracil and angiotensin-converting enzyme inhibitor via anti-angiogenic activities. Oncol Rep. 2007;17:441–6.
105. Ohnuma Y, Toda M, Fujita M, et al. Blockade of an angiotensin type I receptor enhances effects of radiation on tumor growth and tumor-associated angiogenesis by reducing vascular endothelial growth factor expression. Biomed Pharmacother. 2009;63:136–45.
106. Noguchi R, Yoshiji H, Ikenaka Y, et al. Synergistic inhibitory effect of gemcitabine and angiotensin type-1 receptor blocker, losartan, on murine pancreatic tumor growth via anti-angiogenic activities. Oncol Rep. 2009;22:355–60.
107. Bergers G, Benjamin LE. Tumorigenesis and the angiogenic switch. Nat Rev Cancer. 2003;3:401–10.
108. Bergers G, Javaherian K, Lo KM, et al. Effects of angiogenesis inhibitors on multistage carcinogenesis in mice. Science. 1999;284:808–12.
109. Bolontrade MF, Stern MC, Binder RL, et al. Angiogenesis is an early event in the development of chemically induced skin tumors. Carcinogenesis. 1998;19:2107–13.
110. Staton CA, Chetwood AS, Cameron IC, et al. The angiogenic switch occurs at the adenoma stage of the adenoma-carcinoma sequence in colorectal cancer. Gut. 2007;56:1426.
111. Yoshiji H, Yoshii J, Ikenaka Y, et al. Suppression of the renin-angiotensin system attenuates vascular endothelial growth factor-mediated tumor development and angiogenesis in murine hepatocellular carcinoma cells. Int J Oncol. 2002;20:1227–31.
112. Yoshiji H, Kuriyama S, Noguchi R, et al. Combination of vitamin K(2) and the angiotensin-converting enzyme inhibitor, perindopril, attenuates the liver enzyme-altered preneoplastic lesions in rats via angiogenesis suppression. J Hepatol. 2005;42:687–93.
113. Yoshiji H, Noguchi R, Toyohara M, et al. Combination of vitamin K2 and angiotensin-converting enzyme inhibitor ameliorates cumulative recurrence of hepatocellular carcinoma. J Hepatol. 2009;51:315–21.
114. Yoshiji H, Noguchi R, Yamazaki M, et al. Combined treatment of vitamin K2 and angiotensin-converting enzyme inhibitor ameliorates hepatic dysplastic nodule in a patient with liver cirrhosis. World J Gastroenterol. 2007;13:3259–61.
115. Yoshiji H, Noguchi R, Ikenaka Y, et al. Impact of renin-angiotensin system in hepatocellular carcinoma. Curr Cancer Drug Targets. 2011;11:431–41.
116. Folkman J. Angiogenesis in cancer, vascular, rheumatoid and other disease. Nat Med. 1995;1:27–31.
117. Carmeliet P. Angiogenesis in health and disease. Nat Med. 2003;9:653–60.
118. Carmeliet P, Jain RK. Angiogenesis in cancer and other diseases. Nature. 2000;407:249–57.
119. Chaturvedi N, Sjolie AK, Stephenson JM, et al. Effect of lisinopril on progression of retinopathy in normotensive people with type 1 diabetes. The EUCLID Study Group. EURODIAB Controlled Trial of Lisinopril in Insulin-Dependent Diabetes Mellitus. Lancet. 1998;351:28–31.
120. Gilbert RE, Kelly DJ, Cox AJ, et al. Angiotensin converting enzyme inhibition reduces retinal overexpression of vascular endothelial growth factor and hyperpermeability in experimental diabetes. Diabetologia. 2000;43:1360–7.
121. Otani A, Takagi H, Suzuma K, et al. Angiotensin II potentiates vascular endothelial growth factor-induced angiogenic activity in retinal microcapillary endothelial cells. Circ Res. 1998;82:619–28.

122. Sjolie AK, Klein R, Porta M, et al. Effect of candesartan on progression and regression of retinopathy in type 2 diabetes (DIRECT-Protect 2): a randomised placebo-controlled trial. Lancet. 2008;372:1385–93.
123. Nacak M, Nacak I, Sanli M, et al. Association of angiotensin converting enzyme gene insertion/deletion polymorphism with lung cancer in Turkey. Cancer Genet Cytogenet. 2010;198:22–6.
124. Srivastava K, Srivastava A, Mittal B. Angiotensin I-converting enzyme insertion/deletion polymorphism and increased risk of gall bladder cancer in women. DNA Cell Biol. 2010;29:417–22.
125. Gaddam KK, Pimenta E, Husain S, et al. Aldosterone and cardiovascular disease. Curr Probl Cardiol. 2009;34:51–84.
126. Williams GH. Aldosterone biosynthesis, regulation, and classical mechanism of action. Heart Fail Rev. 2005;10:7–13.
127. Funder JW. Minireview: aldosterone and mineralocorticoid receptors: past, present, and future. Endocrinology. 2010;151:5098–102.
128. Jeong Y, Chaupin DF, Matsushita K, et al. Aldosterone activates endothelial exocytosis. Proc Natl Acad Sci U S A. 2009;106:3782–7.
129. Kaji K, Yoshiji H, Kitade M, et al. Selective aldosterone blocker, eplerenone, attenuates hepatocellular carcinoma growth and angiogenesis in mice. Hepatol Res. 2010;40:540–9.
130. Noguchi R, Yoshiji H, Ikenaka Y, et al. Selective aldosterone blocker ameliorates the progression of non-alcoholic steatohepatitis in rats. Int J Mol Med. 2010;26:407–13.
131. Wilkinson-Berka JL, Tan G, Jaworski K, et al. Identification of a retinal aldosterone system and the protective effects of mineralocorticoid receptor antagonism on retinal vascular pathology. Circ Res. 2009;104:124–33.
132. Noguchi R, Yoshiji H, Ikenaka Y, et al. Dual blockade of angiotensin-II and aldosterone suppresses the progression of a non-diabetic rat model of steatohepatitis. Hepatol Res. 2012;43:765–74.
133. Aihara Y, Yoshiji H, Noguchi R, et al. Direct renin inhibitor, aliskiren, attenuates the progression of non-alcoholic steatohepatitis in the rat model. Hepatol Res. 2013;43:1241–50.
134. Okita K, Sakaida I, Hino K. Current strategies for chemoprevention of hepatocellular carcinoma. Oncology. 2002;62 Suppl 1:24–8.
135. Sakaida I, Hironaka K, Uchida K, et al. Fibrosis accelerates the development of enzyme-altered lesions in the rat liver. Hepatology. 1998;28:1247–52.
136. Yoshiji H, Kuriyama S, Yoshii J, et al. Extracellular matrix remodeling may predominate over hepatocyte injury in hepatocellular carcinoma development. Oncol Rep. 2003;10:957–62.
137. Boudreau N, Bissell MJ. Extracellular matrix signaling: integration of form and function in normal and malignant cells. Curr Opin Cell Biol. 1998;10:640–6.
138. Theret N, Musso O, Turlin B, et al. Increased extracellular matrix remodeling is associated with tumor progression in human hepatocellular carcinomas. Hepatology. 2001;34:82–8.
139. Friedman SL. Liver fibrosis – from bench to bedside. J Hepatol. 2003;38 Suppl 1:S38–53.
140. Friedman SL. Molecular mechanisms of hepatic fibrosis and principles of therapy. J Gastroenterol. 1997;32:424–30.
141. Friedman SL. Cytokines and fibrogenesis. Semin Liver Dis. 1999;19:129–40.
142. Bataller R, Gines P, Nicolas JM, et al. Angiotensin II induces contraction and proliferation of human hepatic stellate cells. Gastroenterology. 2000;118:1149–56.
143. Arthur MJ, Mann DA, Iredale JP. Tissue inhibitors of metalloproteinases, hepatic stellate cells and liver fibrosis. J Gastroenterol Hepatol. 1998;13(Suppl):S33–8.
144. Arthur MJ. Degradation of matrix proteins in liver fibrosis. Pathol Res Pract. 1994;190:825–33.
145. Yoshiji H. Anti-fibrotic therapy: are matrix metalloproteinases friends or foes? Hepatol Res. 2009;39:748–50.

146. Iredale JP. Tissue inhibitors of metalloproteinases in liver fibrosis. Int J Biochem Cell Biol. 1997;29:43–54.
147. Iredale JP, Benyon RC, Arthur MJ, et al. Tissue inhibitor of metalloproteinase-1 messenger RNA expression is enhanced relative to interstitial collagenase messenger RNA in experimental liver injury and fibrosis. Hepatology. 1996;24:176–84.
148. Iredale JP, Goddard S, Murphy G, et al. Tissue inhibitor of metalloproteinase-I and interstitial collagenase expression in autoimmune chronic active hepatitis and activated human hepatic lipocytes. Clin Sci (Colch). 1995;89:75–81.
149. Nakatsukasa H, Ashida K, Higashi T, et al. Cellular distribution of transcripts for tissue inhibitor of metalloproteinases 1 and 2 in human hepatocellular carcinomas. Hepatology. 1996;24:82–8.
150. Yoshiji H, Kuriyama S, Yoshii J, et al. Tissue inhibitor of metalloproteinases-1 attenuates spontaneous liver fibrosis resolution in the transgenic mouse. Hepatology. 2002;36:850–60.
151. Yoshiji H, Kuriyama S, Miyamoto Y, et al. Tissue inhibitor of metalloproteinases-1 promotes liver fibrosis development in a transgenic mouse model. Hepatology. 2000;32:1248–54.
152. Murawaki Y, Ikuta Y, Idobe Y, et al. Tissue inhibitor of metalloproteinase-1 in the liver of patients with chronic liver disease. J Hepatol. 1997;26:1213–19.
153. Murawaki Y, Yamamoto H, Kawasaki H, et al. Serum tissue inhibitor of metalloproteinases in patients with chronic liver disease and with hepatocellular carcinoma. Clin Chim Acta. 1993;218:47–58.
154. Yoshiji H, Kuriyama S, Fukui H. Blockade of renin-angiotensin system in antifibrotic therapy. J Gastroenterol Hepatol. 2007;22 Suppl 1:S93–5.
155. Yoshiji H, Kuriyama S, Yoshii J, et al. Angiotensin-II type 1 receptor interaction is a major regulator for liver fibrosis development in rats. Hepatology. 2001;34:745–50.
156. Ohishi T, Saito H, Tsusaka K, et al. Anti-fibrogenic effect of an angiotensin converting enzyme inhibitor on chronic carbon tetrachloride-induced hepatic fibrosis in rats. Hepatol Res. 2001;21:147–58.
157. Paizis G, Gilbert RE, Cooper ME, et al. Effect of angiotensin II type 1 receptor blockade on experimental hepatic fibrogenesis. J Hepatol. 2001;35:376–85.
158. Jonsson JR, Clouston AD, Ando Y, et al. Angiotensin-converting enzyme inhibition attenuates the progression of rat hepatic fibrosis. Gastroenterology. 2001;121:148–55.
159. Hirose A, Ono M, Saibara T, et al. Angiotensin II type 1 receptor blocker inhibits fibrosis in rat nonalcoholic steatohepatitis. Hepatology. 2007;45:1375–81.
160. Ueki M, Koda M, Yamamoto S, et al. Preventive and therapeutic effects of angiotensin II type 1 receptor blocker on hepatic fibrosis induced by bile duct ligation in rats. J Gastroenterol. 2006;41:996–1004.
161. Yoshiji H, Fukui H. Renin-angiotensin system and progression of chronic liver diseases. J Gastroenterol. 2006;41:1020–2.
162. Yoshiji H, Noguchi R, Ikenaka Y, et al. Losartan, an angiotensin-II type 1 receptor blocker, attenuates the liver fibrosis development of non-alcoholic steatohepatitis in the rat. BMC Res Notes. 2009;2:70.
163. Terui Y, Saito T, Watanabe H, et al. Effect of angiotensin receptor antagonist on liver fibrosis in early stages of chronic hepatitis C. Hepatology. 2002;36:1022.
164. Yokohama S, Yoneda M, Haneda M, et al. Therapeutic efficacy of an angiotensin II receptor antagonist in patients with nonalcoholic steatohepatitis. Hepatology. 2004;40:1222–5.
165. Georgescu EF, Ionescu R, Niculescu M, et al. Angiotensin-receptor blockers as therapy for mild-to-moderate hypertension-associated non-alcoholic steatohepatitis. World J Gastroenterol. 2009;15:942–54.
166. Ueki M, Koda M, Shimizu T, et al. Effect of an angiotensin-II type-1 receptor blocker, candesartan on hepatic fibrosis in chronic hepatitis C: a prospective study. Hepatogastroenterology. 2009;56:1100–4.
167. Corey KE, Shah N, Misdraji J, et al. The effect of angiotensin-blocking agents on liver fibrosis in patients with hepatitis C. Liver Int. 2009;29:748–53.

168. Kitade M, Yoshiji H, Kojima H, et al. Neovascularization and oxidative stress in the progression of nonalcoholic steatohepatitis. Mol Med Rep. 2008;1:543–8.
169. Liu Z. The renin-angiotensin system and insulin resistance. Curr Diab Rep. 2007;7:34–42.
170. Rimola A, Londono MC, Guevara G, et al. Beneficial effect of angiotensin-blocking agents on graft fibrosis in hepatitis C recurrence after liver transplantation. Transplantation. 2004;78:686–91.
171. Yoshiji H, Kuriyama S, Noguchi R, et al. Combination of interferon-beta and angiotensin-converting enzyme inhibitor, perindopril, attenuates the murine liver fibrosis development. Liver Int. 2005;25:153–61.
172. Yoshiji H, Noguchi R, Kuriyama S, et al. Imatinib mesylate (STI-571) attenuates liver fibrosis development in rats. Am J Physiol Gastrointest Liver Physiol. 2005;288:G907–13.
173. Yoshiji H, Noguchi R, Kojima H, et al. Interferon augments the anti-fibrotic activity of an angiotensin-converting enzyme inhibitor in patients with refractory chronic hepatitis C. World J Gastroenterol. 2006;12:6786–91.
174. Yoshiji H, Kuriyama S, Noguchi R, et al. Angiotensin-II and vascular endothelial growth factor interaction plays an important role in rat liver fibrosis development. Hepatol Res. 2006;36:124–9.
175. Kaji K, Yoshiji H, Ikenaka Y, et al. Possible involvement of angiogenesis in chronic liver diseases: interaction among renin-angiotensin-aldosterone system, insulin resistance and oxidative stress. Curr Med Chem. 2012;19:1889–98.
176. Marchesini G, Bianchi G, Merli M, et al. Nutritional supplementation with branched-chain amino acids in advanced cirrhosis: a double-blind, randomized trial. Gastroenterology. 2003;124:1792–801.
177. Muto Y, Sato S, Watanabe A, et al. Effects of oral branched-chain amino acid granules on event-free survival in patients with liver cirrhosis. Clin Gastroenterol Hepatol. 2005;3:705–13.
178. Muto Y, Sato S, Watanabe A, et al. Overweight and obesity increase the risk for liver cancer in patients with liver cirrhosis and long-term oral supplementation with branched-chain amino acid granules inhibits liver carcinogenesis in heavier patients with liver cirrhosis. Hepatol Res. 2006;35:204–14.
179. Nishitani S, Ijichi C, Takehana K, et al. Pharmacological activities of branched-chain amino acids: specificity of tissue and signal transduction. Biochem Biophys Res Commun. 2004;313:387–9.
180. Nishitani S, Takehana K, Fujitani S, et al. Branched-chain amino acids improve glucose metabolism in rats with liver cirrhosis. Am J Physiol Gastrointest Liver Physiol. 2005;288: G1292–300.
181. Kawaguchi T, Taniguchi E, Itou M, et al. Branched-chain amino acids improve insulin resistance in patients with hepatitis C virus-related liver disease: report of two cases. Liver Int. 2007;27:1287–92.
182. Kawaguchi T, Nagao Y, Matsuoka H, et al. Branched-chain amino acid-enriched supplementation improves insulin resistance in patients with chronic liver disease. Int J Mol Med. 2008;22:105–12.
183. Yoshiji H, Noguchi R, Kitade M, et al. Branched-chain amino acids suppress insulin-resistance-based hepatocarcinogenesis in obese diabetic rats. J Gastroenterol. 2009;44:483–91.
184. Tsuchiya K, Asahina Y, Sato T, et al. Oral supplementation with branched-chain amino acid (BCAA) improves survival and decreases the third time recurrence after successful treatment of hepatocellular carcinoma (HCC). J Hepatol (EASL Proc). 2009;48(suppl No2):S160.
185. Hagiwara A, Nishiyama M, Ishizaki S. Branched-chain amino acids prevent insulin-induced hepatic tumor cell proliferation by inducing apoptosis through mTORC1 and mTORC2-dependent mechanisms. J Cell Physiol. 2012;227:2097–105.
186. Minischetti M, Vacca A, Ribatti D, et al. TNP-470 and recombinant human interferon-alpha2a inhibit angiogenesis synergistically. Br J Haematol. 2000;109:829–37.

187. Llovet JM, Bruix J. Novel advancements in the management of hepatocellular carcinoma in 2008. J Hepatol. 2008;48 Suppl 1:S20–37.
188. Kitade M, Yoshiji H, Noguchi R, et al. Crosstalk between angiogenesis, cytokeratin-18, and insulin resistance in the progression of non-alcoholic steatohepatitis. World J Gastroenterol. 2009;15:5193–9.
189. Hickman IJ, Macdonald GA. Impact of diabetes on the severity of liver disease. Am J Med. 2007;120:829–34.
190. Nielsen MF, Caumo A, Aagaard NK, et al. Contribution of defects in glucose uptake to carbohydrate intolerance in liver cirrhosis: assessment during physiological glucose and insulin concentrations. Am J Physiol Gastrointest Liver Physiol. 2005;288:G1135–43.
191. Kawaguchi T, Yoshida T, Harada M, et al. Hepatitis C virus down-regulates insulin receptor substrates 1 and 2 through up-regulation of suppressor of cytokine signaling 3. Am J Pathol. 2004;165:1499–508.
192. Cusi K. Role of insulin resistance and lipotoxicity in non-alcoholic steatohepatitis. Clin Liver Dis. 2009;13:545–63.
193. Sanyal AJ, Campbell-Sargent C, Mirshahi F, et al. Nonalcoholic steatohepatitis: association of insulin resistance and mitochondrial abnormalities. Gastroenterology. 2001;120:1183–92.
194. El-Serag HB, Richardson PA, Everhart JE. The role of diabetes in hepatocellular carcinoma: a case-control study among United States Veterans. Am J Gastroenterol. 2001;96:2462–7.
195. Siddique A, Kowdley KV. Insulin resistance and other metabolic risk factors in the pathogenesis of hepatocellular carcinoma. Clin Liver Dis. 2011;15:281–96, vii–x.
196. Alexia C, Fallot G, Lasfer M, et al. An evaluation of the role of insulin-like growth factors (IGF) and of type-I IGF receptor signalling in hepatocarcinogenesis and in the resistance of hepatocarcinoma cells against drug-induced apoptosis. Biochem Pharmacol. 2004;68:1003–15.
197. Natarajan R, Bai W, Lanting L, et al. Effects of high glucose on vascular endothelial growth factor expression in vascular smooth muscle cells. Am J Physiol. 1997;273:H2224–31.
198. Donadon V, Balbi M, Mas MD, et al. Metformin and reduced risk of hepatocellular carcinoma in diabetic patients with chronic liver disease. Liver Int. 2010;30:750–8.
199. Khattab M, Emad M, Abdelaleem A, et al. Pioglitazone improves virological response to peginterferon alpha-2b/ribavirin combination therapy in hepatitis C genotype 4 patients with insulin resistance. Liver Int. 2010;30:447–54.
200. El-Serag HB, Johnson ML, Hachem C, et al. Statins are associated with a reduced risk of hepatocellular carcinoma in a large cohort of patients with diabetes. Gastroenterology. 2009;136:1601–8.
201. Holst JJ, Vilsboll T, Deacon CF. The incretin system and its role in type 2 diabetes mellitus. Mol Cell Endocrinol. 2009;297:127–36.
202. Toft-Nielsen MB, Damholt MB, Madsbad S, et al. Determinants of the impaired secretion of glucagon-like peptide-1 in type 2 diabetic patients. J Clin Endocrinol Metab. 2001;86:3717–23.
203. Farilla L, Hui H, Bertolotto C, et al. Glucagon-like peptide-1 promotes islet cell growth and inhibits apoptosis in Zucker diabetic rats. Endocrinology. 2002;143:4397–408.
204. Li Y, Hansotia T, Yusta B, et al. Glucagon-like peptide-1 receptor signaling modulates beta cell apoptosis. J Biol Chem. 2003;278:471–8.
205. Drucker DJ, Nauck MA. The incretin system: glucagon-like peptide-1 receptor agonists and dipeptidyl peptidase-4 inhibitors in type 2 diabetes. Lancet. 2006;368:1696–705.
206. Lambeir AM, Durinx C, Scharpe S, et al. Dipeptidyl-peptidase IV from bench to bedside: an update on structural properties, functions, and clinical aspects of the enzyme DPP IV. Crit Rev Clin Lab Sci. 2003;40:209–94.
207. Gorrell MD, Wang XM, Park J, et al. Structure and function in dipeptidyl peptidase IV and related proteins. Adv Exp Med Biol. 2006;575:45–54.

208. Piazza GA, Callanan HM, Mowery J, et al. Evidence for a role of dipeptidyl peptidase IV in fibronectin-mediated interactions of hepatocytes with extracellular matrix. Biochem J. 1989;262:327–34.
209. Brill S, Zvibel I, Halpern Z, et al. The role of fetal and adult hepatocyte extracellular matrix in the regulation of tissue-specific gene expression in fetal and adult hepatocytes. Eur J Cell Biol. 2002;81:43–50.
210. Stecca BA, Nardo B, Chieco P, et al. Aberrant dipeptidyl peptidase IV (DPP IV/CD26) expression in human hepatocellular carcinoma. J Hepatol. 1997;27:337–45.
211. Perner F, Gyuris T, Rakoczy G, et al. Dipeptidyl peptidase activity of CD26 in serum and urine as a marker of cholestasis: experimental and clinical evidence. J Lab Clin Med. 1999;134:56–67.
212. Lakatos PL, Firneisz G, Rakoczy G, et al. Elevated serum dipeptidyl peptidase IV (CD26, EC 3.4.14.5) activity in patients with primary biliary cirrhosis. J Hepatol. 1999;30:740.
213. Firneisz G, Lakatos PL, Szalay F. Serum dipeptidyl peptidase IV (DPP IV, CD26) activity in chronic hepatitis C. Scand J Gastroenterol. 2001;36:877–80.
214. Stone SF, Lee S, Keane NM, et al. Association of increased hepatitis C virus (HCV)-specific IgG and soluble CD26 dipeptidyl peptidase IV enzyme activity with hepatotoxicity after highly active antiretroviral therapy in human immunodeficiency virus-HCV-coinfected patients. J Infect Dis. 2002;186:1498–502.
215. Levy MT, McCaughan GW, Abbott CA, et al. Fibroblast activation protein: a cell surface dipeptidyl peptidase and gelatinase expressed by stellate cells at the tissue remodelling interface in human cirrhosis. Hepatology. 1999;29:1768–78.
216. Levy MT, McCaughan GW, Marinos G, et al. Intrahepatic expression of the hepatic stellate cell marker fibroblast activation protein correlates with the degree of fibrosis in hepatitis C virus infection. Liver. 2002;22:93–101.
217. Wang XM, Yu DM, McCaughan GW, et al. Fibroblast activation protein increases apoptosis, cell adhesion, and migration by the LX-2 human stellate cell line. Hepatology. 2005;42:935–45.
218. Kaji K, Yoshiji H, Ikenaka Y, et al. Dipeptidyl peptidase-4 inhibitor attenuates hepatic fibrosis via suppression of activated hepatic stellate cell in rats. J Gastroenterol. 2013.
219. Miele L, Valenza V, La Torre G, et al. Increased intestinal permeability and tight junction alterations in nonalcoholic fatty liver disease. Hepatology. 2009;49:1877–87.
220. Douhara A, Moriya K, Yoshiji H, et al. Reduction of endotoxin attenuates liver fibrosis through suppression of hepatic stellate cell activation and remission of intestinal permeability in a rat non-alcoholic steatohepatitis model. Mol Med Rep. 2015;11:1693–700.
221. Shirai Y, Yoshiji H, Noguchi R, et al. Cross talk between toll-like receptor-4 signaling and angiotensin-II in liver fibrosis development in the rat model of non-alcoholic steatohepatitis. J Gastroenterol Hepatol. 2013;28:723–30.

Chapter 9
Heart Disease and the Liver: Interactions Between the Heart and the Liver

Akiomi Yoshihisa and Yasuchika Takeishi

Abstract Interactive complications between the heart and kidney can result in cardiorenal syndrome. Similar to this, there is also an interaction between the function of the heart and liver as well as a broad spectrum of acute and chronic entities that affect both of these organs, recognized as cardiohepatic syndrome. This chapter seeks to highlight the role of heart failure as a cause of liver dysfunction, the role of liver cirrhosis and nonalcoholic fatty liver disease as a cause of cardiovascular disease and/or heart disease, and finally, chronic alcoholism and systemic disorders, such as hemochromatosis and amyloidosis, which may affect the function of both the heart and liver.

Keyword Cardiohepatic syndrome • Hypoxic hepatopathy • Congestive hepatopathy • Cirrhotic cardiomyopathy • Nonalcoholic fatty liver disease (NAFLD)

9.1 Introduction: Interactions Between the Heart and the Liver

Interactive complications between the heart and kidney can result in cardiorenal syndrome [1]. Similar to this, there is also an interaction between the function of the heart and liver as well as a broad spectrum of acute and chronic entities that affect both of these organs [2, 3], recognized as cardiohepatic syndrome. As shown in Fig. 9.1, these can be classified into heart diseases affecting the liver, liver diseases affecting the heart, and common comorbidities and conditions affecting both the heart and liver at the same time. In acute and chronic liver dysfunction due to heart failure (HF), a combination of reduced arterial perfusion and passive congestion leads to cardiogenic hypoxic hepatopathy and congestive hepatopathy. Dynamic elevation of serum transaminase in relation to cardiogenic shock indicates massive hepatocellular necrosis, which is called ischemic hepatopathy [2–5]. Congestive

A. Yoshihisa (✉) • Y. Takeishi
Department of Cardiology and Hematology, Fukushima Medical University, 1 Hikarigaoka, Fukushima 960-1295, Japan
e-mail: yoshihis@fmu.ac.jp

H. Ohira (ed.), *The Liver in Systemic Diseases*, DOI 10.1007/978-4-431-55790-6_9

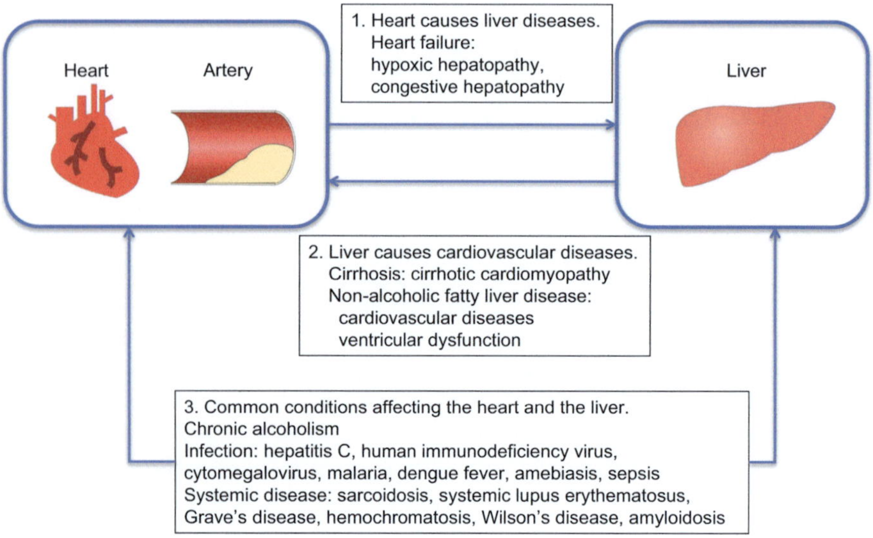

Fig. 9.1 Interactions between the heart and the liver

hepatopathy (cardiac cirrhosis) includes a spectrum of hepatic derangements occurring especially in right HF [2, 3, 6, 7]. Unlike cirrhosis caused by alcoholism or viral hepatitis, the impact of congestive hepatopathy on prognosis has not yet been clearly established [8]. These conditions may cause liver dysfunction, and secured perfusion of vital organs should be performed to manage heart disease complications. On the other hand, liver cirrhosis affects heart function and electrophysiology in the absence of other cardiac diseases [2, 3, 9–11]. Patients with cirrhosis exhibit cardiac systolic and diastolic dysfunction, as well as electrophysical abnormalities, all of which indicate cirrhotic cardiomyopathy. In addition, nonalcoholic fatty liver disease (NAFLD) is reportedly associated with cardiovascular disease (CVD) and HF. Furthermore, numerous comorbidities and conditions such as chronic alcoholism, infections (including hepatitis C virus), inflammatory and systemic diseases, obesity, and sleep-disordered breathing affect both the heart and liver [2, 3]. This chapter seeks to highlight the role of HF as a cause of liver dysfunction and liver cirrhosis, the role of NAFLD as a cause of CVD and/or heart disease, and finally, chronic alcoholism and systemic disorders, such as hemochromatosis and amyloidosis, which may affect the function of both the heart and liver.

9.2 Heart Failure

9.2.1 HF Causes Liver Disorders

In many countries, HF is a major cause of death in the elderly. HF causes low perfusion and congestion in multiple organs such as the kidney, liver, and others. The liver receives up to 25 % of cardiac output and is therefore damaged by reductions in blood flow [2]. In addition, the lack of valves in the hepatic veins allows increased inferior caval pressure to hit the sinusoidal bed without any protection. Though liver damage in HF has long been recognized [11], studies related to congestive hepatopathy are relatively few. There are several potential reasons for variant results: (1) HF etiology has changed over the years, for example, rheumatic valvular disease in the earliest studies [11] and ischemic cardiomyopathy in recent studies [12]; (2) the outcome of HF has dramatically improved [13] due to the increased efficiency of pharmacotherapy, including β-blockers and/or renin-angiotensin-aldosterone inhibitors [14], and non-pharmacotherapy including cardiac resynchronization therapy [13] and positive airway pressure [15–17], not to mention the widespread use of heart transplantation [2]. Further, the vasopressin V_2 antagonist tolvaptan is reportedly useful for management of HF [18] and liver cirrhosis [19]. Thus, the incidence of congestive hepatopathy has recently been reduced due to improvement of HF management [2, 3, 12]. The recognition and diagnosis of cardiac hepatopathy are important, as liver damage can influence the prognosis and outcome of cardiac disease and can only recover through measured improvement of cardiac function. As shown in Fig. 9.2, the fundamental mechanisms of cardiac hepatopathy are reduction of arterial perfusion (forward failure: hypoxic hepatopathy), the deleterious effects of which are amplified by concomitant hypoxia and passive congestion (backward failure: congestive hepatopathy) secondary to increased systemic venous pressure [12, 20]. Arterial hypoperfusion predominates in acute HF, leading to hypoxic hepatopathy, whereas passive congestion prevails in congestive hepatopathy secondary to chronic HF [2, 3]. However, these forward and backward factors often coexist and potentiate each other [21, 22].

9.2.2 *Hypoxic and Ischemic Hepatopathy*

Acute HF (especially, forward failure) most commonly arises in the context of profound shock state from myocardial infarction and worsening of HF. Furthermore, hypoxic hepatopathy has been found in instances of severe hypoxemia, such as obstructive sleep apnea and respiratory failure, as well as in toxic/septic shock under conditions of increased metabolic demand [23–25]. Ischemic hepatopathy is characterized by centrilobular necrosis of zone 3 hepatocytes in the absence of histological inflammation of viral hepatitis [2–4, 26–28]. Oxygen consumption can be easily increased when the hepatic blood flow is decreased. The liver protects itself from hypoxic damage in hypoxia by increasing oxygen extraction via the hepatocytes up to 95 % as the blood passes through the liver [2, 3]. Oxygen should be administered as early as possible in hypoxemic patients to achieve an arterial oxygen saturation >95 %. When inadequate end-organ perfusion and tissue hypoxia are persistent, or when acute shock develops, this protecting mechanism against hypoxic liver damage is overwhelmed. In ischemic hepatopathy, acute

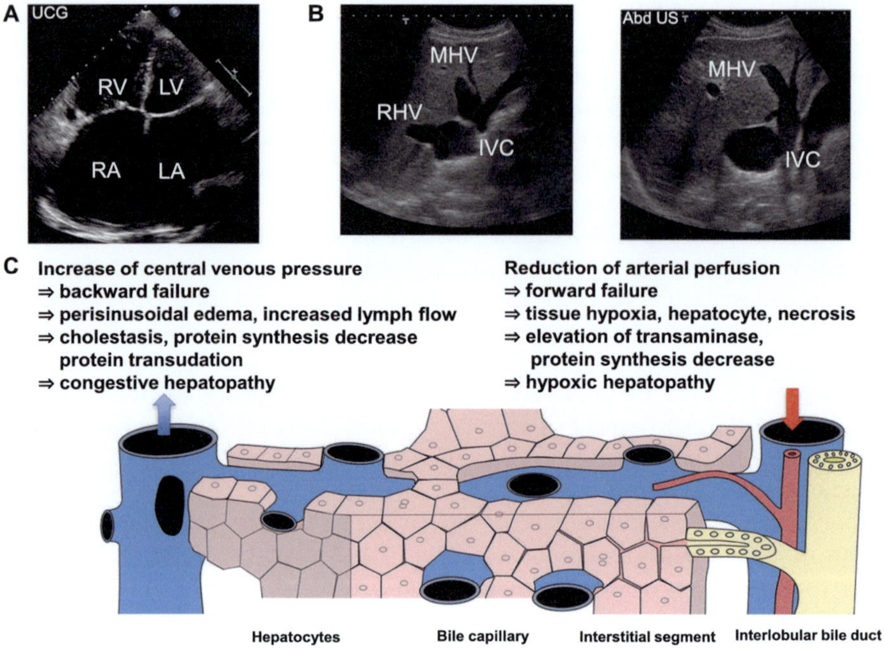

Fig. 9.2 Congestive hepatopathy and hypoxic hepatopathy. Right-heart pressure and volume overload cause liver congestion. (**a**) Echocardiogram shows enlargement of the right atrium by right-heart pressure and volume overload. *RV* right ventricle, *RA* right atrium, *LV* left ventricle, *LA* left atrium. (**b**) Abdominal echogram showing the dilatation of the inferior vena cava (IVC), right hepatic vein (RHV), and middle hepatic vein (MHV). (**c**) Pathophysiology of liver dysfunction in heart failure

increase of serum alanine aminotransferase (ALT), aspartate aminotransferase (AST), and lactic dehydrogenase (LDH), prolongation of the prothrombin time, and, occasionally, functional renal damage occur, followed by an improvement of these conditions brought on by hemodynamic improvement [2, 3, 21, 29]. The time courses can help to distinguish ischemic hepatopathy from acute viral or drug-induced hepatitis [30]. Treatment such as oxygen therapy, inotropic agents and vasopressor with caution, and diuretics for hypervolemia should be considered [3]. Encephalopathy can be present, but other mechanisms, such as cerebral hypoperfusion, likely contribute along with those involved in hepatic encephalopathy [2, 31]. Since hypoxic hepatopathy can be undistinguishable from acute liver failure resulting from other causes, echocardiography is warranted in the diagnosis of unidentified hepatopathy [32]. Compared with other types of hepatitis, once the underlying cardiocirculatory event is corrected, the prognosis of hypoxic hepatopathy is less severe [29].

9.2.3 Congestive Hepatopathy

In chronic HF (especially backward failure), the increased venous pressure caused by right-ventricular volume and pressure overload leads to the atrophy of hepatocytes and causes perisinusoidal edema, which can impair the diffusion of oxygen and nutrients to the hepatocytes [6]. This backward failure is also responsible for the enhanced hepatic lymph formation, leading to ascites when the lymph production rate exceeds the draining capacity of the lymphatic system [2, 3]. Moreover, increased pressure within the hepatic sinusoid favors bile duct damage by disrupting endothelial cells and the interhepatocyctic tight junctions that separate the extravascular space from the bile canaliculus [33]. Esophageal varices rarely develop in cardiac hepatopathy despite the presence of portal hypertension [12]. On the other hand, in portal hypertension due to cirrhosis, the hepatic venous pressure is increased and leads to portosystemic collateral formation and/or pulmonary hypertension. Moreover, increased pressure within the hepatic sinusoid favors bile duct damage by disrupting endothelial cells and the interhepatocyctic tight junctions that separate the extravascular space from the bile canaliculus. Finally, stagnant flow favors thrombosis within sinusoids, hepatic venules, and portal tracts, thereby contributing to liver fibrosis [2, 3, 6, 33]. In congestive hepatopathy, the liver is enlarged, with a purple or reddish hue and prominent hepatic veins [2, 3]. The cut surface shows a classic nutmeg appearance, reflecting an alternating pattern of hemorrhage and necrosis of zone 3 of the Rappaport's acinus with normal or slightly steatotic areas in zones 1 and 2 [3, 21]. Centrilobular liver cell necrosis can extend to peripheral areas if HF persists and worsens and is followed by the deposition and spread of connective tissue bridging one central vein to another, ultimately leading to cirrhosis [2, 11]. Finally, stagnant flow favors thrombosis within sinusoids, hepatic venules, and portal tracts, contributing to liver fibrosis and possibly explaining its uneven distribution [3, 34]. Congestive hepatopathy is often asymptomatic and sometimes shows jaundice, ascites, hepatomegaly with hepatojugular reflux, and a pulsatile liver [2]. Laboratory features mainly reveal cholestasis [22, 29, 35, 36], with increased serum γ-glutamyl transpeptidase (GGT), alkaline phosphatase (ALP), and bilirubin, while transaminases are often normal or moderately increased, unless severe HF with a significant forward component coexists. The degree of cholestasis is related to the severity of HF, as assessed by an increase in right atrial pressure, pulmonary hypertension, and the presence of tricuspid regurgitation [22, 35]. Increased serum ALP or bilirubin predicts all-cause mortality [36], cardiovascular death, or hospitalization for HF [22, 37]. Congestive hepatopathy also leads to synthetic function impairment, prolonged prothrombin time, and reduced serum albumin concentration, which are also associated with mortality in HF patients [22, 38]. Furthermore, congestive hepatopathy occurs especially in patients with right-heart overload, such as shunt-related disease, congenital heart disease, constrictive pericarditis, mitral stenosis, tricuspid regurgitation, cor pulmonale, and pulmonary hypertension. Long-term survivors who undergo the Fontan operation, which is a radical operation for tricuspid stenosis using the right-pulmonary artery bypass, can develop liver damage as a result of the interplay between hypoxia and central venous hypertension that is due to the passive, nonpulsatile flow through the pulmonary arterial bed [2, 39]. Indeed, hepatomegaly and liver dysfunction have been reported in many cases, being related to a reduced cardiac index and increased right atrial pressure [40]. In addition, chronic constrictive pericarditis leads to a sustained elevation of systemic venous pressure and liver damage [41]. As the usual physical signs of HF may be inconspicuous, patients presenting a clinical picture of liver cirrhosis, including ascites, but also distended jugular veins, pericardial calcifications, or thickening, should be examined by echocardiography, computed tomography, or magnetic resonance imaging. Doppler echocardiography or right cardiac catheterization is needed for the differential diagnosis of restrictive cardiomyopathy. Although this is not always easy, the recognition of chronic constrictive pericarditis is of paramount importance, as it can be cured by cardiac surgery. Treatments such as ACE inhibitor, β-blocker, and diuretics should be considered [3].

9.2.4 Model for End-Stage Liver Disease Scoring Series in HF

Liver dysfunction often exists in cases of HF as cardiac or congestive hepatopathy and is associated with adverse clinical outcomes in advanced HF patients [8, 36, 37, 42, 43]. Congestive hepatopathy and subsequent cirrhosis in patients with advanced HF have been recognized [44]. Recently, a composite model for end-stage liver disease (MELD) scoring series, using models including MELD (including total bilirubin, creatinine, and prothrombin time international normalized ratio [INR]), MELD Na (MELD with sodium), and MELD-XI (MELD excluding INR), has been developed. They are established scoring systems of liver or hepatorenal function, and a high score is associated with poor prognosis, not only in patients who had undergone liver transplantation [45] but also those with advanced HF in which heart transplantation and/or ventricular assist devices are considered [42, 46–48]. In HF patients, the MELD scoring series indicates multiple organ dysfunction secondary to impaired cardiac function. Shinagawa et al. reported that a high total bilirubin level is an independent predictor of cardiac events in HF patients [43]. Abe et al. reported that MELD-XI was an independent predictor of cardiac death and all-cause mortality in general HF patients whose conditions were associated with right-heart volume overload and higher pulmonary arterial pressure [22]. HF results in various abnormal liver functions, such as the elevation of serum bilirubin, ALP, GGT, and ALT [22]. Other hemodynamic data suggest that elevated central venous pressure and right atrial pressure may contribute to cholestatic abnormalities and impairment of hepatocyte function in patients with HF [7, 49]. Several metabolic processes of bilirubin, such as secretion of direct bilirubin into bile [50], are attenuated by hepatocellular hypoxia. In addition, biliary obstruction caused by elevated hepatic venous pressure leads to an increase of serum total bilirubin. Several studies so far have shown that serum bilirubin correlates with various hemodynamic and cardiac parameters, such as right atrial pressure [7, 35], severity of tricuspid regurgitation [7, 22, 35], pulmonary artery wedge pressure [7, 22, 43], cardiac output [7, 43], and left-ventricular ejection fraction [35]. HF with a high MELD-XI score is accompanied by poorer nutrition, cholestatic state, cardiac volume overload, and higher pulmonary arterial pressure [22]. Pulmonary arterial pressure is a reported predictor of prognosis in HF patients [51, 52].

9.3 Liver Cirrhosis

9.3.1 Liver Cirrhosis Causes Heart Disease: Cirrhotic Cardiomyopathy

Patients with liver cirrhosis frequently experience autonomic cardiovascular dysfunction, increased activity of the sympathetic nervous system, and reduced vagal cardiac function, which have important implications for liver dysfunction and poor survival [53, 54]. A hyperdynamic state has been described in patients with cirrhosis [55]. Cardiac dysfunction, also known as cirrhotic cardiomyopathy, has also been reported [2, 3, 56–58]. The relationship between the myocardial changes and the development of cirrhosis and its clinical course are presented in Fig. 9.3 [2]. Cirrhotic cardiomyopathy includes a reduced cardiac systolic and diastolic dysfunction as well as electrophysiological abnormalities (Fig. 9.3) [2, 3, 10, 59–61]. Cirrhotic cardiomyopathy has recently been defined as follows: (1) systolic dysfunction (blunted increase in cardiac output with exercise, volume challenge, or pharmacological stimuli) and/or resting left-ventricular ejection fraction $<55\,\%$, (2) diastolic dysfunction, and (3) supportive criteria (electrophysiological abnormalities, abnormal chronotropic response, electromechanical dyssynchrony, prolonged QT interval, enlarged left atrium, increased myocardial mass, increase of B-type natriuretic peptide, and troponins) [58]. A number of pathogenetic mechanisms for the impaired contractility in cirrhotic cardiomyopathy have been described as follows: desensitization and downregulation of cardiac β-adrenergic receptors with a decreased content of G-protein and following impaired intracellular signaling; alterations in particular in M1 muscarinic receptors; upregulation of cannabinoid 1-receptor stimulation; altered plasma membrane cholesterol/phospholipid ratio; increased inhibitory effects of hemeoxygenase, carbon monoxide, nitric oxide, and tumor necrosis-α; reduced density of potassium channels; changed function and fluxes through L-type calcium channels; and altered ratio and function of collagens and titins [2, 3]. Systolic dysfunction can be demonstrated by pharmacological or physical stress and has recently been implicated in the development of renal failure in advanced disease [62]. Diastolic dysfunction in cirrhosis may reflect ventricular hypertrophy and altered collagen structure, and it seems to be

	Compensated cirrhosis	Compensated/mild uncompensated cirrhosis with ascites	Decompensated liver cirrhosis with ascites and renal dysfunction
Systemic circulation	vasodilation	hyperdynamic state Cardiac output ↑	hyperdynamic sate/ cardiac output
Cardiac function	normal	diastolic dysfunction	systolic dysfunction/ cardiac failure
Cardiac findings	QT↑	QT↑↑, abnormal transmitral inflow, deceleration time↑, left ventricular ejection fraction ↑	QT↑, dyssynchronised electrical and mechanical systole, left atrium volume and left ventricular end diastolic volume↑, left ventricular ejection fraction
Cardiac morphology	normal	hypertrophy (fibrosis, edema)	hypertrophy/dilatation

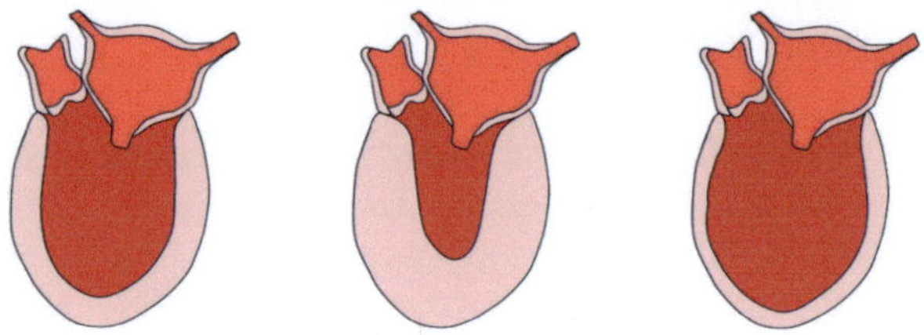

Fig. 9.3 Cirrhosis cardiac systolic and diastolic dysfunction and QT interval prolongation in liver cirrhosis

related to prognosis [3, 10, 60]. The electrocardiographic QT interval is prolonged in about half of cirrhotic patients and may be related to patient characteristics and survival [61].

9.3.2 Cardiac Systolic and Diastolic Dysfunction and QT Interval Prolongation in Liver Cirrhosis

As shown in Fig. 9.3, hyperdynamic state with increased cardiac output is seen in advanced cirrhosis. Pathogenetic hallmarks are the pronounced splanchnic arterial vasodilatation and reduced systemic vascular resistance [58]. In this setting, cardiac pressures are largely normal, at least in part because the reduced afterload protects systolic function. High-output states result from increased blood volume and are defined as hyperdynamic-state HF [63]. Despite the characteristic high-cardiac output, systolic dysfunction is present [58] and is associated with the inability of the heart to meet its demands with respect to the generation of an adequate arterial blood pressure and cardiac output [2, 64]. This can be unveiled by physical exercise that increases left-ventricular pressure and volume as well as left-ventricular ejection fraction and heart rate in cirrhotic patients [64–66]. Angiotensin-converting enzyme inhibitors and other vasodilators should be used with caution because of the risk of further aggravation of the vasodilatory state [2]. Systolic dysfunction may have an impact on the development of complications, such as sodium and water retention as well as ascites formation, and the development of renal dysfunction and prognosis [2, 3, 58, 66–68].

Diastolic dysfunction in cirrhosis is associated with increased myocardial wall stiffness due to myocardial hypertrophy, fibrosis, and subendothelial edema [67, 69]. Combinations of myocardial hypertrophy, contractile dysfunction, changes in heart volumes, and diastolic dysfunction may represent an essential element in cirrhotic cardiomyopathy [66]. Diastolic dysfunction, which is characterized by abnormal transmitral inflow using echocardiography, is seen in about half of patients with cirrhosis [58, 70]. Diastolic dysfunction is an essential element in cirrhotic cardiomyopathy and is furthermore associated with a higher mortality after transjugular intrahepatic portosystemic shunt insertion and reduced ascites mobilization [3, 10, 71]. Diastolic dysfunction in cirrhosis may be associated with poor prognosis, in the setting of rapid increases in preload, such as in transjugular intrahepatic portosystemic shunt insertion, etc. [2].

The prolongation of the electrocardiographic QT interval, which is a marker of cardiac repolarization and a predictor of ventricular arrhythmias and sudden death [72, 73], is common (over 60 %) in advanced cirrhosis [72]. To date, the pathophysiology of QT prolongation in cirrhosis is not yet fully understood. The presence of portal hypertension; portosystemic shunts [74, 75]; potential cardiotoxins, such as endotoxins, cytokines, and bile salts [76]; and increased sympathoadrenergic tone may affect the QT interval prolongation [2, 3]. Increased adrenergic drive would prolong QT interval in the setting of impaired function of K^+ channels [77]. Concordant with this, β-blockers shorten a prolonged QT in cirrhosis [78, 79], whereas stressful events such as gastrointestinal bleeding further prolong QT interval [80]. QT prolongation in cirrhosis is also associated with poor survival [72]. The impact of drugs on the QT interval also should be considered when evaluating electrocardiography [61].

9.4 NAFLD

9.4.1 Relationship of NAFLD and CVD

NAFLD is a common cause of chronic liver disease in the general population. NAFLD is recognized as fatty infiltration that affects >5 % of hepatocytes, in the presence of <20 g/day of alcohol consumption, without evidence of other causes of liver disease [81]. NAFLD progresses slowly and represents a spectrum of varying liver disease severity, ranging from simple steatosis to coexistent inflammation with hepatocyte ballooning and necrosis, variable grades of fibrosis, and ultimately cirrhosis with an increased risk of hepatocellular carcinoma [81, 82]. NAFLD encompasses a spectrum of pathological conditions such as inflammation, ranging from simple steatosis to nonalcoholic steatohepatitis (NASH), and cirrhosis [83]. The presence of NASH/NAFLD is also recognized as a phenotype of metabolic syndrome (MetS) in the liver and indicates risk of insulin resistance, dyslipidemia, and hypertension, all of which are reportedly associated with cardiovascular events. There is still abundant evidence linking only NAFLD itself to increased CVD risk and accelerated atherogenesis regardless of other comorbid conditions, such as MetS [84]. Although the relationship between NAFLD and an increased prevalence of CVD seems to be robust and consistently replicated across populations of different ethnicities, the contribution of NAFLD to the increased incidence of CVD is more controversial [85–87]. Both retrospective and prospective studies have assessed the relationship between NAFLD, as diagnosed by biopsy or imaging, and the risk of incidental CVD events [85, 86, 88]. There is bias with respect to diagnostic methods of NAFLD, cohort and event observation. Additional large-scale prospective studies are needed to draw firm conclusions about any independent hepatic contribution to the increased cardiovascular risk observed among patients with NAFLD.

In patients with biopsy-proven NAFLD, several retrospective studies have shown that the presence and severity of hepatic fibrosis are the main determinants of all-cause and liver-related mortality and that CVD is a very common cause of death among NAFLD patients [88–92]. Ekstedt et al. [88] and Soderberg et al. [91] also reported that patients with NASH, but not those with simple steatosis, had an increased risk of mortality attributable to CVD compared with the matched general population. However, a recent meta-analysis concluded that patients with NAFLD (as detected by biopsy or ultrasonography) have a substantially higher risk of mortality and morbidity as a result of CVD than the matched general population, but the histological severity of NAFLD does not increase CVD mortality [85, 92]. Thus, CVD is a serious threat to patients with NASH. However, these studies, which examined the natural history of biopsy-proven NAFLD, were retrospective cohort studies with relatively small numbers of patients who were seen at tertiary-care referral centers [85, 88–91, 93, 94].

In patients with ultrasonography-proven NAFLD, large prospective studies showed an increased incidence of CVD events, independent of several CVD risk factors [95–100]. Ultrasonography-proven NAFLD in a community-based cohort of healthy adults was associated with an increased risk of nonfatal cardiovascular events including coronary artery disease (CAD), ischemic stroke, and cerebral hemorrhage, also independent of other risk factors [97]. More recently, Haring et al. found that liver ultrasonography was useful in patients with increased levels of GGT not only for the diagnosis of NAFLD but also for better cardiovascular risk stratification in a population-based study [98]. On the other hand, Stepanova et al. [101] and Lazo et al. [102] have reported that although NAFLD was independently associated with an increased prevalence of CVD, it did not predict the risk of all-cause and cause-specific (cardiovascular, cancer, or liver) mortality over a 14-year period [85].

In patients with serum enzyme-suspected NAFLD using elevated serum enzyme levels as surrogate markers of NAFLD (which should therefore be interpreted cautiously), many large population-based studies have shown that serum enzyme-suspected NAFLD is associated with an increased risk of CVD, independently of alcohol consumption and several established cardiovascular risk factors [84–86, 103–112]. Additionally, in a systematic review and meta-analysis, Fraser et al. confirmed that an elevated serum GGT level was an independent, long-term predictor of incident cardiovascular events [107]. Some studies [109, 110], but not all [105, 108, 111], have confirmed that an increased serum ALT level is less predictive of incident CVD than an increased serum GGT level, which is thought to be a marker of not only NAFLD but also oxidative stress [84, 113, 114]. ALT has been reported to be more closely related to liver fat content than GGT [113]. Similarly, several cohort studies have reported an independent association between elevated ALT and CVD mortality after adjusting for other CVD risk factors [85, 86, 105, 108, 111]. The meta-analysis of the only two prospective studies that used an elevated serum ALT level as a surrogate marker of NAFLD failed to show any independent association with CVD outcomes [107].

9.4.2 *Underlying Pathophysiological Mechanisms of CAD, CVD, and NAFLD*

Patients with NAFLD typically meet the diagnostic criteria for MetS (i.e., abdominal obesity, hypertension, dyslipidemia, and insulin resistance) and therefore have multiple risk factors for CVD [84, 112–114]. In addition, patients with NAFLD are independently associated with having a higher risk of diabetes [115], hypertension [116], and chronic kidney disease [117–119], which are established risk factors of CVD and independent predictors of poor prognosis in HF. Histological severity of NASH (i.e., fibrosis stage) was independently associated with either decreasing renal function or increasing albuminuria [118]. Sleep-disordered breathing, which is an obesity-related disease, is also associated with liver dysfunction, NAFLD [120], CAD [121, 122], and HF [122].

As shown in Fig. 9.4, several mechanisms of NAFLD and CVD (including HF) are assumed, such as insulin resistance, visceral fat, epicardial fat, inflammation, and lipid disorders. The visceral adipose tissue appears to have a strong independent positive correlation with liver fat [123]. Liver fat is an independent predictor of insulin resistance in the skeletal muscle, the adipose tissue, and the liver [124]. Alterations in cellular free fatty acid transport are involved in the pathogenesis of ectopic fat distribution by diverting the accumulation of triglyceride away from the adipose tissue and toward other key metabolic organs, such as skeletal muscle and the liver [85, 86]. Apart from being a fat storage organ and/or tissue, visceral fat is also metabolically active, secreting several adipokines, cytokines, and hormones that serve to regulate inflammation, liver fat, and insulin resistance and modify CVD outcome [82, 85, 86, 125]. The presence of liver fat and/or NASH is associated with lower adiponectin levels and higher levels of C-reactive protein, fibrinogen, and plasminogen activator inhibitor-1 [126–128]. The epicardial adipose tissue is linked with the myocardium and adventitial layer of the coronary

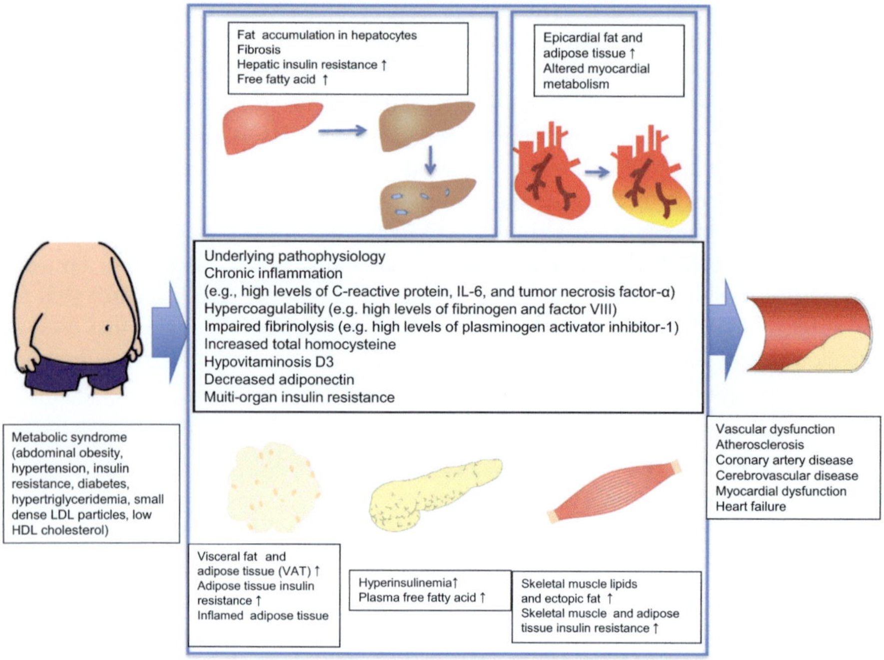

Fig. 9.4 Underlying pathophysiology between MetS, NAFLD, and CVD

arteries and shares the same microcirculation or paracrine route and vasocrine effect on the heart and its blood vessels [129]. Increased myocardial fat represents abnormal ectopic fat storage and may indeed be a marker of the cumulative effects of NAFLD and insulin resistance in the setting of pathological adiposity [130, 131], with consequent associated adverse CVD events [132]. Furthermore, the liver is a key metabolic organ and is central to the regulation of systemic inflammation. Nuclear factor kappa-B is a hepatocellular transcription factor that plays a key role in intrahepatic inflammation [85]. That mitochondrial dysfunction and damage are associated with insulin resistance, and atherosclerosis has been reported in several studies [133], representing a plausible link between NAFLD and increased CVD risk [85, 86].

9.4.3 CAD in NAFLD

CAD is a disease which occurs as a result of an increase and rupture of plaque brought on by risk factors such as diabetes, dyslipidemia, hypertension, and obesity, which are also associated with NAFLD. It has been reported that, compared with control subjects who do not have steatosis, patients with NAFLD have impaired coronary flow reserve [134], flow-mediated vasodilatation [135, 136], arterial stiffness [137, 138], and increased carotid artery intimal media thickness [135, 139–143]; these are established markers for detecting subclinical atherosclerosis. Lower flow-mediated vasodilatation, which is a marker of endothelial function, was observed in NASH compared with simple steatosis, again confirming the graded association of CVD risk with severity of NAFLD [135]. Targher et al. found that carotid artery intimal medial thickness was greatest in patients with NASH, intermediate in those with simple steatosis, and lowest in healthy controls after adjusting for risk factors [139]. Several studies have demonstrated a significantly increased coronary atherosclerotic burden in the presence of NAFLD [85, 86, 144–146], with one study also reporting a significant association between "vulnerable plaque" and NAFLD in patients undergoing multislice computed tomography for clinical suspicion of CAD [145]. A strong association between NAFLD and the prevalence of significant CAD determined by coronary angiography has also been reported, albeit with variable thresholds of significant CAD between studies [147–150].

9.4.4 Altered Cardiac Function and Myocardial Metabolism in NAFLD

Only a few studies have reported that abnormal left-ventricular geometry and diastolic dysfunction were evident in patients with NAFLD [85, 86, 151–153]. It has been reported that positive correlations exist between the degree of diastolic dysfunction and amount of liver fat, with diastolic dysfunction and insulin resistance being the only independent parameters associated with NAFLD [151]. The consistent findings of subclinical cardiac dysfunction in an asymptomatic population with NAFLD are perhaps not surprising, given that left-ventricular dysfunction and left-ventricular mass are strongly correlated with insulin resistance and its subsequent prognosis [154]. To gain further insight into the causes of subclinical cardiac dysfunction in NAFLD, the effects of hepatic steatosis on myocardial metabolism have also been examined [155, 156]. One study found a positive association between hepatic fat content and myocardial insulin resistance; patients with high liver fat content not only showed significantly lower whole-body insulin sensitivity as expected but also reduced myocardial glucose uptake and extraction rate, reduced coronary flow reserve, as well as increased plasma levels of inflammatory markers and vascular adhesion molecules. Only liver fat content remained significantly associated with impaired myocardial metabolism even after adjusting for insulin resistance, visceral fat mass, and other important variables [155]. Impaired left-ventricular energy metabolism has been reported as well as increased epicardial fat in NAFLD compared with controls [156, 157]. This suggests that in patients with hepatic steatosis, abnormalities in myocardial metabolism may precede functional and structural cardiac remodeling, leading to increased left-ventricular mass and diastolic dysfunction [85, 86]. Patients with NAFLD have left-ventricular diastolic dysfunction [152] and impaired left-ventricular energy metabolism, as measured on cardiac phosphorus-31 magnetic resonance spectroscopy [156]. This produces inefficient energy metabolism by cardiomyocytes, switching to fat rather than glucose oxidation in physiologically demanding states and yielding less adenosine triphosphate per oxygen molecule consumed [85, 86]. The excess free fatty acid supply also leads to cardiac lipotoxicity by causing intracellular lipid accumulation and overwhelming normal cardiomyocyte oxidative capacity, resulting in increased oxidative stress and consequent cardiac apoptosis and dysfunction [125, 154].

9.5 Common Conditions

9.5.1 Common Conditions Affecting Both the Liver and the Heart

There are several systemic diseases that affect both the liver and the heart, including not only chronic alcoholism but also congenital, autoimmune, metabolic, infection, and inflammatory disorders [2, 3].

9.5.2 Chronic Alcoholism

Chronic alcoholism can reveal both liver and heart complications. Even though genetic and environmental factors, types of beverages, and drinking patterns play a role, the amount of alcohol consumed is crucial in leading to disease [2, 3, 158, 159]. In a meta-analysis of daily consumption levels in relation to cirrhosis, patients taking >25 g/day were at higher risk of cirrhosis than nondrinkers [160]. Alcohol consumption had a larger impact on the mortality of liver cirrhosis compared with its morbidity [161]. A recent meta-analysis found increased risks of mortality from liver cirrhosis among women and men drinking 12–24 g/day [161]. While chronic consumption of amounts of ethanol >25 g/day in males and 12 g/day in females is associated with an increased risk of cirrhosis, >90 g/day for at least 5 years appears to be needed to induce detectable changes in cardiac structure and function [162]. In contrast, there is a J-shaped relationship between wine intake and vascular risk, indicating that moderate alcohol consumption (about 25 g/day) is cardioprotective [163]. Active alcohol consumption by patients with cirrhosis reveals lower left-ventricular ejection fraction, as well as greater end-diastolic diameter and left-ventricular mass, compared to cirrhosis subjects abstaining from alcohol. Most heavy drinkers remain asymptomatic in the earlier stages of disease progression, and many never develop the familiar clinical manifestations that typify HF [158]. Patients with alcoholic cirrhosis should be screened for cardiomyopathy. There is a correlation between the development of alcoholic heart muscle disease and alcoholic cirrhosis [159], a combination of which carries a worse prognosis than either disease alone [2, 3, 158].

9.5.3 *Infections and Inflammatory Disorders*

Hepatitis C virus causes chronic inflammation not only of the liver but also of the myocardium and, later, dilated cardiomyopathy attributable to necrosis and loss of myocytes. However, because myocytes do not replicate, the proliferative stimuli induced by hepatitis C infection may promote myocyte hypertrophy and hypertrophic cardiomyopathy [164]. A role of the direct effect of hepatitis C virus core proteins was suggested in the pathogenesis of cardiomyopathy [165]. Chronic hepatitis C virus-associated steatosis was suggested as a leading cause of CADs [166, 167].

Human immunodeficiency virus is known to cause hepatitis, hepatic granulomas, myocarditis, cardiomyopathy, and pulmonary hypertension [168]. *Cytomegalovirus* infection in immunocompetent hosts rarely leads to severe organ complications such as myopericarditis concomitant with hepatitis [169]. Tropical diseases also affect both organs [2, 3]. For example, dengue fever may lead to hepatic necroses combined with myocarditis [170], and malaria can cause massive hepatic involvement and cardiac failure [171]. Sarcoidosis is a systemic disease characterized by non-caseating granulomas in multiple organs (lung, skin, heart, and liver, etc.). Hepatic sarcoidosis may lead to cholestasis as well as portal hypertension and its associated complications [172]. Hyperthyroidism, which is based on autoimmune Grave's disease, may present with jaundice and atrial fibrillation, pulmonary hypertension, and HF [173].

9.5.4 *Systemic Disorders*

Hemochromatosis is an autosomal recessive disorder of iron metabolism characterized by tissue iron overload and may cause multiorgan disease with liver cirrhosis, hepatocellular carcinoma, endocrine disorders like diabetes, skin pigmentation, and cardiac disease. Although hemochromatosis causes electrocardiographic changes and hypertrophy, and increases end-diastolic and end-systolic volumes, HF is rarely caused [174]. Wilson's disease is caused by abnormal accumulation of copper. Hepatic manifestations include a broad clinical picture from asymptomatic biochemistry dysfunction to chronic hepatitis and cirrhosis. In Wilson's disease, concentric left-ventricular remodeling and diastolic dysfunction, with a relatively high frequency of benign supraventricular extrasystolic beats, are present [2, 175]. Amyloidosis affects multiple organs including the liver, intestinal tract, skin, and heart. Hepatic amyloid deposition leads to elevation of liver enzymes in early stages and, later, increased serum bilirubin and jaundice. Amyloidosis may lead to restrictive cardiomyopathy [176]. Amyloid light-chain amyloidosis primarily infiltrates the liver, and transthyretin amyloidosis mainly affects the heart.

References

1. Ronco C, McCullough P, Anker SD, Anand I, Aspromonte N, Bagshaw SM, et al. Cardio-renal syndromes: report from the consensus conference of the acute dialysis quality initiative. Eur Heart J. 2010;31(6):703–11.
2. Moller S, Bernardi M. Interactions of the heart and the liver. Eur Heart J. 2013;34(36):2804–11.
3. Fouad YM, Yehia R. Hepato-cardiac disorders. World J Hepatol. 2014;6(1):41–54.
4. Seeto RK, Fenn B, Rockey DC. Ischemic hepatitis: clinical presentation and pathogenesis. Am J Med. 2000;109(2):109–13.
5. Henrion J, Schapira M, Luwaert R, Colin L, Delannoy A, Heller FR. Hypoxic hepatitis: clinical and hemodynamic study in 142 consecutive cases. Medicine. 2003;82(6):392–406.
6. Dunn GD, Hayes P, Breen KJ, Schenker S. The liver in congestive heart failure: a review. Am J Med Sci. 1973;265(3):174–89.
7. Kubo SH, Walter BA, John DH, Clark M, Cody RJ. Liver function abnormalities in chronic heart failure. Influence of systemic hemodynamics. Arch Intern Med. 1987;147(7):1227–30.
8. Batin P, Wickens M, McEntegart D, Fullwood L, Cowley AJ. The importance of abnormalities of liver function tests in predicting mortality in chronic heart failure. Eur Heart J. 1995;16(11):1613–18.
9. Mohamed R, Forsey PR, Davies MK, Neuberger JM. Effect of liver transplantation on QT interval prolongation and autonomic dysfunction in end-stage liver disease. Hepatology. 1996;23(5):1128–34.
10. Cazzaniga M, Salerno F, Pagnozzi G, Dionigi E, Visentin S, Cirello I, et al. Diastolic dysfunction is associated with poor survival in patients with cirrhosis with transjugular intrahepatic portosystemic shunt. Gut. 2007;56(6):869–75.
11. Sherlock S. The liver in heart failure; relation of anatomical, functional, and circulatory changes. Br Heart J. 1951;13(3):273–93.
12. Myers RP, Cerini R, Sayegh R, Moreau R, Degott C, Lebrec D, et al. Cardiac hepatopathy: clinical, hemodynamic, and histologic characteristics and correlations. Hepatology. 2003;37(2):393–400.
13. Fonarow GC, Albert NM, Curtis AB, Gheorghiade M, Liu Y, Mehra MR, et al. Incremental reduction in risk of death associated with use of guideline-recommended therapies in patients with heart failure: a nested case-control analysis of IMPROVE HF. J Am Heart Assoc. 2012;1(1):16–26.
14. McAlister FA, Wiebe N, Ezekowitz JA, Leung AA, Armstrong PW. Meta-analysis: beta-blocker dose, heart rate reduction, and death in patients with heart failure. Ann Intern Med. 2009;150(11):784–94.
15. Ware LB, Matthay MA. Clinical practice. Acute pulmonary edema. N Engl J Med. 2005;353(26):2788–96.
16. Kasai T, Floras JS, Bradley TD. Sleep apnea and cardiovascular disease: a bidirectional relationship. Circulation. 2012;126(12):1495–510.
17. Yoshihisa A, Suzuki S, Yamaki T, Sugimoto K, Kunii H, Nakazato K, et al. Impact of adaptive servo-ventilation on cardiovascular function and prognosis in heart failure patients with preserved left ventricular ejection fraction and sleep-disordered breathing. Eur J Heart Fail. 2013;15(5):543–50.

18. Suzuki S, Yoshihisa A, Yamaki T, Sugimoto K, Kunii H, Nakazato K, et al. Long-term effects and prognosis in acute heart failure treated with tolvaptan: the AVCMA trial. BioMed Res Int. 2014;2014:704289.
19. Akiyama S, Ikeda K, Sezaki H, Fukushima T, Sorin Y, Kawamura Y, et al. Therapeutic effects of short- and intermediate-term tolvaptan administration for refractory ascites in patients with advanced liver cirrhosis. Hepatol Res: Off J Jpn Soc Hepatol. 2014;45 (11):1062–70.
20. Kavoliuniene A, Vaitiekiene A, Cesnaite G. Congestive hepatopathy and hypoxic hepatitis in heart failure: a cardiologist's point of view. Int J Cardiol. 2013;166(3):554–8.
21. Birrer R, Takuda Y, Takara T. Hypoxic hepatopathy: pathophysiology and prognosis. Intern Med. 2007;46(14):1063–70.
22. Abe S, Yoshihisa A, Takiguchi M, Shimizu T, Nakamura Y, Yamauchi H, et al. Liver dysfunction assessed by model for end-stage liver disease excluding INR (MELD-XI) scoring system predicts adverse prognosis in heart failure. PLoS One. 2014;9(6):e100618.
23. Taylor RM, Tujios S, Jinjuvadia K, Davern T, Shaikh OS, Han S, et al. Short and long-term outcomes in patients with acute liver failure due to ischemic hepatitis. Dig Dis Sci. 2012;57 (3):777–85.
24. Henrion J, Minette P, Colin L, Schapira M, Delannoy A, Heller FR. Hypoxic hepatitis caused by acute exacerbation of chronic respiratory failure: a case-controlled, hemodynamic study of 17 consecutive cases. Hepatology. 1999;29(2):427–33.
25. Mathurin P, Durand F, Ganne N, Mollo JL, Lebrec D, Degott C, et al. Ischemic hepatitis due to obstructive sleep apnea. Gastroenterology. 1995;109(5):1682–4.
26. Ellenberg M, Osserman KE. The role of shock in the production of central liver cell necrosis. Am J Med. 1951;11(2):170–8.
27. Killip 3rd T, Payne MA. High serum transaminase activity in heart disease. Circulatory failure and hepatic necrosis. Circulation. 1960;21:646–60.
28. Clarke WT. Centrilobular hepatic necrosis following cardiac infarction. Am J Pathol. 1950;26(2):249–55.
29. Myers RP, Lee SS. Cirrhotic cardiomyopathy and liver transplantation. Liver Transplant. 2000;6(4 Suppl 1):S44–52.
30. Fuhrmann V, Kneidinger N, Herkner H, Heinz G, Nikfardjam M, Bojic A, et al. Hypoxic hepatitis: underlying conditions and risk factors for mortality in critically ill patients. Intensive Care Med. 2009;35(8):1397–405.
31. Weisberg IS, Jacobson IM. Cardiovascular diseases and the liver. Clin Liver Dis. 2011;15 (1):1–20.
32. de Leeuw K, Meertens JH, van der Horst IC, van der Berg AP, Ligtenberg JJ, Tulleken JE, et al. "Acute liver failure": the heart may be the matter. Acta Clin Belg. 2011;66(3):236–9.
33. Cogger VC, Fraser R, Le Couteur DG. Liver dysfunction and heart failure. Am J Cardiol. 2003;91(11):1399.
34. Wanless IR, Liu JJ, Butany J. Role of thrombosis in the pathogenesis of congestive hepatic fibrosis (cardiac cirrhosis). Hepatology. 1995;21(5):1232–7.
35. Lau GT, Tan HC, Kritharides L. Type of liver dysfunction in heart failure and its relation to the severity of tricuspid regurgitation. Am J Cardiol. 2002;90(12):1405–9.
36. Poelzl G, Ess M, Mussner-Seeber C, Pachinger O, Frick M, Ulmer H. Liver dysfunction in chronic heart failure: prevalence, characteristics and prognostic significance. Eur J Clin Invest. 2012;42(2):153–63.
37. Allen LA, Felker GM, Pocock S, McMurray JJ, Pfeffer MA, Swedberg K, et al. Liver function abnormalities and outcome in patients with chronic heart failure: data from the Candesartan in Heart Failure: assessment of Reduction in Mortality and Morbidity (CHARM) program. Eur J Heart Fail. 2009;11(2):170–7.
38. Ambrosy AP, Vaduganathan M, Huffman MD, Khan S, Kwasny MJ, Fought AJ, et al. Clinical course and predictive value of liver function tests in patients hospitalized for worsening heart failure with reduced ejection fraction: an analysis of the EVEREST trial. Eur J Heart Fail. 2012;14(3):302–11.

39. Asrani SK, Asrani NS, Freese DK, Phillips SD, Warnes CA, Heimbach J, et al. Congenital heart disease and the liver. Hepatology. 2012;56(3):1160–9.
40. Wu FM, Ukomadu C, Odze RD, Valente AM, Mayer Jr JE, Earing MG. Liver disease in the patient with Fontan circulation. Congenit Heart Dis. 2011;6(3):190–201.
41. Bergman M, Vitrai J, Salman H. Constrictive pericarditis: a reminder of a not so rare disease. Eur J Intern Med. 2006;17(7):457–64.
42. Kim MS, Kato TS, Farr M, Wu C, Givens RC, Collado E, et al. Hepatic dysfunction in ambulatory patients with heart failure: application of the MELD scoring system for outcome prediction. J Am Coll Cardiol. 2013;61(22):2253–61.
43. Shinagawa H, Inomata T, Koitabashi T, Nakano H, Takeuchi I, Naruke T, et al. Prognostic significance of increased serum bilirubin levels coincident with cardiac decompensation in chronic heart failure. Circ J. 2008;72(3):364–9.
44. van Deursen VM, Damman K, Hillege HL, van Beek AP, van Veldhuisen DJ, Voors AA. Abnormal liver function in relation to hemodynamic profile in heart failure patients. J Card Fail. 2010;16(1):84–90.
45. Wiesner R, Edwards E, Freeman R, Harper A, Kim R, Kamath P, et al. Model for end-stage liver disease (MELD) and allocation of donor livers. Gastroenterology. 2003;124(1):91–6.
46. Matthews JC, Pagani FD, Haft JW, Koelling TM, Naftel DC, Aaronson KD. Model for end-stage liver disease score predicts left ventricular assist device operative transfusion requirements, morbidity, and mortality. Circulation. 2010;121(2):214–20.
47. Chokshi A, Cheema FH, Schaefle KJ, Jiang J, Collado E, Shahzad K, et al. Hepatic dysfunction and survival after orthotopic heart transplantation: application of the MELD scoring system for outcome prediction. J Heart Lung Transplant. 2012;31(6):591–600.
48. Yang JA, Kato TS, Shulman BP, Takayama H, Farr M, Jorde UP, et al. Liver dysfunction as a predictor of outcomes in patients with advanced heart failure requiring ventricular assist device support: use of the Model of End-stage Liver Disease (MELD) and MELD eXcluding INR (MELD-XI) scoring system. J Heart Lung Transplant. 2012;31(6):601–10.
49. Giallourakis CC, Rosenberg PM, Friedman LS. The liver in heart failure. Clin Liver Dis. 2002;6(4):947–67, viii-ix.
50. Shorey J, Schenker S, Combes B. Effect of acute hypoxia on hepatic excretory function. Am J Physiol. 1969;216(6):1441–52.
51. Szwejkowski BR, Elder DH, Shearer F, Jack D, Choy AM, Pringle SD, et al. Pulmonary hypertension predicts all-cause mortality in patients with heart failure: a retrospective cohort study. Eur J Heart Fail. 2012;14(2):162–7.
52. Ghio S, Temporelli PL, Klersy C, Simioniuc A, Girardi B, Scelsi L, et al. Prognostic relevance of a non-invasive evaluation of right ventricular function and pulmonary artery pressure in patients with chronic heart failure. Eur J Heart Fail. 2013;15(4):408–14.
53. Valeriano V, Funaro S, Lionetti R, Riggio O, Pulcinelli G, Fiore P, et al. Modification of cardiac function in cirrhotic patients with and without ascites. Am J Gastroenterol. 2000;95 (11):3200–5.
54. Ates F, Topal E, Kosar F, Karincaoglu M, Yildirim B, Aksoy Y, et al. The relationship of heart rate variability with severity and prognosis of cirrhosis. Dig Dis Sci. 2006;51 (9):1614–18.
55. Kowalski HJ, Abelmann WH. The cardiac output at rest in Laennec's cirrhosis. J Clin Invest. 1953;32(10):1025–33.
56. Lee RF, Glenn TK, Lee SS. Cardiac dysfunction in cirrhosis. Best Pract Res Clin Gastroenterol. 2007;21(1):125–40.
57. Liu H, Lee SS. Nuclear factor-kappaB inhibition improves myocardial contractility in rats with cirrhotic cardiomyopathy. Liver Int. 2008;28(5):640–8.
58. Moller S, Henriksen JH. Cardiovascular complications of cirrhosis. Gut. 2008;57(2):268–78.
59. Krag A, Bendtsen F, Mortensen C, Henriksen JH, Moller S. Effects of a single terlipressin administration on cardiac function and perfusion in cirrhosis. Eur J Gastroenterol Hepatol. 2010;22(9):1085–92.

60. Glenn TK, Honar H, Liu H, ter Keurs HE, Lee SS. Role of cardiac myofilament proteins titin and collagen in the pathogenesis of diastolic dysfunction in cirrhotic rats. J Hepatol. 2011;55 (6):1249–55.
61. Bernardi M, Maggioli C, Dibra V, Zaccherini G. QT interval prolongation in liver cirrhosis: innocent bystander or serious threat? Expert Rev Gastroenterol Hepatol. 2012;6(1):57–66.
62. Krag A, Bendtsen F, Burroughs AK, Moller S. The cardiorenal link in advanced cirrhosis. Med Hypotheses. 2012;79(1):53–5.
63. Schrier RW. Decreased effective blood volume in edematous disorders: what does this mean? J Am Soc Nephrol. 2007;18(7):2028–31.
64. Moller S, Henriksen JH. Cirrhotic cardiomyopathy. J Hepatol. 2010;53(1):179–90.
65. Wong F, Girgrah N, Graba J, Allidina Y, Liu P, Blendis L. The cardiac response to exercise in cirrhosis. Gut. 2001;49(2):268–75.
66. Wong F. Cirrhotic cardiomyopathy. Hepatol Int. 2009;3(1):294–304.
67. Gaskari SA, Honar H, Lee SS. Therapy insight: cirrhotic cardiomyopathy. Nat Clin Pract Gastroenterol Hepatol. 2006;3(6):329–37.
68. Sola E, Gines P. Renal and circulatory dysfunction in cirrhosis: current management and future perspectives. J Hepatol. 2010;53(6):1135–45.
69. Saner FH, Neumann T, Canbay A, Treckmann JW, Hartmann M, Goerlinger K, et al. High brain-natriuretic peptide level predicts cirrhotic cardiomyopathy in liver transplant patients. Transplant Int. 2011;24(5):425–32.
70. Kazankov K, Holland-Fischer P, Andersen NH, Torp P, Sloth E, Aagaard NK, et al. Resting myocardial dysfunction in cirrhosis quantified by tissue Doppler imaging. Liver Int. 2011;31 (4):534–40.
71. Rabie RN, Cazzaniga M, Salerno F, Wong F. The use of E/A ratio as a predictor of outcome in cirrhotic patients treated with transjugular intrahepatic portosystemic shunt. Am J Gastroenterol. 2009;104(10):2458–66.
72. Bernardi M, Calandra S, Colantoni A, Trevisani F, Raimondo ML, Sica G, et al. Q-T interval prolongation in cirrhosis: prevalence, relationship with severity, and etiology of the disease and possible pathogenetic factors. Hepatology. 1998;27(1):28–34.
73. Day CP, James OF, Butler TJ, Campbell RW. QT prolongation and sudden cardiac death in patients with alcoholic liver disease. Lancet. 1993;341(8858):1423–8.
74. Ytting H, Henriksen JH, Fuglsang S, Bendtsen F, Moller S. Prolonged Q-T(c) interval in mild portal hypertensive cirrhosis. J Hepatol. 2005;43(4):637–44.
75. Trevisani F, Merli M, Savelli F, Valeriano V, Zambruni A, Riggio O, et al. QT interval in patients with non-cirrhotic portal hypertension and in cirrhotic patients treated with transjugular intrahepatic porto-systemic shunt. J Hepatol. 2003;38(4):461–7.
76. Zambruni A, Trevisani F, Caraceni P, Bernardi M. Cardiac electrophysiological abnormalities in patients with cirrhosis. J Hepatol. 2006;44(5):994–1002.
77. Ward CA, Ma Z, Lee SS, Giles WR. Potassium currents in atrial and ventricular myocytes from a rat model of cirrhosis. Am J Physiol. 1997;273(2 Pt 1):G537–44.
78. Henriksen JH, Bendtsen F, Hansen EF, Moller S. Acute non-selective beta-adrenergic blockade reduces prolonged frequency-adjusted Q-T interval (QTc) in patients with cirrhosis. J Hepatol. 2004;40(2):239–46.
79. Zambruni A, Trevisani F, Di Micoli A, Savelli F, Berzigotti A, Bracci E, et al. Effect of chronic beta-blockade on QT interval in patients with liver cirrhosis. J Hepatol. 2008;48 (3):415–21.
80. Trevisani F, Di Micoli A, Zambruni A, Biselli M, Santi V, Erroi V, et al. QT interval prolongation by acute gastrointestinal bleeding in patients with cirrhosis. Liver Int. 2012;32(10):1510–15.
81. Neuschwander-Tetri BA, Caldwell SH. Nonalcoholic steatohepatitis: summary of an AASLD single topic conference. Hepatology. 2003;37(5):1202–19.
82. Tiniakos DG, Vos MB, Brunt EM. Nonalcoholic fatty liver disease: pathology and pathogenesis. Annu Rev Pathol. 2010;5:145–71.

83. Targher G, Arcaro G. Non-alcoholic fatty liver disease and increased risk of cardiovascular disease. Atherosclerosis. 2007;191(2):235–40.
84. Targher G, Marra F, Marchesini G. Increased risk of cardiovascular disease in non-alcoholic fatty liver disease: causal effect or epiphenomenon? Diabetologia. 2008;51(11):1947–53.
85. Bhatia LS, Curzen NP, Calder PC, Byrne CD. Non-alcoholic fatty liver disease: a new and important cardiovascular risk factor? Eur Heart J. 2012;33(10):1190–200.
86. Brea A, Puzo J. Non-alcoholic fatty liver disease and cardiovascular risk. Int J Cardiol. 2013;167(4):1109–17.
87. Targher G, Day CP, Bonora E. Risk of cardiovascular disease in patients with nonalcoholic fatty liver disease. N Engl J Med. 2010;363(14):1341–50.
88. Ekstedt M, Franzen LE, Mathiesen UL, Thorelius L, Holmqvist M, Bodemar G, et al. Long-term follow-up of patients with NAFLD and elevated liver enzymes. Hepatology. 2006;44 (4):865–73.
89. Adams LA, Lymp JF, St Sauver J, Sanderson SO, Lindor KD, Feldstein A, et al. The natural history of nonalcoholic fatty liver disease: a population-based cohort study. Gastroenterology. 2005;129(1):113–21.
90. Rafiq N, Bai C, Fang Y, Srishord M, McCullough A, Gramlich T, et al. Long-term follow-up of patients with nonalcoholic fatty liver. Clin Gastroenterol Hepatol. 2009;7(2):234–8.
91. Soderberg C, Stal P, Askling J, Glaumann H, Lindberg G, Marmur J, et al. Decreased survival of subjects with elevated liver function tests during a 28-year follow-up. Hepatology. 2010;51 (2):595–602.
92. Musso G, Gambino R, Cassader M, Pagano G. Meta-analysis: natural history of non-alcoholic fatty liver disease (NAFLD) and diagnostic accuracy of non-invasive tests for liver disease severity. Ann Med. 2011;43(8):617–49.
93. Matteoni CA, Younossi ZM, Gramlich T, Boparai N, Liu YC, McCullough AJ. Nonalcoholic fatty liver disease: a spectrum of clinical and pathological severity. Gastroenterology. 1999;116(6):1413–19.
94. Dam-Larsen S, Franzmann M, Andersen IB, Christoffersen P, Jensen LB, Sorensen TI, et al. Long term prognosis of fatty liver: risk of chronic liver disease and death. Gut. 2004;53(5):750–5.
95. Targher G, Bertolini L, Rodella S, Tessari R, Zenari L, Lippi G, et al. Nonalcoholic fatty liver disease is independently associated with an increased incidence of cardiovascular events in type 2 diabetic patients. Diabetes Care. 2007;30(8):2119–21.
96. Jepsen P, Vilstrup H, Moller JK, Sorensen HT. Prognosis of patients with liver cirrhosis and spontaneous bacterial peritonitis. Hepatogastroenterology. 2003;50(54):2133–6.
97. Hamaguchi M, Kojima T, Takeda N, Nagata C, Takeda J, Sarui H, et al. Nonalcoholic fatty liver disease is a novel predictor of cardiovascular disease. World J Gastroenterol. 2007;13 (10):1579–84.
98. Haring R, Wallaschofski H, Nauck M, Dorr M, Baumeister SE, Volzke H. Ultrasonographic hepatic steatosis increases prediction of mortality risk from elevated serum gamma-glutamyl transpeptidase levels. Hepatology. 2009;50(5):1403–11.
99. Zhou YJ, Li YY, Nie YQ, Huang CM, Cao CY. Natural course of nonalcoholic fatty liver disease in southern China: a prospective cohort study. J Dig Dis. 2012;13(3):153–60.
100. Treeprasertsuk S, Leverage S, Adams LA, Lindor KD, St Sauver J, Angulo P. The Framingham risk score and heart disease in nonalcoholic fatty liver disease. Liver Int. 2012;32 (6):945–50.
101. Stepanova M, Younossi ZM. Independent association between nonalcoholic fatty liver disease and cardiovascular disease in the US population. Clin Gastroenterol Hepatol. 2012;10(6):646–50.
102. Lazo M, Hernaez R, Bonekamp S, Kamel IR, Brancati FL, Guallar E, et al. Non-alcoholic fatty liver disease and mortality among US adults: prospective cohort study. BMJ. 2011;343: d6891.

103. Ruttmann E, Brant LJ, Concin H, Diem G, Rapp K, Ulmer H, et al. Gamma-glutamyltransferase as a risk factor for cardiovascular disease mortality: an epidemiological investigation in a cohort of 163,944 Austrian adults. Circulation. 2005;112(14):2130–7.
104. Lee DH, Silventoinen K, Hu G, Jacobs Jr DR, Jousilahti P, Sundvall J, et al. Serum gamma-glutamyltransferase predicts non-fatal myocardial infarction and fatal coronary heart disease among 28,838 middle-aged men and women. Eur Heart J. 2006;27(18):2170–6.
105. Schindhelm RK, Dekker JM, Nijpels G, Bouter LM, Stehouwer CD, Heine RJ, et al. Alanine aminotransferase predicts coronary heart disease events: a 10-year follow-up of the Hoorn Study. Atherosclerosis. 2007;191(2):391–6.
106. Wannamethee SG, Lennon L, Shaper AG. The value of gamma-glutamyltransferase in cardiovascular risk prediction in men without diagnosed cardiovascular disease or diabetes. Atherosclerosis. 2008;201(1):168–75.
107. Fraser A, Harris R, Sattar N, Ebrahim S, Smith GD, Lawlor DA. Gamma-glutamyltransferase is associated with incident vascular events independently of alcohol intake: analysis of the British Women's Heart and Health study and meta-analysis. Arterioscler Thromb Vasc Biol. 2007;27(12):2729–35.
108. Dunn W, Xu R, Wingard DL, Rogers C, Angulo P, Younossi ZM, et al. Suspected nonalcoholic fatty liver disease and mortality risk in a population-based cohort study. Am J Gastroenterol. 2008;103(9):2263–71.
109. Goessling W, Massaro JM, Vasan RS, D'Agostino Sr RB, Ellison RC, Fox CS. Aminotransferase levels and 20-year risk of metabolic syndrome, diabetes, and cardiovascular disease. Gastroenterology. 2008;135(6):1935–44, 44 e1.
110. Ruhl CE, Everhart JE. Elevated serum alanine aminotransferase and gamma-glutamyltransferase and mortality in the United States population. Gastroenterology. 2009;136(2):477–85 e11.
111. Yun KE, Shin CY, Yoon YS, Park HS. Elevated alanine aminotransferase levels predict mortality from cardiovascular disease and diabetes in Koreans. Atherosclerosis. 2009;205 (2):533–7.
112. Angulo P. Nonalcoholic fatty liver disease. N Engl J Med. 2002;346(16):1221–31.
113. Kotronen A, Yki-Jarvinen H. Fatty liver: a novel component of the metabolic syndrome. Arterioscler Thromb Vasc Biol. 2008;28(1):27–38.
114. de Alwis NM, Day CP. Non-alcoholic fatty liver disease: the mist gradually clears. J Hepatol. 2008;48 Suppl 1:S104–12.
115. Bae JC, Rhee EJ, Lee WY, Park SE, Park CY, Oh KW, et al. Combined effect of nonalcoholic fatty liver disease and impaired fasting glucose on the development of type 2 diabetes: a 4-year retrospective longitudinal study. Diabetes Care. 2011;34(3):727–9.
116. Lopez-Suarez A, Guerrero JM, Elvira-Gonzalez J, Beltran-Robles M, Canas-Hormigo F, Bascunana-Quirell A. Nonalcoholic fatty liver disease is associated with blood pressure in hypertensive and nonhypertensive individuals from the general population with normal levels of alanine aminotransferase. Eur J Gastroenterol Hepatol. 2011;23(11):1011–17.
117. Yilmaz Y, Alahdab YO, Yonal O, Kurt R, Kedrah AE, Celikel CA, et al. Microalbuminuria in nondiabetic patients with nonalcoholic fatty liver disease: association with liver fibrosis. Metabolism. 2010;59(9):1327–30.
118. Targher G, Bertolini L, Rodella S, Lippi G, Zoppini G, Chonchol M. Relationship between kidney function and liver histology in subjects with nonalcoholic steatohepatitis. Clin J Am Soc Nephrol. 2010;5(12):2166–71.
119. Arase Y, Suzuki F, Kobayashi M, Suzuki Y, Kawamura Y, Matsumoto N, et al. The development of chronic kidney disease in Japanese patients with non-alcoholic fatty liver disease. Intern Med. 2011;50(10):1081–7.
120. Chin K, Nakamura T, Takahashi K, Sumi K, Ogawa Y, Masuzaki H, et al. Effects of obstructive sleep apnea syndrome on serum aminotransferase levels in obese patients. Am J Med. 2003;114(5):370–6.

121. Marin JM, Carrizo SJ, Vicente E, Agusti AG. Long-term cardiovascular outcomes in men with obstructive sleep apnoea-hypopnoea with or without treatment with continuous positive airway pressure: an observational study. Lancet. 2005;365(9464):1046–53.
122. Gottlieb DJ, Yenokyan G, Newman AB, O'Connor GT, Punjabi NM, Quan SF, et al. Prospective study of obstructive sleep apnea and incident coronary heart disease and heart failure: the sleep heart health study. Circulation. 2010;122(4):352–60.
123. Kotronen A, Westerbacka J, Bergholm R, Pietilainen KH, Yki-Jarvinen H. Liver fat in the metabolic syndrome. J Clin Endocrinol Metab. 2007;92(9):3490–7.
124. Korenblat KM, Fabbrini E, Mohammed BS, Klein S. Liver, muscle, and adipose tissue insulin action is directly related to intrahepatic triglyceride content in obese subjects. Gastroenterology. 2008;134(5):1369–75.
125. Peterson LR. Obesity and insulin resistance: effects on cardiac structure, function, and substrate metabolism. Curr Hypertens Rep. 2006;8(6):451–6.
126. Fabbrini E, Magkos F, Mohammed BS, Pietka T, Abumrad NA, Patterson BW, et al. Intrahepatic fat, not visceral fat, is linked with metabolic complications of obesity. Proc Natl Acad Sci U S A. 2009;106(36):15430–5.
127. Sung KC, Ryan MC, Kim BS, Cho YK, Kim BI, Reaven GM. Relationships between estimates of adiposity, insulin resistance, and nonalcoholic fatty liver disease in a large group of nondiabetic Korean adults. Diabetes Care. 2007;30(8):2113–18.
128. Petersen KF, Dufour S, Savage DB, Bilz S, Solomon G, Yonemitsu S, et al. The role of skeletal muscle insulin resistance in the pathogenesis of the metabolic syndrome. Proc Natl Acad Sci U S A. 2007;104(31):12587–94.
129. Sacks HS, Fain JN. Human epicardial adipose tissue: a review. Am Heart J. 2007;153 (6):907–17.
130. Kankaanpaa M, Lehto HR, Parkka JP, Komu M, Viljanen A, Ferrannini E, et al. Myocardial triglyceride content and epicardial fat mass in human obesity: relationship to left ventricular function and serum free fatty acid levels. J Clin Endocrinol Metab. 2006;91(11):4689–95.
131. Iacobellis G, Pellicelli AM, Grisorio B, Barbarini G, Leonetti F, Sharma AM, et al. Relation of epicardial fat and alanine aminotransferase in subjects with increased visceral fat. Obesity. 2008;16(1):179–83.
132. Iacobellis G, Lonn E, Lamy A, Singh N, Sharma AM. Epicardial fat thickness and coronary artery disease correlate independently of obesity. Int J Cardiol. 2011;146(3):452–4.
133. Semenkovich CF. Insulin resistance and atherosclerosis. J Clin Invest. 2006;116(7):1813–22.
134. Yilmaz Y, Kurt R, Yonal O, Polat N, Celikel CA, Gurdal A, et al. Coronary flow reserve is impaired in patients with nonalcoholic fatty liver disease: association with liver fibrosis. Atherosclerosis. 2010;211(1):182–6.
135. Villanova N, Moscatiello S, Ramilli S, Bugianesi E, Magalotti D, Vanni E, et al. Endothelial dysfunction and cardiovascular risk profile in nonalcoholic fatty liver disease. Hepatology. 2005;42(2):473–80.
136. Senturk O, Kocaman O, Hulagu S, Sahin T, Aygun C, Konduk T, et al. Endothelial dysfunction in Turkish patients with non-alcoholic fatty liver disease. Intern Med J. 2008;38 (3):183–9.
137. Vlachopoulos C, Manesis E, Baou K, Papatheodoridis G, Koskinas J, Tiniakos D, et al. Increased arterial stiffness and impaired endothelial function in nonalcoholic fatty liver disease: a pilot study. Am J Hypertens. 2010;23(11):1183–9.
138. Salvi P, Ruffini R, Agnoletti D, Magnani E, Pagliarani G, Comandini G, et al. Increased arterial stiffness in nonalcoholic fatty liver disease: the Cardio-GOOSE study. J Hypertens. 2010;28(8):1699–707.
139. Targher G, Bertolini L, Padovani R, Rodella S, Zoppini G, Zenari L, et al. Relations between carotid artery wall thickness and liver histology in subjects with nonalcoholic fatty liver disease. Diabetes Care. 2006;29(6):1325–30.

140. Kim HC, Kim DJ, Huh KB. Association between nonalcoholic fatty liver disease and carotid intima-media thickness according to the presence of metabolic syndrome. Atherosclerosis. 2009;204(2):521–5.
141. Fracanzani AL, Burdick L, Raselli S, Pedotti P, Grigore L, Santorelli G, et al. Carotid artery intima-media thickness in nonalcoholic fatty liver disease. Am J Med. 2008;121(1):72–8.
142. Volzke H, Robinson DM, Kleine V, Deutscher R, Hoffmann W, Ludemann J, et al. Hepatic steatosis is associated with an increased risk of carotid atherosclerosis. World J Gastroenterol. 2005;11(12):1848–53.
143. Targher G, Bertolini L, Padovani R, Zenari L, Zoppini G, Falezza G. Relation of nonalcoholic hepatic steatosis to early carotid atherosclerosis in healthy men: role of visceral fat accumulation. Diabetes Care. 2004;27(10):2498–500.
144. Chen CH, Nien CK, Yang CC, Yeh YH. Association between nonalcoholic fatty liver disease and coronary artery calcification. Dig Dis Sci. 2010;55(6):1752–60.
145. Akabame S, Hamaguchi M, Tomiyasu K, Tanaka M, Kobayashi-Takenaka Y, Nakano K, et al. Evaluation of vulnerable coronary plaques and non-alcoholic fatty liver disease (NAFLD) by 64-detector multislice computed tomography (MSCT). Circ J. 2008;72 (4):618–25.
146. Assy N, Djibre A, Farah R, Grosovski M, Marmor A. Presence of coronary plaques in patients with nonalcoholic fatty liver disease. Radiology. 2010;254(2):393–400.
147. Arslan U, Turkoglu S, Balcioglu S, Tavil Y, Karakan T, Cengel A. Association between nonalcoholic fatty liver disease and coronary artery disease. Coron Artery Dis. 2007;18 (6):433–6.
148. Acikel M, Sunay S, Koplay M, Gundogdu F, Karakelleoglu S. Evaluation of ultrasonographic fatty liver and severity of coronary atherosclerosis, and obesity in patients undergoing coronary angiography. Anadolu Kardiyoloji Dergisi: AKD Anatol J Cardiol. 2009;9 (4):273–9.
149. Mirbagheri SA, Rashidi A, Abdi S, Saedi D, Abouzari M. Liver: an alarm for the heart? Liver Int. 2007;27(7):891–4.
150. Alper AT, Hasdemir H, Sahin S, Onturk E, Akyol A, Nurkalem Z, et al. The relationship between nonalcoholic fatty liver disease and the severity of coronary artery disease in patients with metabolic syndrome. Turk Kardiyoloji Dernegi Arsivi: Turk Kardiyoloji Derneginin Yayin Organidir. 2008;36(6):376–81.
151. Fallo F, Dalla Pozza A, Sonino N, Lupia M, Tona F, Federspil G, et al. Non-alcoholic fatty liver disease is associated with left ventricular diastolic dysfunction in essential hypertension. Nutr Metab Cardiovasc Dis: NMCD. 2009;19(9):646–53.
152. Goland S, Shimoni S, Zornitzki T, Knobler H, Azoulai O, Lutaty G, et al. Cardiac abnormalities as a new manifestation of nonalcoholic fatty liver disease: echocardiographic and tissue Doppler imaging assessment. J Clin Gastroenterol. 2006;40(10):949–55.
153. Fotbolcu H, Yakar T, Duman D, Karaahmet T, Tigen K, Cevik C, et al. Impairment of the left ventricular systolic and diastolic function in patients with non-alcoholic fatty liver disease. Cardiol J. 2010;17(5):457–63.
154. Witteles RM, Fowler MB. Insulin-resistant cardiomyopathy clinical evidence, mechanisms, and treatment options. J Am Coll Cardiol. 2008;51(2):93–102.
155. Lautamaki R, Borra R, Iozzo P, Komu M, Lehtimaki T, Salmi M, et al. Liver steatosis coexists with myocardial insulin resistance and coronary dysfunction in patients with type 2 diabetes. Am J Physiol Endocrinol Metab. 2006;291(2):E282–90.
156. Perseghin G, Lattuada G, De Cobelli F, Esposito A, Belloni E, Ntali G, et al. Increased mediastinal fat and impaired left ventricular energy metabolism in young men with newly found fatty liver. Hepatology. 2008;47(1):51–8.
157. Fraser A, Harris R, Sattar N, Ebrahim S, Davey Smith G, Lawlor DA. Alanine aminotransferase, gamma-glutamyltransferase, and incident diabetes: the British Women's Heart and Health Study and meta-analysis. Diabetes Care. 2009;32(4):741–50.

158. George A, Figueredo VM. Alcoholic cardiomyopathy: a review. J Card Fail. 2011;17(10):844–9.
159. Gramenzi A, Caputo F, Biselli M, Kuria F, Loggi E, Andreone P, et al. Review article: alcoholic liver disease--pathophysiological aspects and risk factors. Aliment Pharmacol Ther. 2006;24(8):1151–61.
160. Corrao G, Bagnardi V, Zambon A, Torchio P. Meta-analysis of alcohol intake in relation to risk of liver cirrhosis. Alcohol Alcohol. 1998;33(4):381–92.
161. Rehm J, Taylor B, Mohapatra S, Irving H, Baliunas D, Patra J, et al. Alcohol as a risk factor for liver cirrhosis: a systematic review and meta-analysis. Drug Alcohol Rev. 2010;29(4):437–45.
162. European Association for the Study of L. EASL clinical practical guidelines: management of alcoholic liver disease. J Hepatol. 2012;57(2):399–420.
163. Costanzo S, Di Castelnuovo A, Donati MB, Iacoviello L, de Gaetano G. Wine, beer or spirit drinking in relation to fatal and non-fatal cardiovascular events: a meta-analysis. Eur J Epidemiol. 2011;26(11):833–50.
164. Matsumori A. Hepatitis C, virus infection and cardiomyopathies. Circ Res. 2005;96(2):144–7.
165. Omura T, Yoshiyama M, Hayashi T, Nishiguchi S, Kaito M, Horiike S, et al. Core protein of hepatitis C virus induces cardiomyopathy. Circ Res. 2005;96(2):148–50.
166. Adinolfi LE, Restivo L, Zampino R, Guerrera B, Lonardo A, Ruggiero L, et al. Chronic HCV infection is a risk of atherosclerosis. Role of HCV and HCV-related steatosis. Atherosclerosis. 2012;221(2):496–502.
167. Miyajima I, Kawaguchi T, Fukami A, Nagao Y, Adachi H, Sasaki S, et al. Chronic HCV infection was associated with severe insulin resistance and mild atherosclerosis: a population-based study in an HCV hyperendemic area. J Gastroenterol. 2013;48(1):93–100.
168. Patane S, Marte F, Sturiale M, Dattilo G, Albanese A. Myocarditis and cardiomyopathy HIV associated. Int J Cardiol. 2011;146(3):e56–7.
169. Zubiaurre L, Zapata E, Bujanda L, Castillo M, Oyarzabal I, Gutierrez-Stampa MA, et al. Cytomegalovirus hepatitis and myopericarditis. World J Gastroenterol. 2007;13(4):647–8.
170. Malavige GN, Fernando S, Fernando DJ, Seneviratne SL. Dengue viral infections. Postgrad Med J. 2004;80(948):588–601.
171. Herr J, Mehrfar P, Schmiedel S, Wichmann D, Brattig NW, Burchard GD, et al. Reduced cardiac output in imported Plasmodium falciparum malaria. Malar J. 2011;10:160.
172. Kitamura Y, Motoi M, Terada T. An autopsy case of ancient sarcoidosis associated with severe fibrosis in the liver and heart. Pathol Int. 1998;48(7):536–41.
173. Hegazi MO, Ahmed S. Atypical clinical manifestations of graves' disease: an analysis in depth. J Thyroid Res. 2012;2012:768019.
174. Ripoll C, Yotti R, Bermejo J, Banares R. The heart in liver transplantation. J Hepatol. 2011;54(4):810–22.
175. Hlubocka Z, Marecek Z, Linhart A, Kejkova E, Pospisilova L, Martasek P, et al. Cardiac involvement in Wilson disease. J Inherit Metab Dis. 2002;25(4):269–77.
176. Dungu JN, Anderson LJ, Whelan CJ, Hawkins PN. Cardiac transthyretin amyloidosis. Heart. 2012;98(21):1546–54.

Chapter 10
Liver and Lung Diseases: Hepatopulmonary Syndrome and Portopulmonary Hypertension

Mitsuru Munakata

Abstract Interactions of the liver and lung are observed in several pathological conditions. These interactions are classified into three types. In such as hypoxic hepatitis and nonalcoholic fatty liver disorder in the patients with obstructive sleep apnea, the functional abnormalities of the respiratory system, hypoxemia in this disorder, cause liver abnormalities. In sarcoidosis and α1-antitrypsin deficiency, both the lung and liver are affected together by the common underlying pathologies. And, the well-known and most unique interactions between the lung and liver are observed in hepatopulmonary syndrome and portopulmonary hypertension. Hepatopulmonary syndrome is characterized by the presence of liver disease and/or portal hypertension, increased alveolar-arterial oxygen gradient, and the evidence of intrapulmonary vascular dilatations. Portopulmonary hypertension is characterized by the combination of pulmonary hypertension and portal hypertension with or without liver diseases. Since these two diseases have very unique pathophysiology and significantly affect the quality of life and prognosis of the patients, in this chapter, recent understanding of their clinical manifestation, pathophysiology, diagnostic strategy, and treatment will be discussed.

Keywords Portal hypertension • Liver cirrhosis • Hypoxemia • Pulmonary hypertension

10.1 Introduction

The basic function of the lung is to extract and uptake oxygen from the atmosphere and to eliminate carbon dioxide, by-product of energy production using oxygen, to the atmosphere. To maintain its function, ambient air must pass deep through the airways to reach the alveoli. In addition, it must come very close to the alveolar wall

M. Munakata (✉)
Department of Pulmonary Medicine, School of Medicine, Fukushima Medical University, Hikarigaoka-1, Fukushima City 960-1295, Japan
e-mail: munakata@fmu.ac.jp

H. Ohira (ed.), *The Liver in Systemic Diseases*, DOI 10.1007/978-4-431-55790-6_10

for oxygen to be transferred to the hemoglobin contained in red blood cells (RBC). The distance between alveolar air and RBC is several angstroms, and this is the width between outer gaseous environment and our inner aqueous environment. Because of such structures, the lung is quite vulnerable to the stimuli both from outer environment and inner aqueous environment. And, large amount of fresh air, roughly estimated as 9,000 L, must come into and go out of the lung every day. In addition, almost all the blood pumped out from the left heart must pass the lung during each cycle.

These characteristics connect the lung and liver tightly and cause several comorbidities. Such relations are classified into three types. First is that the functional abnormality of the lung, such as hypoxemia, affects the liver. Hypoxic hepatitis, also known as ischemic hepatitis, is well recognized during acute and chronic respiratory failure and congestive heart failure [1]. Recently, obstructive sleep apnea (OSA) has been known to associate with nonalcoholic fatty liver disorder (NAFLD) [2]. Second is that both the lung and liver are affected together by common underlying pathologies. α1-Antitrypsin deficiency is a genetic disorder clinically characterized by liver disease and early onset pulmonary emphysema [3]. In sarcoidosis, systemic granulomatous disease affects a variety of organs including the lung and liver [4]. The final one is that the functional abnormality of hepatobiliary system affects the respiratory system. The well-known and the most unique interactions are hepatopulmonary syndrome and portopulmonary hypertension seen in patients with liver diseases and portal hypertension. In this section, these two very unique interactions between the lung and liver will be discussed.

10.2 Hepatopulmonary Syndrome (HPS)

10.2.1 Definition and Epidemiology

Since the first case report by Fluckiger M. in 1884, it has been recognized that the patients with liver cirrhosis and portal hypertension were sometimes associated with clubbed fingers and severe hypoxemia without overt ventilator abnormality. In 1977, Kennedy and Knudson reported a similar case and proposed the term hepatopulmonary syndrome (HPS) for such combination of signs, by analogy to hepatorenal syndrome [5]. Now, it is usually defined as an arterial oxygenation defect induced by intrapulmonary vascular dilatations (IPVD) associated with hepatic disease [6, 7]. Diagnostic criteria consisted of the following three characteristics: the presence of liver disease and/or portal hypertension, increased alveolar-arterial oxygen gradient (A-aDO2 $>$15 mmHg), and the evidence of IPVD [7].

Several underling abnormalities of hepatobiliary systems are known to be associated with HPS. The most common abnormality is portal hypertension with or without liver cirrhosis. However, HPS is also associated with portal hypertension with extrahepatic obstruction, acute or chronic hepatitis, and Budd-Chiari syndrome [8–10]. Reported incidences of HSP in patients with liver diseases have wide variation, in the range of 4–47 %. Fairly reliable data were reported by Abrams et al. [11]. They examined 40 consecutive patients with biopsy-proven liver cirrhosis by microbubble transthoracic echocardiography (MTTE), lung perfusion scan, pulmonary function tests, and arterial blood gas analysis. Fifteen of 40 patients (38 %) had positive MTTE, and 11 of 15 MTTE positive patients had abnormal A-aDO2 (>15 mmHg), but 4 of these 11 patients showed abnormal ventilator function, suggesting coexisting lung diseases such as chronic obstructing lung disease and interstitial pneumonia. Accordingly, the incidence of pure HPS was 17.5 % (7 out of 40 patients with liver cirrhosis).

10.2.2 Pathophysiology

10.2.2.1 Pulmonary Functional Abnormality

The major functional abnormality in the lung is impaired pulmonary gas exchange, especially oxygen extraction, resulting in hypoxemia and increased A-aDO2. This is estimated to be caused mainly by intrapulmonary arteriovenous shunting and capillary vasodilation. Theoretically, such structural changes can cause right to left shunt, ventilation-perfusion (V/Q) mismatch, and diffusion limitation. Melot et al. examined ten patients with liver cirrhosis, although all of them were smokers, applying multiple inert gas exchange method, and revealed that the major cause of hypoxemia is due to V/A mismatching [12]. However, hypoxemia seen in HPS, especially the severe one, usually shows only limited responses to oxygen supplementation therapy, suggesting the importance of right to left shunt as a mechanism of pulmonary exchange abnormality [13]. In some cases, a lack of hypoxic constriction of pulmonary vascular system was reported [14]. It is speculated to be due to the existence of vasodilatory substances in the blood of these patients. Interestingly, such defect in hypoxic vasoconstriction can be reversed by the time [15].

Some patients show reduced diffusion capacity of carbon monoxide (DLco), and it is caused by expanded distance from alveolar air to red blood cells due to severe capillary dilatation. Other pulmonary function tests including spirogram and lung volume are typically normal in HPS. Abnormalities in these tests suggest possible existence of concomitant pulmonary diseases.

10.2.2.2 Structural Abnormality of the Lung

In the lung of the patients with HPS, several pathological abnormalities have been reported, although limited number of report are available [16, 17]. The most characteristic finding is the dilatation of capillary vessels in alveolar regions (Fig. 10.1). Other findings include diffuse or localized dilatation of alveolar

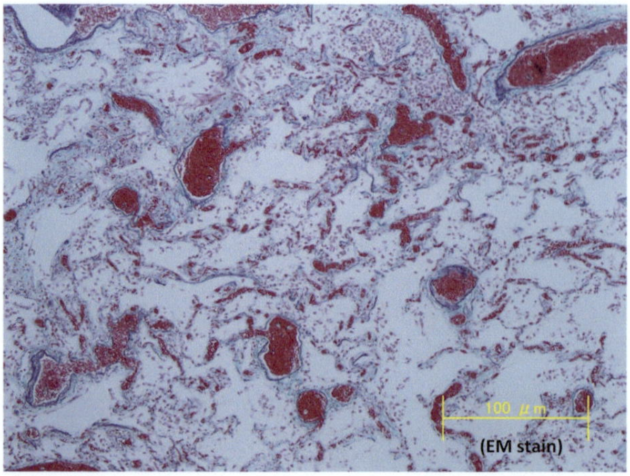

Fig. 10.1 Histopathological findings observed in the lung of the patient with HPS. The dilatations of capillary and precapillary vessels filled with red blood cells are observed in alveolar regions

precapillary and post-capillary vessels, pleural surface and intrapulmonary arterio-venous communications, and portopulmonary venous anastomosis [16]. In addition, pulmonary architecture is usually intact, and no thickening of the connective tissue of the lung and fibrosis is observed [17].

10.2.2.3 Pathogenesis

Although basic mechanism of HPS has not been clarified fully, it is believed to be due to modulation of pulmonary vasculature by the factors either produced or metabolized in the liver. This mechanism is suggested by the facts that underling hepatobiliary disease is not only liver cirrhosis but also portal hypertension without cirrhosis and acute liver dysfunction due to hepatitis. Mechanisms of HPS have been studied by animal models mainly chronic common bile duct ligation (CBDL) in rodents. Results of such experiments suggested that nitric oxide (NO)- and carbon monoxide (CO)-mediated vasodilation and vascular endothelial growth factor (VEGF)-mediated angiogenesis play important roles in the development of HPS [18].

There are evidences suggesting the increase in circulating endothelin-1 (ET-1) levels in both experimental and human HPS. The main source of overproduced ET-1 is estimated to be biliary epithelium (cholangiocytes) [19]. ET-1 binds to ET-1B receptors of pulmonary endothelial cells to induce endothelial nitric oxide synthase (eNOS) activation and release of NO, resulting in pulmonary vasodilation. Endotoxemia due to intestinal bacterial translocation with impaired liver endotoxin clearance leads to recruitment and activation of pulmonary vascular monocytes and macrophages to produce pro-inflammatory cytokine such as tumor necrosis factor alpha (TNF-α) and activation of VEGF pathways. TNF-α activates inducible nitric oxide synthase (iNOS) in macrophages to produce NO, a potent vasodilator. It is also known that, in rodent model of HPS, heme oxygenase (HO) is activated and releases CO, which is also a potent vasodilator [20]. In HPS patients, elevated exhaled NO and arterial carboxyhemoglobin levels have been reported [21, 22]. These gasomediators are believed to play a major role in pulmonary vasodilatation seen in HPS patients.

In rodent CBDL model, pulmonary angiogenesis is also observed and the following mechanisms are suggested. Increased TNF-α signaling results in the accumulation of pulmonary intravascular monocytes. This leads to the activation of VEGF-dependent signal pathways to increase endothelial cell survival and proliferation and results in pulmonary angiogenesis.

10.2.3 Diagnosis

10.2.3.1 Symptom and Sign

Dyspnea on exertion (DOE) is the most common symptom of HPS with hypoxemia. However, sensation of dyspnea during hypoxemia and hypoxic ventilatory responses is variable among each individual, and there are some patients with severe hypoxemia without complaining dyspnea. Characteristically, dyspnea is increased in their upright position (called "platypnea"). This is due to the decrease in PaO2 after changing position from supine to upright (called "orthodeoxia"). It is caused by the heterogeneous redistribution of blood flow to lower lung zones with prominent IPVD in upright position, resulting in an increase in intrapulmonary shunt and in areas with low V/Q ratio [23]. In advanced HPS patients, spider naevi, digital clubbing, and cyanosis of nail beds are frequently observed.

10.2.3.2 Diagnostic Strategy

Diagnosis of HPS is made by confirming the presence of three characteristics, the presence of liver disease and/or portal hypertension, increased alveolar-arterial oxygen gradient (A-aDO2 >15 mmHg), and the evidence of IPVD [7]. The presence of IPVD can be detected by perfusion lung scanning using ^{99m}Tc-macroaggregated albumin (MAA) and contrast-enhanced echocardiography using microbubbles (microbubble transthoracic echocardiography; MTTE). Due to the high sensitivity and specificity of MTTE, it is considered to be the gold standard for the detection of IPVD. Pulmonary angiography and chest computed tomography (CT) are also used to detect vascular abnormalities in HPS [7].

In the bedside, an approximate estimate of alveolar-arterial oxygen gradient (A-aDO2) can be obtained from arterial blood gas values (PaO2 and PaCO2) in the following way. Alveolar oxygen pressure (PAO2) = PIO2 – PaCO2/R, where PIO2 is the inhaled oxygen pressure. In usual ambient air breathing, PIO2 = [atmospheric pressure (760 mmHg) – saturated vapor pressure (47 mmHg)] × 0.21 = 150 mmHg. R is the respiratory exchange ratio and is around 0.8 in normal stable condition. So, **A-aDO2** = PAO2 – PaO2 = PIO2 – PaCO2/0.8 – PaO2 = **150 – PaCO2/0.8 – PaO2**. Recent blood gas analyzers can automatically calculate and report A-aDO2 values. For the diagnosis of HPS, A-aDO2 should be more than 15 mmHg. Severity grading of HPS was proposed by the European Respiratory Society Task Force and is determined by PaO2 values: mild (PaO2 >80 mmHg), moderate (PaO2 = 60–79- mmHg), severe (PaO2 = 59–50 mmHg), and very severe (PaO2 < 50 mmHg) [7].

In MAA scan, ^{99m}Tc-labeled MAA is injected in vein and whole-body scan is made. Particle size of MAA is generally between 10 and 90 μm (90 % of particles) and no particle is larger than 150 μm. Since the sizes of particles exceed those of alveolar capillary beds, normally, they are trapped in the pulmonary vascular network. In patients with IPVD, the particles pass through the pulmonary vascular beds and address to extrapulmonary organ such as the brain, kidneys, spleen, and liver (Fig. 10.2). A fraction of shunt can be also calculated by comparing the whole body and lung counts. It should be noticed that, from the methodological principles, it is not possible to differentiate intrapulmonary and intracardiac shunts.

In MTTE, usually, 10 ml of normal saline with microbubbles (made by hand agitation) is injected into peripheral vein. In normal subjects, microbubbles are trapped and absorbed by alveoli during the first pass and do not reach left heart. In contrast, in patients with IPVD, microbubbles are detected in the left atrium and ventricle within greater than three cardiac cycles (Fig. 10.3). In patients with intracardiac right to left shunt, microbubbles can be detected immediately after venous injection. So, MTTE can differentiate intrapulmonary and intracardiac shunts.

In pulmonary angiography, two types of abnormalities (minimal and advanced pattern) were reported [24]. In minimal pattern, diffuse spidery dilatation of peripheral lung was observed, and in advanced pattern, diffuse spongy appearance was observed. In some patients, discrete arteriovenous communications were also detected. In chest CT, the presence of significantly dilated peripheral pulmonary vasculature was reported (Fig. 10.4) and suggested to be helpful in the diagnosis of HSP [25].

10.2.4 Treatment

10.2.4.1 Pharmacological Treatment

Only few randomized control studies for HPS have been done, and no effective drug with high level of clinical evidence has been reported. On the basis of understanding of its pathophysiological mechanisms, several potentially useful drugs have been examined their effectiveness for small number of patients with HPS, and there are some agents showing clinical benefits [26].

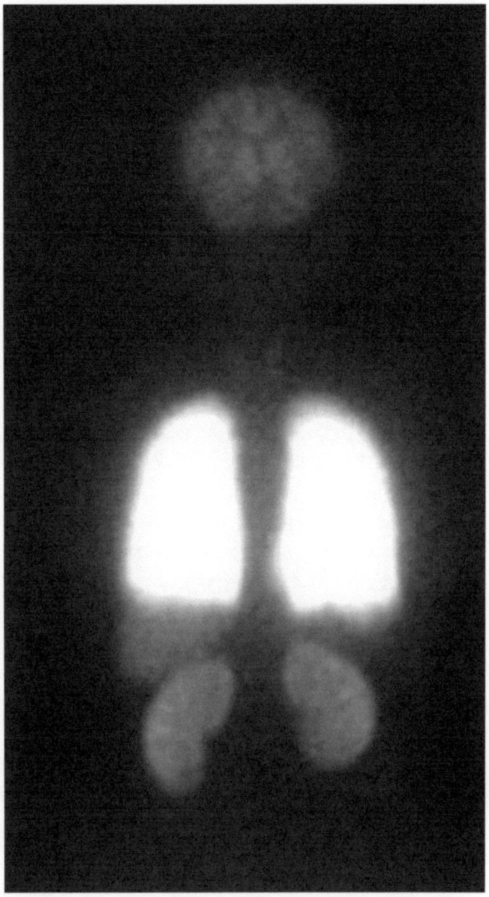

Fig. 10.2 ^{99m}Tc-labeled MAA scan of the patient with HPS. The particles pass through the pulmonary vascular beds and address to the brain and kidneys. In this case, calculated shunt fraction was 25 %

Pentoxifylline (PTX), a nonspecific phosphodiesterase inhibitor, has been suggested in rodent model of HPS to have anti-inflammatory properties by inhibiting several inflammatory cytokines including TNF-α, iNOS, and VEGF-A. There are three studies examining the effect of 400–1,200 mg per day of PTX on nine to ten patients with HPS. Improvement of PaO2 and A-aDO2 was observed in two studies, and improvement of clinical symptoms was observed in one of the two studies. In another study, neither improvement of PaO2 nor clinical symptom was observed.

Methylene blue (MB) inhibits the effect of NO by inhibiting soluble guanylate cyclase activity and has been reported to be useful in rodent model of HPS. There are three case reports showing some effect of bolus injection of MB in patients with HPS. Schenk et al. examined the effect of MB in seven patients with HSP whose PaO2 were less than 60 mmHg [27]. The patients received intravenously administration of 3 mg/kg of MB over 15 min. Five hours after MB administration, their PaO2 were increased significantly from 58 ± 2.5SD mmHg to 74 ± 11.5 mmHg.

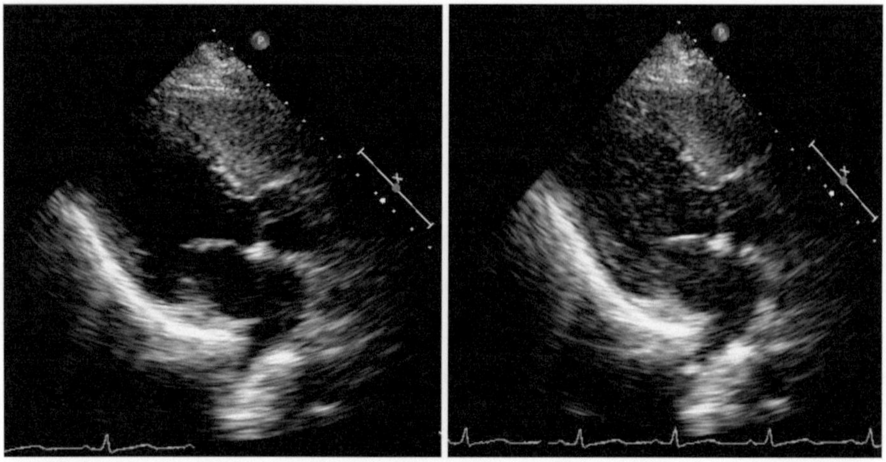

Fig. 10.3 Microbubble transthoracic echocardiography (MTTE) findings of the patients with HPS. Before the injection of microbubbles, the left atrium and ventricle are clearly observed (*right*). Three beats after injection, microbubbles are detected in the left atrium and ventricle (*left*)

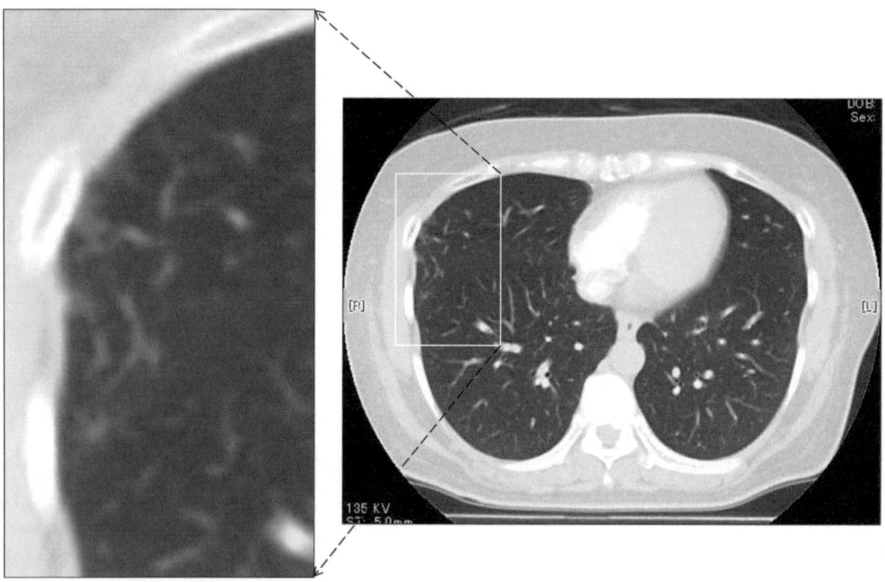

Fig. 10.4 Chest CT of the patients with HPS. Significantly dilated peripheral pulmonary vasculature was observed

In addition, improvement in A-aDO2 and reduction in shunt fraction were also observed. Although the result was quite encouraging, a randomized control trial examining the effect of MB in HPS has not been conducted.

Gomez et al. also looked at the effect of inhaled N^G-nitro-L-arginine methyl ester (L-NAME), a well-known inhibitor of NOSs (order of potency, iNOS > eNOS > nNOS), in patients with HPS [28]. They could demonstrate significant reduction in fractional exhaled nitric oxide (FeNO) and cardiac output and significant increase in systemic and pulmonary vascular resistance. However, there was no change in pulmonary gas exchange parameters including PaO2 and A-aDO2.

Garlic (*Allium sativum*), known as food or old herbal medicine, has been attracting some interests as a therapeutic option for HPS. In 1992, Caldwell et al. reported a case of HPS [29]. The patient was a 60-year-old female with HPS, who failed somatostatin therapy and also declined OLT. Instead of such treatment, she took large daily doses of garlic powder and experienced significant improvement of HPS. This case report stimulated clinical researchers to perform clinical trials. In 2010, a randomized controlled trial for garlic in HPS was conducted and reported by De et al. [30]. Twenty-one and 20 patients with HPS were randomly assigned to receive either oral garlic supplementation or placebo, respectively, and evaluated monthly over 9–18 months. After 9 months, PaO2 was significantly higher and A-aDO2 was significantly lower among patients with garlic compared to placebo. Reversal of HPS was observed in 14 of 21 patients (66.7 %) on garlic and in 1 of 20 patients (5 %) on placebo, suggesting beneficial effect of garlic supplementation for HPS. Since the chance of receiving liver transplantation is quite limited, further clinical trials are awaited to confirm such hopeful effects of garlic.

Other possible candidates for medical treatment for HPS are somatostatin analog, caffeic acid phenethyl ester (CAPE), mycophenolate mofetil (MMF), quercetin, sorafenib, iloprost, N-acetyl cysteine, etc. [26].

10.2.4.2 Non-pharmacological Treatment

Orthotopic Liver Transplantation (OLT)

So far, the most reliable treatment for HPS is orthotopic liver transplantation (OLT). In 2004 ERS Task Force Report for HPS, OLT was recommended for both adult and pediatric patients with HPS, and complete resolution of HPS was observed in more than 80 % of patients with HPS received OLT [7]. In a study of large series of HPS patients at Mayo Clinic [31], 5-year survival of the patients with HPS who did and did not undergo OLT were 76 % and 23 %, respectively, and that for control cirrhotic patients without HPS who did not undergo OLT was 63 %. Survival from the time of HPS diagnosis in those who subsequently underwent OLT was similar to control cirrhotic patients (having no HPS). These results suggest that the complication of HPS significantly affects survival of the patients with liver diseases, and OLT is the very effective treatment for HPS [31]. In recent large prospective study, Pascasio et al. analyzed 316 patients with liver cirrhosis who were evaluated for OLT in 2002–2007 [32]. The prevalence of HPS was 25.6 % (81/316 patients), although diagnostic criteria for HPS were slightly different: PaO2

<70 mmHg, A-aDO2 >20 mmHg at supine position, and positive MTTE. Forty-nine of 81 HPS patients and 128 of 235 patients without HPS received OLT. There was no significant difference in post-OLT survival between two groups. Improvement of pulmonary gas exchange abnormalities was observed in all of the patients 1 year after OLT, and in 96 % of the patients in the first 6 months after OLT, it suggested the reversibility of HPS by OLT [33].

Long-Term Oxygen Therapy (Home Oxygen Therapy)

In patients with severe HPS (PaO2 <60 mmHg), long-term oxygen therapy (or home oxygen therapy; HOT) should be considered [7]. Since right to left shunt through IPVD is one of the mechanisms of hypoxemia, improvement of hypoxemia by oxygen therapy may not be prominent in some patients. However, no systematic clinical trial to demonstrate the usefulness of HOT has been done. There was a report of two cases of HPS showing improvement of liver function after long-term oxygen therapy [33].

10.3 Portopulmonary Hypertension (PPHTN)

10.3.1 Definition an Epidemiology

Portopulmonary hypertension (PPHTN) is the combination of pulmonary hypertension and portal hypertension with or without liver diseases. Portal hypertension is defined by the presence of portal venous pressure more than 15 mmHg or portocaval gradient more than 5 mmHg [34]. Clinically, it is speculated by the presence of splenomegaly, portosystemic shunts, thrombocytopenia, or esophageal and gastric varices. The pulmonary hypertension observed in PPHTN is classified to the subtype of Group 1 pulmonary arterial hypertensions (PAH) (1.4.3) according to the 2013 Niece classification of pulmonary hypertension [35]. It is characterized by the presence of mean pulmonary pressure (mPAP)≥25 mmHg, mean pulmonary artery occlusion pressure (mPAOP) or pulmonary capillary wedge pressure (PCWP)<15 mmHg, and pulmonary vascular resistance (PVR)≥ 240 dyn•s•cm^{-5}.

Badesch et al. reported that 136 patients with PPHTN (10.6 %) were observed in 2,525 patients with all Group 1 PAH from the data of REVEAL registry, a large registry for pulmonary hypertension in the United States of America [36]. Similar incidence (10.4 %) of PPHTN in Group1 PHA was also reported from the data of pulmonary hypertension registry in France [37]. On the other hand, the incidence of PPHTN in the patients with portal hypertension has been reported to be 4–10 % [37, 38].

10.3.2 Pathophysiology

10.3.2.1 Histopathological Findings

The histopathological findings seen in pulmonary vasculature of PPHTN are similar to those of Group 1 pulmonary arterial hypertension, and it is not possible to distinguish PPHTN from other types of PAH. They include muscularization of small pulmonary arteries, intimal thickening, smooth muscle hypertrophy, in situ thrombosis, and plexiform lesions (a dilated pulmonary artery with the normal structure replaced by an intraluminal plexus of endothelial cells and slit-like vascular channels) [7, 39].

10.3.2.2 Pathophysiology

Precise mechanisms of PPHTN have not been clarified. Pulmonary circulation is a low-pressure system compared to the systemic one, and there are large reserves of capillary beds which are not usually recruited. Because of such large capillary reserve, the increase in cardiac output seen in patients with liver cirrhosis usually does not directly associated with pulmonary hypertension. Therefore, an imbalance between vasoconstrictors and vasodilators has been suggested one of the main mechanisms of PPTHN. Vasoproliferative process and vascular remodeling are also observed pathologically in PPHTN, and PPHTN is observed in the patients having portal hypertension with or without liver dysfunction; vasoactive factors bypassing the liver through portosystemic shunt have been speculated to play significantly roles [40]. Such factors include nitric oxide (NO), prostacyclin (prostaglandin I2; PGI2), endothelin-1 (ET-1), glucagon, serotonin, interleukin-1, and interleukin-6. In addition, only a small proportion of patients with portal hypertension develop PPHTN, and contribution of genetic factors associated with susceptibility to PPHTN has been speculated [41]. Furthermore, Lee et al. reported monoclonal endothelial cell proliferation in PPH and suggested the contribution of somatic genetic alteration similar to neoplastic process [42].

Coexistence of HPS and PPHTN is also noticed. Fussner et al. reported that IPVDs were detected in 20 of 34 patients (59 %) with HPS [43]. This suggested the existence of shared background mechanisms in HPS and PPHTN. Actually, the case reported by Kobayashi et al. [14] and Tanino et al. [15] was the same patient. He was a 52-year-old patient with liver cirrhosis and diagnosed as having HSP. At the first diagnosis of HPS, mPAP was 12 mmHg and PVR was 29 dyn•s•cm^{-5}. But both mPAP and PVR gradually increased, and 5 years after the diagnosis of HPS, they became 48 mmHg and 534 dyn•s•cm^{-5}, respectively, and he was diagnosed as having PPHTN. During his HPS periods, his PaO2 was around 60 mmHg with PaCO2 around 25 mmHg, but his hypoxemia was improved, and it was 83 mmHg when he was diagnosed as having PPHTN, suggesting the disappearance of IPVDs during this process.

10.3.3 Diagnosis

10.3.3.1 Symptoms and Signs

Clinical symptoms of PPHTN are similar to those of primary pulmonary hypertension except for those related to underling hepatobiliary abnormalities and portal hypertension. Relatively common symptoms include dyspnea on exertion and general fatigue. In advanced cases, chest pain or discomfort and syncope are sometimes observed. Physical signs of PPTHP are derived from pulmonary hypertension, right cardiac failure, and portal hypertension with or without liver dysfunction. An accentuated second heart sound and holosystolic murmur at the lower left sternal border due to tricuspid regurgitation are the signs of pulmonary hypertension. Typically, the murmur is enhanced during inspiration (called "Rivero-Carvallo sign"). A gallop rhythm, jugular venous distension, and peripheral edema are the signs of right heart failure. Hematemesis due to the rupture of esophageal and gastric varices and ascites are the signs of portal hypertension with or without liver dysfunction.

Transthoracic Doppler Echocardiography (TDE)

TDE is the most commonly used procedures to screen PPHTN. Major findings are enlarged right ventricle and atrium and left-side shift and/or paradoxical movement of ventricular septum. It is possible to estimate right ventricular systolic pressure (RSPV) from peak tricuspid regurgitant jet velocity by applying the modified Bernoulli's equation. There is a relatively good correlation between estimated RSPV by TDE and true RSPV measured by right heart catheterization (RHC). However, it is not possible to confirm the existence of pulmonary hypertension by TDE. In 2004 ERS Task Force Report, all patients with estimated RSPV more than 50 mmHg have been recommended to proceed to RHC [7]. Colle et al. proposed a cutoff value of estimated RSPV of 30 mmHg to detect PPHTN at an early stage [44]. Since the status of pulmonary hemodynamics may change over time and it also affects the indication of liver transplantation (LT), LT candidates are recommended to receive TDE annually [7, 45]. Recently, tricuspid annular plane systolic excursion (TAPSE) has also been recommended as a good marker reflecting the severity of PAH.

Right Heart Catheterization (RHC)

RHC is the most reliable examination to detect PPHTN. Using Swan-Ganz catheter inserted through the right or left jugular vein, systolic/diastolic/mean pulmonary arterial pressures, pulmonary capillary wedge pressure (PCWP), and mean right atrial pressure can be measured. Pulmonary vascular resistance (PVR) is calculated by the following formula: PVR = (mPAP − PCWP) × 80/cardiac output (CO). Staging of severity is proposed by ERS Task Force as follows: mild (25<mPAP<35 mmHg), moderate (35≤mPAP<45 mmHg), and severe (mPAP≥45 mmHg) [7].

Others

In chest roentgenogram, dilatation of the pulmonary artery trunk, the right and left main branches, and their larger central subdivisions are observed. The more peripheral vessels typically decrease abruptly in caliber. Signs of right ventricular hypertrophy are also observed. In electrocardiography, signs of right ventricular overload such as right axis deviation, increased R/S ratio (more than 1) in V1 and decreased R/S ratio (less than 1) in V5-6, and pulmonary P (increase in P wave height more than 0.25 mV) are observed. In chest CT, dilatation of the pulmonary artery trunk and the right and left main branches are also observed, and in the lung field, mosaic perfusion patterns are sometimes observed. It is important to confirm the absence of thrombus in the trunk and central pulmonary artery to distinguish from pulmonary hypertension owing to chronic thrombotic and/or embolic disease. Lung perfusion scanning (MAA scan) is normal or shows non-segmental low-perfusion areas and mottled pattern. Segmental perfusion defects with normal ventilation scanning indicate pulmonary hypertension due to chronic pulmonary thromboembolism.

10.3.4 Treatment

PPHTN has very poor prognosis without treatment. Its mean survival rate is about 15 months and the 6-month survival rate is around 50 %. Liver transplantation (LT) can reverse PAP, but mortality rate is high in patients with PPHTN [46]. For these reasons, LT is indicated only for the limited part of the patients with PPHTN. On the other hand, several new drugs have been developed for PAH, and high level clinical evidences have been accumulated gradually. They were also considered applicable for the patients with PPHTN. Although there is no randomized control study of such drug in patients with PPHTN, the prognosis and the quality of life of the patients seem to be improving.

10.3.4.1 Pharmacological Treatment

Prostacyclin and Its Derivatives

Intravenous prostacyclin (epoprostenol) induces pulmonary vascular dilation and also has antiplatelet-aggregating property and antiproliferative effect of vascular endothelium and smooth muscle. Improved pulmonary hemodynamics and increased exercise tolerance are reported in patients with PAH treated with epoprostenol [47]. Intravenous epoprostenol has been shown to improve pulmonary hemodynamics also in patients with PPHTN [48, 49]. But, significant improvement of long-term survival has not been demonstrated [49]. The requirement of a permanent central venous rout and continuous infusion pump and a risk of infection and hypotension raise the hurdle for the application of epoprostenol. For these reasons, prostacyclin is not recommended as a first-line treatment for PPHTN [18]. Recently, inhaled iloprost, a stable analog of prostacyclin having longer vasodilatory effect, was shown to be effective in patients with PAH [50]. In addition, beraprost, an orally active prostacyclin analog, has been shown to be effective for PAH [51]. However, the effect of inhaled iloprost and oral beraprost in patients with PPHTN has not been reported.

Endothelin Receptor Antagonist

Endothelin is a peptide derived from vascular endothelial cells and has potent vascular smooth muscle contractive and proliferative activities. Two types of receptors for endothelin-1, ET_A and ET_B, are known. Vascular smooth muscle cells have both ET_A and ET_B, and vascular endothelial cells have only ET_B. Bosentan, a dual inhibitor of endothelin-1 receptor (20:1 ET_A/ET_B selectivity) which can be administered orally, has been demonstrated to be effective in patients with PAH [52]. It shows significant improvement in NYHA functional class, 6-min walk distance, and pulmonary hemodynamics in patients with PPHTN without proving long-term effectiveness [53]. Ambrisentan, a more selective ET_A antagonist (100:1 ET_A/ET_B selectivity), was also reported to be useful for the patients with PPHTN [54]. It can be orally administered and its side effects, especially liver functional damage, are less than those of bosentan.

Modifiers of Nitric Oxide (NO) System

There are two types of modifiers of NO system available for the treatment of PAH. One is phosphodiesterase type 5 (PDE5) inhibitor. PDE5 inhibitor suppresses the degradation of cGMP produced through the activation of guanylate cyclase by NO. It can inhibit vascular smooth muscle contraction and proliferation. As PDE5 inhibitor, three types of drugs (sildenafil, vardenafil, and tadalafil) are available for PAH in Japan. In 2006, Reichenberger reported the usefulness of sildenafil with or without inhaled prostacyclin analogs in 14 patients with PPHTN [55]. So far, several case series supporting the effectiveness of vardenafil and tadalafil have also been reported [56, 57]. It is noteworthy that both vardenafil and tadalafil may improve portal hypertension in addition to pulmonary arterial pressure.

Riociguat is a soluble guanylate cyclase stimulator which has two action mechanisms in NO system. It acts in synergy with endogenous NO and also directly stimulates soluble guanylate cyclase. In clinical study for patients with PAH including those with PPHTN (11 of 309 PAH patients), it was shown to improve exercise capacity [58].

Others

For the patients with right-side heart failure, diuretics may be useful to reduce intravascular volume and hepatic congestion. Cardiac glycosides such as digoxin and β-blockers have some role in PAH, but their usefulness in PPHTN has not been clarified.

10.3.4.2 Non-pharmacological Treatment

Long-Term Oxygen Therapy (Home Oxygen Therapy (HOT))

For the patients with hypoxemia, long-term oxygen therapy (or HOT) is recommended. Hypoxemia induces hypoxic pulmonary vasoconstriction which increases pulmonary arterial pressure. Oxygen supplement is expected to reduce such vasoconstriction and pulmonary arterial pressure.

Orthotopic Liver Transplantation (OLT)

In general, OLT is not indicated or contraindicated for the patients with advanced PPHTN [7]. Krowka et al. reported the outcome of 43 patients with PPHTN who receive OLT [59]. Cardiopulmonary mortality in patients with mPAP≥50 mmHg was 100 %, and that in patients with 35≤mPAP<50 mmHg is 50 %. In patients with mPAP<35 mmHg, the mortality rate was 0 %. From these date, now OLT was indicated for the patients with mPAP<35 mmHg [7]. For the patients with mPAP≥35 mmHg, if medical treatments with vasodilatory agents reduce their mPAP under 35 mmHg, OLT may be indicated [34].

References

1. Henrion J, Schapira M, Luwaert R, Colin L, Delannoy A, Heller FR. Hypoxic hepatitis: clinical and hemodynamic study in 142 consecutive cases. Medicine. 2003;82:392–406.
2. Paschetta E, Belci P, Alisi A, Licccardo D, Cutrera R, Musso G, Nobili V. OSAS-related inflammatory mechanisms of the liver injury in nonalcoholic fatty liver disease. Mediators Inflamm. 2015. doi:10.1155/2015/815721.
3. Stoller JK, Aboussouan LS. α1-antitrypsin deficiency. Lancet. 2005;365:2225–36.
4. Kahi CJ, Saxena R, Temkit M, Canlas K, Roberts S, Knox K, Wilkes D, Kwo PY. Hepatobiliary disease in sarcoidosis. Sarcoidosis Vasc Diffuse Lung Dis. 2006;23:117–23.

5. Kennedy TC, Knudson RJ. Exercise-aggrevated hypoxemia and orthodeoxia in cirrhosis. Chest. 1997;72:305–9.
6. Lange PA, Stoller JK. The hepatopulmonary syndrome. Ann Intern Med. 1995;122:521–9.
7. Rodriguez-Roisin R, Krowka MJ, Herve P, Fallon MB. Pulmonary-hepatic vascular disorders (PHD). Eur Respir J. 2004;24:861–80.
8. Teuber G, Teupe C, Dietrich CF, Caspary WF, Buhl R, Zeuzem S. Pulmonary dysfunction in non-cirrhotic patients with chronic viral hepatitis. Eur J Intern Med. 2002;13:311–8.
9. Gupta D, Vijaya DR, Gupta R, Dhiman RK, Bhargava M, Vema J, Chawla YK. Prevalence of hepatopulmonary syndrome in cirrhosis an extrahepatic portal venous obstruction. Am J Gastroenterol. 2001;96:3395–9.
10. Regev A, Yeshurun M, Rodrigues M, Sagie A, Neff GW, Molina EG, Schiff ER. Transient hepatopulmonary syndrome in a patient with acute hepatitis. J Viral Hepat. 2001;8:83–6.
11. Abrams GA, Jaffe CC, Hoffer PB, Binder HJ, Fallon MB. Diagnostic utility of contrast echocardiography and lung perfusion scan in patients with hepatopulmonary syndrome. Gastroenterology. 1995;109:1283–8.
12. Melot C, Naeije R, Dechamps P, Hallemans R, Lejeune P. Pulmonary and extrapulmonary factors to hypoxemia in liver cirrhosis. Am Rev Respir Dis. 1989;139:632–40.
13. Edell ES, Cortese DA, Krowka MJ, Rehder K. Sever hypoxemia and live disease. Am Rev Respir Dis. 1989;140:1631–5.
14. Kobayashi S, Aida A, Aoi K, Nishimura M, Kawakami Y. Liver cirrhosis with severe hypoxemia and paradoxic pulmonary vascular response to graded inspiratory oxygen tension. Chest. 1993;103:958–60.
15. Tanino Y, Makita H, Tsujino I, Shinano H, Nishimura M. Chronological change in pulmonary vascular response to hypoxia in hepatopulmonary syndrome. Respiration. 2012;84:242–5.
16. Berthelot P, Wakler JG, Sherlock S, Reid L. Arterial changes in lung in cirrhosis of the liver – lung spider neve. N Engl J Med. 1966;274:291–8.
17. Schraufangel D, Kay J. Structural and pathologic changes in the lung vasculature in chronic liver disease. Clin Chest Med. 1996;17:1–15.
18. Raevens S, Geerts A, Van Steenkiste C, Verhelst X, Van Vlierberghe H, Colle I. Hepatopulmonary syndrome and portopulmonary hypertension: recent knowledge in pathogenesis and overview of clinical assessment. Liver Int. 2015;35:1646–60.
19. Yang W, Zhang J, Hu B, Wu W, Venter J, Aplini G, Fallon MB. The role of receptor tyrosine kinase activation in cholangiocytes and pulmonary vascular endothelium in experimental hepatopulmonary syndrome. Am J Physiol Gastrointest Liver Physiol. 2014;306:G72–80.
20. Zhang J, Ling Y, Luo B, Tang L, Ryter SW, Stockard CR, Grizzle WE, Fallon MB. Analysis of pulmonary heme oxygenase-1 and nitric oxide synthase alterations in experimental hepatopulmonary syndrome. Gastroenterology. 2003;125:1441–51.
21. Rolla G, Brussino L, Colagrande P, Dutto L, Polizzi S, Scappaticci E, Bergerone S, Morello M, Marzano A, Martinasso G, Salizzoni M, Bucca C. Exhaled nitric oxide and oxygenation abnormalities in hepatic cirrhosis. Hepatology. 1997;26:842–7.
22. Aruedas MR, Drake BB, Kapoor A, Fallon MB. Carbon oxyhemoglobin levels in cirrhotic patients with and without hepatopulmonary syndrome. Gastroenterology. 2005;128:328–33.
23. Gomez FP, Martinez-Palli G, Barbera JA, Roca J, Navasa M, Rodriguez-Roisin R. Gas exchange mechanism of orthodeoxia in hepatopulmonary syndrome. Hepatology. 2004;40:660–6.
24. Krowka MJ, Dickson R, Cortes D. Hepatopulmonary syndrome: clinical observations and lack of therapeutic response to somatostatin analogue. Chest. 1993;104:515–21.
25. Lee KN, Lee HJ, Shin WW, Webb WR. Hypoxemia and liver cirrhosis (hepatopulmonary syndrome) in eight patients: comparison of the central and peripheral pulmonary vasculature. Radiology. 1999;211:549–53.
26. Eshraghian A, Kamyab AA, Yoon SK. Pharmacological treatment of hepatopulmonary syndrome. Biomed Res Int. 2013. doi:10.1155/2013/670139.

27. Schnek P, Madl C, Rezaie-Majd S, Lehr S, Muller C. Methylene blue improves the hepatopulmonary syndrome. Ann Int Med. 2000;133:701–6.
28. Gomez FP, Barbera JA, Roca J, Burgos F, Gistau C, Rodrigues-Roisin R. Effects of nebulized N^G-nitro-L-Arginine methyl ester in patients with hepatopulmonary syndrome. Hepatology. 2006;43:1084–91.
29. Caldwell SH, Jeffers LJ, Narula OS, Lang EA, Reddy KR, Schiff ER. Ancient remedies revisited: does Allium sativum (Garlic) palliate the hepatopulmonary syndrome? J Clin Gastroentrol. 1992;15:248–50.
30. De BK, Dutta D, Pal SK, Gangopadhyay S, Baksi SD, Pani A. The role of garlic in hepatopulmonary syndrome: a randomized control trial. Can J Gastroenterol. 2010;24:183–8.
31. Swanson KL, Wiesener RH, Krowka MJ. Natural history of hepatopulmonary syndrome: impact of liver transplantation. Hepatology. 2005;41:1122–9.
32. Pascasio JM, Grilo I, Lopez-Pardo FJ, Ortega-Ruiz F, Tirado JL, Sousa JM, Rodrigues-Puras MJ, Ferrer MT, Sayago M, Gomez-Bravo MA, Grilo A. Prevalence and severity of hepatopulmonary syndrome and its influence on survival in cirrhotic patients evaluated for liver transplantation. Am J Transplant. 2014;14:1391–9.
33. Fukushima KY, Yatsuhashi H, Kinoshita A, et al. Two cases of hepatopulmonary syndrome with improved liver function following long-term oxygen therapy. J Gastroenterol. 2007;42:176–80.
34. Aldenkortt F, Aldenkortt M, Caviezel L, Waeber JL, Weber A, Schiffer E. Portopulmonary hypertension and hepatopulmonary syndrome. World Gastroenterol. 2014;20:8072–81.
35. Simonneau G, Gatzoulis A, Adatia I, Celemajer D, Denton C, Ghofrani A, Sanchez MAG, Kumar RK, Landzberg M, Machado RF, Olschewski H, Robbins IM, Souza R. Update clinical classification of pulmonary hypertension. J Am Coll Cardiol. 2013;25(supl):D34–41.
36. Badesch DB, Raskob GE, Elliott C, Krichman AM, Farber HW, Frost AE, Barst RJ, Benza RL, Liou TG, Turner M, Giles S, Feldkircher K, Miller DP, McGoon MD. Pulmonary arterial hypertension: baseline characteristics from the REVEAL registry. Chest. 2010;137:376–87.
37. Humbert M, Sitbon O, Chaouat A, Bertocchi M, Habib G, Gressin V, Yaichi A, Weitzemblum E, Cordier JF, Chabot F, Dromer C, Pison C, Reynaud-Gaubert M, Haloun A, Laurent M, Hachulla E, Simonneau G. Pulmonary arterial hypertension in France: results from a National registry. Am J Respir Crit Care Med. 2006;173:1023–30.
38. Castro M, Krowka MJ, Schroeder DR, Beck KC, Plevak DJ, Rettke SR, Cortes DA, Wiesner RH. Frequency and clinical implications of increased pulmonary artery pressures in liver transplant patients. Mayo Clin Proc. 1996;71:543–51.
39. Ruttner JR, Bartschi JP, Niedermann R, Schneider J. Plexogenic pulmonary arteriopathy and liver cirrhosis. Thorax. 1980;25:133–6.
40. Bubrock HM, Channik RN, Krowka MJ. What's new in the treatment of portopulmonary hypertension? Expert Rev Gastroenterol Hepatol. 2015;9:983–92.
41. Roberts KE, Falon MB, Krowka MJ, Brown RS, Trote JF, Peter I, Tighiouart H, Knowles JA, Rabinowitz D, Benza RL, Badesch DB, Taichman DB, Horn EM, Zacks S, Kaplowitz N, Kawut SM. Genetic risk factors for portopulmonary hypertension in patients with advanced liver disease. Am J Respir Crit Care Med. 2009;179:835–42.
42. Lee SD, Shroyere KR, Markhan NE, Cool CD, Voeklel NF, Tuder RM. Monoclonal endothelial cell proliferation is present in primary but not secondary pulmonary hypertension. J Clin Invest. 1998;101:927–34.
43. Fussner LA, Lyer VN, Cartin-Ceba R, Lin G, Watt KD, Krowka MJ. Intrapulmonary vascular dilatations are common in portopulmonary hypertension and may be associated with decreased survival. Liver Transpl. 2015;21:1355–64.
44. Colle IO, Moreau R, Godinho E, Belghiti J, Ettori F, Cohen-Solal A, Mal H, Bernuau J, Marty J, Lebrec D, Valla D, Durand F. Diagnosis of portopulmonary hypertension in candidates for live transplantation: a prospective study. Hepatology. 2003;37:401–9.

45. Bozbas SS, Eyuboglu FO, Arslan NG, Ergur FO, Karakayali H, Haberal M. The prevalence and the impact of portopulmonary hypertension on postoperative course in patients undergoing liver transplantation. Tranplant Proc. 2009;41:2860–3.
46. Horvatis T, Fuhrmann V. Therapeutic options in pulmonary hepatic vascular diseases. Expert Rev Clin Pharmacol. 2014;7:31–42.
47. Barst RJ, Rubin LJ, Long WA, McGoon MD, Richi S, Badesch DB, Groves BM, Tapson VF, Bourge RC, Brundage GH, Koerner SK, Langeben D, Keller CA, Murali S, Urtesky BF, Clayton LM, Maria PD, Jobsis MM, Blackburn SD, Shortino D, Crow JW. A comparison of continuous intravenous epoprostenol (prostacyclin) with conventional therapy for primary pulmonary hypertension. N Engl J Med. 1996;334:296–301.
48. Krowka MJ, Frants R, McGoon MD, Severson G, Plevak DJ, Wisener RH. Improvement in pulmonary hemodynamics during intravenous epoprostenol (prostacyclin): a study of 15 patients with moderate to severe portopulmonary hypertension. Hepatology. 1999;30:641–8.
49. Fix OK, Bass NM, Morco TD, Merriman RB. Long-term follow-up of portopulmonary hypertension: effect of treatment with epoprostenol. Liver Transpl. 2007;13:875–85.
50. Olschwski H, Simonneau G, Galie N, Higenbottam T, Naeije R, Rubin LJ, Nikkho S, Speich R, Hoepper MM, Winkler BJ, Sitbon O, Popov W, Ghofrani HA, Manes A, Kiely DG, Ewert R, Meyer A, Corris PA, Delcroix M, Gomez-Sanches M, Siedentop H, Seeger W. Inhaled iloprost for sever pulmonary hypertension. N Engl J Med. 2002;347:322–9.
51. Kunieda T, Nakanishi N, Matsubara H, Ohe T, Okano Y, Hondo H, Nishimura M, Shirato K, Tanabe N, Homma S, Yoshida S, Inokuma S, Kodama M, Koike T, Hishida H. Effects of long-acting beraprost sodium (TRK-100STP) in Japanese patients with pulmonary arterial hypertension. Int Heart J. 2009;50:513–29.
52. Rubin LJ, Badesch DB, Barst RJ, Gallie N, Black CM, Keogh A, Pulido T, Frost A, Roux S, Leconte I, Landzberg M, Simonneau G. Bosentan therapy for pulmonary arterial hypertension. N Engl J Med. 2002;346:896–903.
53. Savole L, Magnier R, Pavec JL, Jais X, Montani D, O'Callaghan DS, Humbert M, Dingemanse J, Simonneau G, Sitbon O. Efficacy, safety and pharmacokinetics of bosentan in portopulmonary hypertension. Eur Respir J. 2013;41:96–103.
54. Gartin-Ceba R, Swanson K, Lyer V, Wiesner RH, Krowka MJ. Safety and efficacy of ambrisentan for the treatment of portopulmonary hypertension. Chest. 2011;139:109–14.
55. Reichenberger F, Voswinckel R, Steveling E, Enke B, Kreckeel A, Olschwski H, Grimminger F, Seeger W, Ghofrani HA. Sildenafil treatment for portopulmonary hypertension. Eur Respir J. 2006;28:563–7.
56. Deibert P, Bremer H, Roessle M, Kurz-Schmieg AK, Kreisel W. PDE-5 inhibitors lower portal and pulmonary pressure in portopulmonary hypertension. Eur Respir J. 2007;29:220–1.
57. Deibert P, Schumacher YO, Ruecker G, Optitz OG, Blum HE, Rossel M, Kreisel W. Effect of vardenafil, an inhibitor of phosphodiesterase-5, on portal haemodynamics in normal and cirrhotic liver – results of a pilot study. Aliment Pharmacol Ther. 2006;23:121–8.
58. Ghofrani HA, Galie N, Grimminger F, Grunig E, Humbert M, Jing ZC, Keogh AM, Langelben D, Kilama MO, Fritsch A, Neuser D, Rubin LJ. Riociguat for the treatment of pulmonary arterial hypertension. N Engl J Med. 2013;369:330–40.
59. Krowka MJ, Plevak DJ, Findlay JY, Rosen CB, Wiesner RH, Krom RAF. Pulmonary hemodynamics and perioperative cardiopulmonary-related mortality in patients with portopulmonary hypertension undergoing liver transplantation. Liver Transpl. 2000;6:443–50.

Chapter 11
Physiological and Pathological Interactions Between Liver and Kidney

Tsuyoshi Watanabe

Abstract Physiologically, the liver and kidney are two most crucial organs for maintenance of homeostasis and metabolic regulation in the body. Although both organs possess their unique functions, both are cooperative and/or compensative for some biological regulations such as hepatorenal reflex, glucose metabolism, EPO production, and excretion of exogenous substances. Thus, dysfunction of each organ may cause that of the other such as hepatorenal syndrome. Various types of renal diseases are also caused by various liver diseases; however, the opposite relation is rare. Coexistence of multi-organ diseases is caused by systemic disorders, which may also cause multi-organ interactions such as brain-heart-liver-kidney in metabolic syndrome. So far, treatments of some of these complexed pathological conditions have been established; evidences for benefits of treatments are not enough. Thus, RCTs on treatments of these interactions are needed in the near future.

Keywords Gluconeogenesis • Excretion of exogenous substances • Hepatorenal reflex (HRR) • Hepatorenal syndrome (HRS) • De novo HBV hepatitis • Renal tubular acidosis (RTA) • Hepatic IgA nephropathy • Hepatitis B virus (HBV)-related glomerular diseases • Cryoglobulin nephropathy • Polycystic kidney disease (PKD) • Amyloidosis • Metabolic syndrome (Mets) • Nonalcoholic fatty liver disease (NAFLD)/nonalcoholic steatohepatitis (NASH) • Chronic kidney disease (CKD) • Obesity-related glomerulopathy (ORG) • Multi-organ interactions • Insulin sensitizers • ω-3 polyunsaturated fatty acids (PUFA)

T. Watanabe (✉)
Japan Labour, Health and Welfare Organization Fukushima Rosai Hospital, Iwaki-City, Fukushima, Japan

Fukushima Medical University, Fukushima City, Fukushima, Japan
e-mail: twat0423@fukushima-rosai.jp; twat0423@fmu.ac.jp

H. Ohira (ed.), *The Liver in Systemic Diseases*, DOI 10.1007/978-4-431-55790-6_11

11.1 Preface

The liver and kidney are traditionally thought to be two most crucial organs in the body for maintenance of life in Japan and East Asian countries, where "kan-jin (肝腎)" that means "liver and kidney" in Japanese language is used as meaning of "essential or crucial things." It is also true in some sense in modern medicine, because the liver and kidney are proved to be two key organs for regulation of homeostasis and metabolism in the body, which are also working together through tight communications at physiological state and pathophysiological process of many diseases.

In this chapter, interactions between the liver and kidney in physiological regulation of the body and then in pathological process of typical examples of disease processes are discussed by reviewing related publications.

11.2 Physiological Interactions Between Liver and Kidney (Fig. 11.1)

Generally speaking, the liver and kidney are key organs for regulation of homeostasis and metabolism in the body: the liver is the major player for metabolism of glucose (energy), protein, and lipid, and kidney is that for homeostasis of

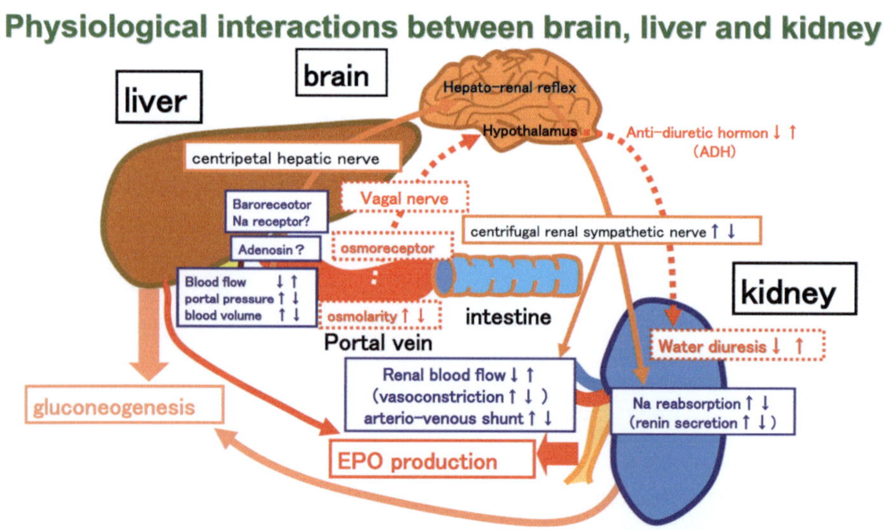

Fig. 11.1 Physiological interaction between liver and kidney: directions of arrows (↑↓) correspond to increase or decrease, respectively, in each category. Abbreviations are as shown in the text

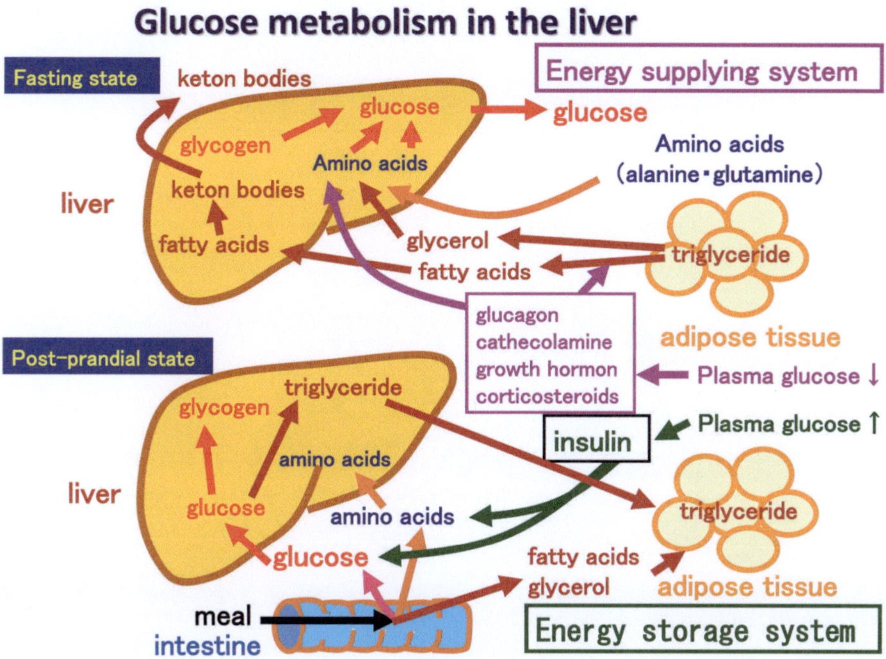

Fig. 11.2 Schematic presentation of glucose metabolism at fasting and postprandial states in the liver

water, electrolytes, and acid-base balance. However, both organs are cooperative and/or compensative for some biological regulations in the body.

In glucose and energy metabolism, the liver plays a major role for gluconeogenesis at fasting state and for energy storage as glycogen at postprandial state (Fig. 11.2), while renal tubular cells in the renal cortex are capable for gluconeogenesis at most 20 % of the total body amount of gluconeogenesis (Fig. 11.3). Insulin is the most important regulator for glucose metabolism in all the organs in the body except for gluconeogenesis in the renal tubular cells. More than half of insulin produced from β cells in the pancreas binds its receptor on the liver after transported via portal vein, which represents a major action for glucose metabolism in the liver, while insulin is catabolized at renal proximal tubules after it plays biological actions in organs such as muscle and adipose tissue in the body and then filtrated through the glomerulus. Thus, liver failure such as liver cirrhosis has tendency to cause postprandial hyperglycemia (hepatic diabetes mellitus) due to decrease of hepatic uptake of glucose and glycogen synthesis and hypoglycemia at fasting or starvation state due to lack of gluconeogenesis (Fig. 11.4). On the other hand, renal failure tends to decrease plasma glucose level and cause hypoglycemia at fasting state even in diabetic patients under hypoglycemic treatment.

Excretion of exogenous substances (drug and toxin) from the body is cooperative functions performed by the liver and kidney: water-soluble materials are

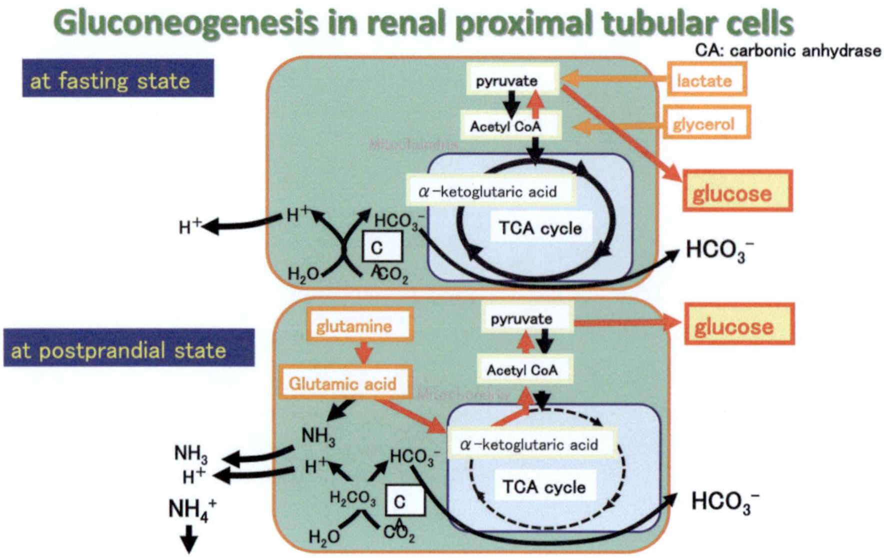

Fig. 11.3 Schematic presentation of glucose metabolism at fasting and postprandial states in the renal proximal tubular cells

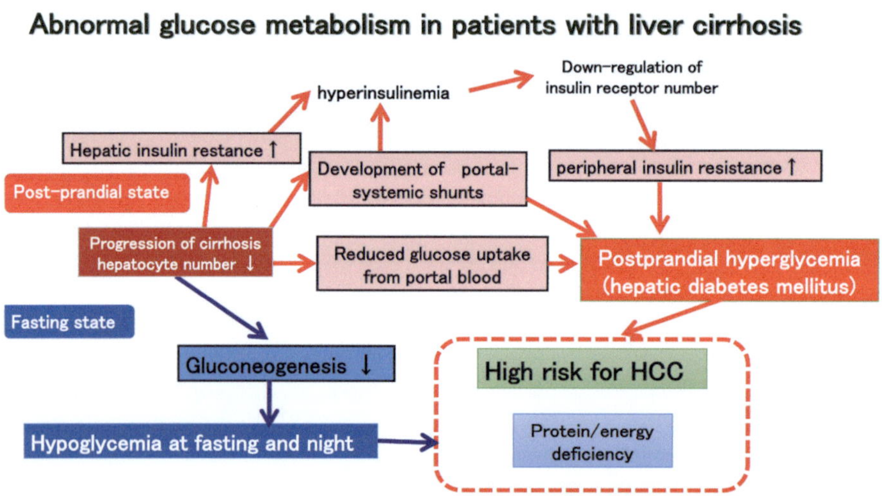

Fig. 11.4 Schematic presentation of abnormal glucose metabolism at fasting and postprandial states in patients with liver cirrhosis

excreted from the body via three renal processes, namely, glomerular filtration, reabsorption in the proximal tubules, and excretion in the distal tubules through various anion and/or cation transporters and channels (renal clearance). On the other hand, lipophilic (fat-soluble) substances are generally metabolized by

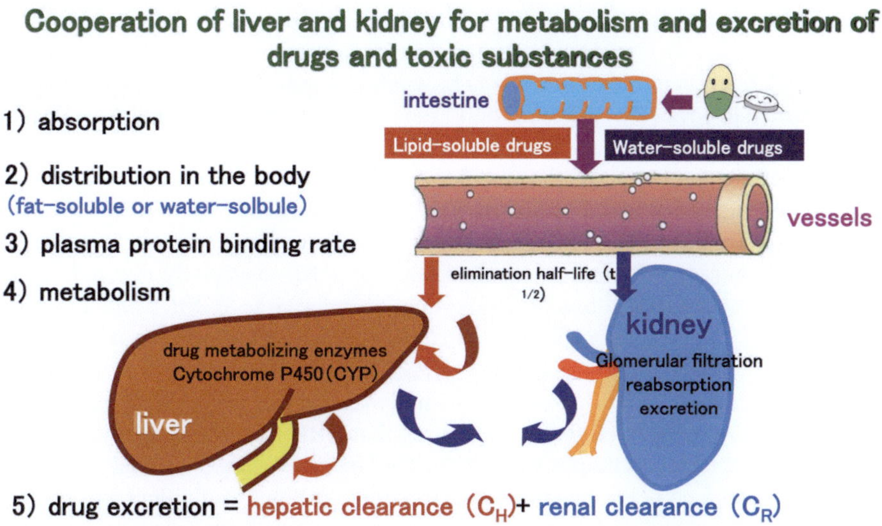

Fig. 11.5 Schematic presentation of cooperation of liver and kidney for metabolism and excretion of drugs and toxic substances

cytochrome P450 enzyme systems in the liver and excreted to the intestine via bile duct (hepatic clearance), some of which are conjugated with sulfate or glucuronate in the liver, and resultant water-soluble substances are excreted by renal clearance. Therefore, doses and intervals of medication should be carefully modulated in the patients with hepatic and/or renal failure depending on the chemical nature of materials and stage of dysfunction of these organs, especially in those with renal failure (Fig. 11.5).

The kidney and liver have endocrine functions which produce erythropoietin (EPO): renal medullary interstitial cell in the kidney is responsible for EPO production in adult; thus, renal anemia develops in renal failure due to insufficient EPO production caused by renal interstitial fibrosis. On the other hand, the liver is the main organ for EPO secretion during fetal development as well as species living in the water before amphibian during evolutional process. However, in human adult, the liver sustains capability to produce EPO and compensate EPO production in renal failure, so that progression of anemia is hampered at the level of around 20 % hematocrit due to compensative EPO production by the liver (Fig. 11.1).

Homeostasis of water (osmolality), volume (sodium), and acid-base balance, which is essentially a main task for kidney, is also regulated partly by functional cooperation between the kidney and liver: the presence of hepatorenal reflex (HRR) is confirmed mainly by animal experiments; changes of osmolality in the portal vein are sensitized by receptor-mediated mechanisms, in which signals regulate antidiuretic hormone (ADH) secretion from hypothalamus by vagal activation in order to rapidly adjust plasma osmolality constant irrespectively of that in portal vein which is reflected by oral sodium intake [1]; infusion of hyperosmotic sodium solution into portal vein causes inhibition of sodium absorption in the renal tubules (sodium diuresis) by signals via decreased activity of centripetal hepatic nerve and centrifugal renal sympathetic nerve [2], which is supposed to be a physiological mechanism to rapidly correct and maintain plasma osmolality constant irrespectively of the amount of sodium intake. On the other hand, reduction of portal blood flow or increase of portal blood pressure (portal hypertension) activates sodium and water reabsorption and then water and sodium retention by enhancement of water and sodium reabsorption through activation of centrifugal renal sympathetic nerve; reduction of renal blood flow (RBF) especially in renal cortex due to vasoconstriction, that of glomerular filtration rate (GFR); and resultant activation of RAS system [3, 4]. In patients with liver cirrhosis, transjugular intrahepatic portosystemic stent-shunt (TIPSS) procedure does not acutely change renal blood flow and cardiopulmonary hemodynamics [5], while acute obstruction of TIPS acutely reduces GFR [6], suggesting that HRR is also functioning even in human and may play pathophysiological roles for onset of hepatorenal syndrome (HRS) as mentioned below. Therefore, liver-kidney pathophysiological interactions are suggested, where signal transduction from osmoreceptor (sodium receptor) and/or baroreceptor in hepatoportal system modulates renal functions via humoral and/or neuronal mechanisms according to biochemical or physiological change in portal vein [7]. Molecular sensing mechanisms of portal blood flow or pressure are still unclear. However, in rats, the role of adenosine increased in portal vein with decreased blood flow for triggering a hepatorenal reflex is suggested [8] (Fig. 11.6).

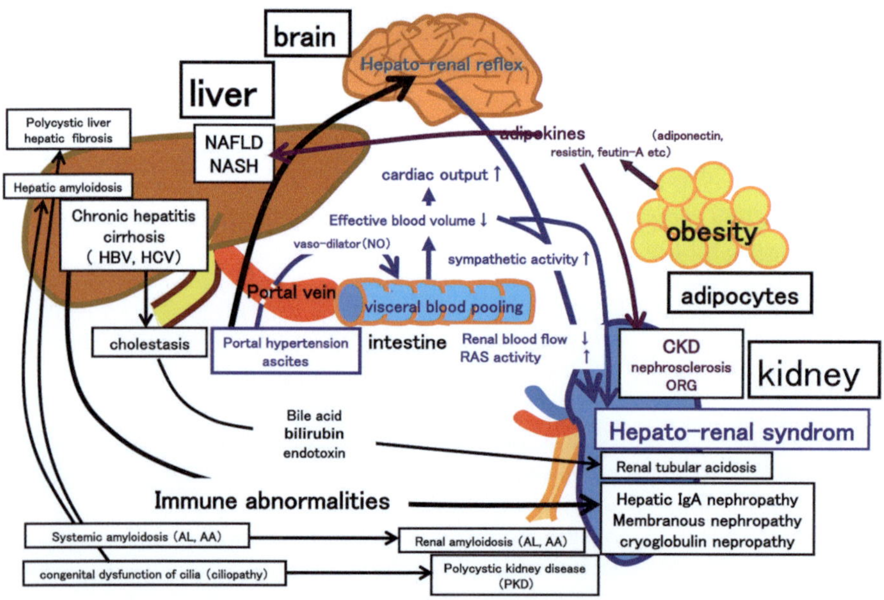

Fig. 11.6 Pathophysiological interactions between liver and kidney in various types of disease processes: abbreviations are shown as in the text

11.3 Hepatorenal Interactions in Various Disease States from Etiological and Pathophysiological Aspects (Fig. 11.6)

11.3.1 Reactivation of Hepatitis Viruses by Immune-Suppressive Treatment on Immunological Renal Diseases: A Special Attention to De Novo HBV Hepatitis (Fig. 11.6)

In patients with chronic kidney diseases (CKD), especially hemodialysis patients, hepatitis B and C infection is more prevalent compared to general population [9], and immunological renal diseases are sometimes therapeutic targets of immune-suppressive treatment such as corticosteroids and other immune-suppressive agents, so that management of hepatitis virus should be paid special attention in patients with renal diseases at carrier state of hepatitis B virus (HBV) or past-infected, clinically cured, or seroconverted state (negative HBs antigen, positive anti-HBs antibody, or anti-HBc antibody) in active hepatitis by reactivation of HBV during or after intensive immune-suppressive or chemotherapeutical treatments. Because hepatitis by HBV reactivation progresses to fulminant hepatitis more frequently compared to acute infection, prediction and prevention of hepatitis are crucial in those treatments, so that clinical guidelines for management of HBV hepatitis in patients treated with immune-suppressive or chemotherapeutic agents are now issued; screening of HBs antigen before immune-suppressive or chemotherapeutic therapy is essential at starting point for management. For patients with positive HBs antigen, quantification of HBV-DNA by real-time PCR method, as well as HBe antigen and antibody testing, should be performed in order to evaluate baseline state of infection of patients and then preventive prescription of nucleic acid analogues, among which entecavir is recommended because of the lowest incidence of acquired drug tolerance, before starting immune-suppressive or chemotherapeutic agents. Even in patients with negative HBs antigen, anti-HBs antibody or anti-HBc antibody should be tested in order to predict incident HBV hepatitis in patients under seroconverted state, so-called de novo HBV hepatitis. When either antibody is positive, quantification of HBV-DNA is mandatory; a nucleic acid analogue should be prescribed for the patient with detectable HBV-DNA. When HBV-DNA is undetectable, quantification of HBV-DNA should be repeated every month during and for 12 months after cessation of treatment, and prescription of a nucleic acid analogue should be started whenever HBV-DNA become detectable. Even though criteria for cessation of a nucleic acid analogue therapy are not determined for HBV carrier, a nucleic acid analogue therapy should be continued for 12 months after cessation of immune-suppressive or chemotherapeutical treatments, and careful observation is necessary for at least 12 months after stopping a nucleic acid analogue therapy in de novo HBV hepatitis [10].

11.3.2 Hepatorenal Syndrome (HRS): A Functional Renal Failure Caused by Hemodynamic Changes in Advanced Liver Disease (Fig. 11.6)

In acute or chronic hepatic failure such as fulminant hepatitis or liver cirrhosis, functional acute kidney injury (AKI), so-called hepatorenal syndrome (HRS), may have occurred, where hemostasis in visceral organs such as the gastrointestinal tract and skin by vasodilatory factors like NO causes reduction of functional systemic blood flow (redistribution of blood flow), followed by simultaneous reduction of RBF, sodium and fluid retention by renal vasoconstriction, and formation of venous-arterial shunt through the mechanism of HRR mentioned above. At compensated stages, blood pressure and RBF are maintained by activated vasoconstrictor such as renin-angiotensin system (RAS) and vasopressin systems. However, at decompensated stages, despite further body fluid retention, further reduction of systemic and renal blood flow resultantly causes AKI. In 2007, diagnostic criteria for HRS were revised, so that diagnosis of HRS has been generalized [11] (Table 11.1). Like AKI in general, for prognostic prediction of AKI in advanced liver cirrhosis, RIFLE (Table 11.2) or AKIN criteria (Table 11.3) based on urine volume and serum creatinine (Cr) titer can be applicable [12]. Serum cystatin C is reported to be more sensitive for early diagnosis of HRS [13]. According to its clinical courses, HRS is classified to two types: type I of acute course (serum Cr titer doubled within 2 weeks from the onset) and type II with somewhat insidious course characterized by less severe tubular damage, osmolality ratio of urine/ plasma >1, and urine/plasma Cr ratio >30. Survival rates after 6 months from diagnosis without liver transplantation are about 10 % and 40 % for types I and II, respectively, which is much worse compared to that in liver cirrhosis patients uncomplicated by HRS that is 80 % [14]. For AKI in advanced liver cirrhosis, treatable etiologies other than HRS such as prerenal renal failure due to intravascular dehydration; acute renal tubular necrosis induced by drugs such as antibiotics, NSAIDs, or anticancer drugs; abdominal compartment syndrome (ACS) induced by vasoconstriction due to elevation of intra-abdominal pressure with massive ascites; and spontaneous bacterial peritonitis (SBP) should be differentiated in every clinical setting; urinary neutrophil gelatinase-associated lipocalin (NGAL),

Table 11.1 New diagnostic hepatorenal syndrome (HRS) criteria (2007) [11]

Cirrhosis with ascites
Serum creatinine >133 μmol/L (1.5 mg/dL)
No improvement of serum creatinine (133 μmol/L (1.5 mg/dL) or lower) after at least 2 days with diuretic withdrawal and volume expansion with albumin
Absence of shock
No current or recent treatment with nephrotoxic drugs
Absence of parenchymal kidney disease as indicated by proteinuria >500 mg/day, microhematuria (>50 RBC per high-power field), and/or abnormal renal ultrasonography

Table 11.2 Rifle criteria for AKI

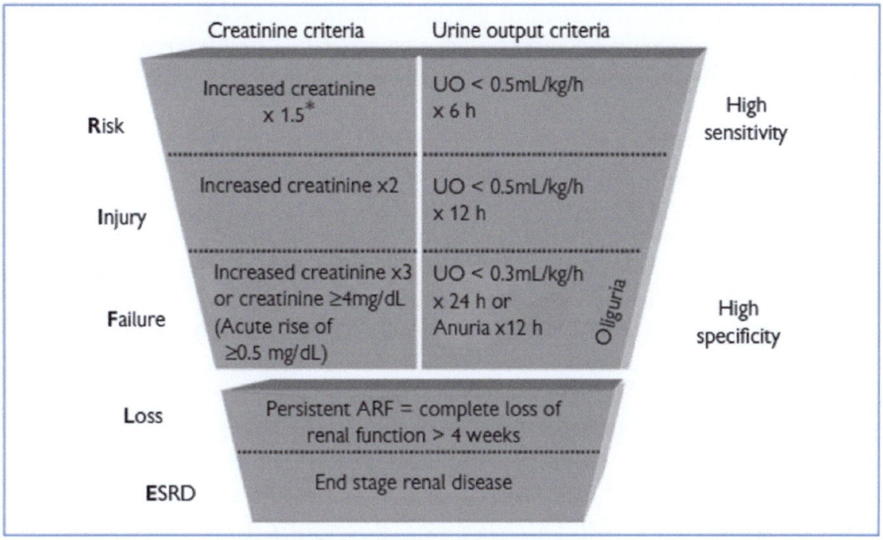

Table 11.3 AKI definition and classification by Acute Kidney Injury Network (AKIN) (Mehta et al. [134])

Definition		
Abrupt (within 48 h) reduction in kidney function currently defined as an absolute increase in serum creatinine of 0.3 mg/dL or more (≥26.4 μmol/L)		
A percentage increase in serum creatinine of 50 % or more (1.5-fold from baseline)		
A reduction in urine output (documented oliguria of <0.5 mL/kg/h for >6 h)		
The AKIN classification/staging system of acute kidney injury [45]		
Stage	**SCr**	**UO**
1	↑ SCr ≥26.5 μmol/L (≥0.3 mg/dL) or ↑SCr ≥150 a 200 % (1.5 a 2×)	<0.5 mL/kg/h (>6 h)
2	↑ SCr >200 a 300 % (>2 a 3×)	<0.5 mL/kg/h (>12 h)
3[a]	↑ SCr >300 % (>3×) or if baseline SCr ≥353.6 μmol/L (≥4 mg/dL) ↑SCr ≥44.2 μmol/L (≥0.5 mg/dL)	<0.3 mL/kg/h (24 h) oranuria (12 h)

SCr serum creatinine, *UO* urine output
[a]Stage 3 also includes patients requiring RRT independent of the stage (defined by SCr and/or UO) they are in at the moment they initiate RRT

interleukin-18 (IL-18), kidney injury molecule-1 (KIM-1), liver-type fatty acid-binding protein (L-FABP), and albumin excretion are relatively higher in ATN, while fractional excretion of sodium (FENa) is lower in HRS compared to other disease entities [15].

For prevention of HRS, in patients with decompensated liver cirrhosis and massive ascites, elimination of ascites with diuretics or paracentesis and improvement of functional systemic blood flow by intravenous infusion of albumin solution are reported to be preventive [16]. For treatments of established HRS, drugs with vasodilatory potential such as dopamine analogues, RAS inhibitors, prostaglandins, and endothelin antagonists are not proved to be effective [17]. Those with vasoconstrictive potential such as a vasopressin V1 agonist (terlipressin) [18], α-adrenergic agonists (norepinephrine, midodrine), or a somatostatin agonist (octreotide) in combination with or without intravenous infusion of albumin solution and also reduction of portal venous pressure by TIPS are proved to be effective for rapid but temporary improvement of GFR [19]. On the other hand, liver transplantation is known as an only way for improvement of long-term renal and life prognosis. However, it should be kept in mind that survival rate after liver transplantation is reversely associated with grade of impairment of renal function [20]. Sometimes hemodialysis therapy is necessitated for replacement of renal function, but is thought not to be clinically relevant when liver transplantation is not premised [21].

11.3.3 Renal Tubular Damage in Cholestatic Liver Diseases (Fig. 11.6)

Renal tubular acidosis (RTA) may be caused by tubular damage (inhibition of H-ATPase, H-K-ATPase) due to accumulated bile acids (direct), bilirubin, or endotoxins in plasma in cholestatic liver disease [22], which is classified to type I (distal type), type II (proximal type), and a mixed type of both, according to localization of tubular damage. In addition to normal anion gap metabolic acidosis and hypokalemia, type I RTA is clinically characterized by urinary stone formation (related to alkaline urine, hypercalciuria, and low urinary citrate), nephrocalcinosis, and bone demineralization (causing rickets in children and osteomalacia in adults), while type II is characterized by increased excretion of urinary β2 microglobulin and presence of Fanconi syndrome (glycosuria, aminoaciduria, hyperphosphaturia/hypophosphatemia, and hyperuricosuria). RTA is highly common (30–50 % prevalence) in cholestatic patients, which, however, is usually incomplete form, thus, rarely causes clinical problems [22].

RTA of different types and tubule-interstitial nephritis (TIN) are rare but one of the important extrahepatic complications of primary biliary cholangitis (PBC), and distal tubular acidosis (type I) is the main renal complication of PBC [23]. TIN with Fanconi syndrome have been reported rarely, where anti-mitochondrial antibodies against mitochondrial enzymes such as pyruvate dehydrogenase and alpha-ketoglutarate dehydrogenase may play pathogenetic roles [24]. Steroid therapy is reported to be beneficial in treating PBC patients with these renal complications [23].

11.3.4 Renal Diseases Related to Immune Abnormalities in Liver Diseases (Fig. 11.7)

Liver diseases are often associated with immune abnormalities, in which immune complex deposited mainly in the glomerulus may sequentially cause cytokine formation, inflammation, complement activation, cell death (apoptosis and necrosis), regeneration, and/or fibrosis in the kidney. Regular follow-up urinalysis is important for early detection of these changes in chronic liver diseases.

11.3.4.1 Hepatic IgA Nephropathy/Hepatic Glomerular IgA Deposition

In chronic hepatitis or liver cirrhosis, histological IgA deposition is frequently detected at mesangial and subendothelial region in the glomerulus [25]. Clinically silent IgA deposition without mesangial proliferation (hepatic glomerular IgA deposition) is quite common, part of which develop a typical form of IgA nephropathy (mesangial proliferation and matrix formation). IgA nephropathy associated with liver disease (hepatic IgAN) is the commonest form of secondary IgAN particularly in alcoholic liver disease, which itself is associated with disorders of the IgA immune system, but also occurs in other forms of cirrhosis and chronic hepatitis. Even though it presents characteristics of IgA nephropathy (microscopic

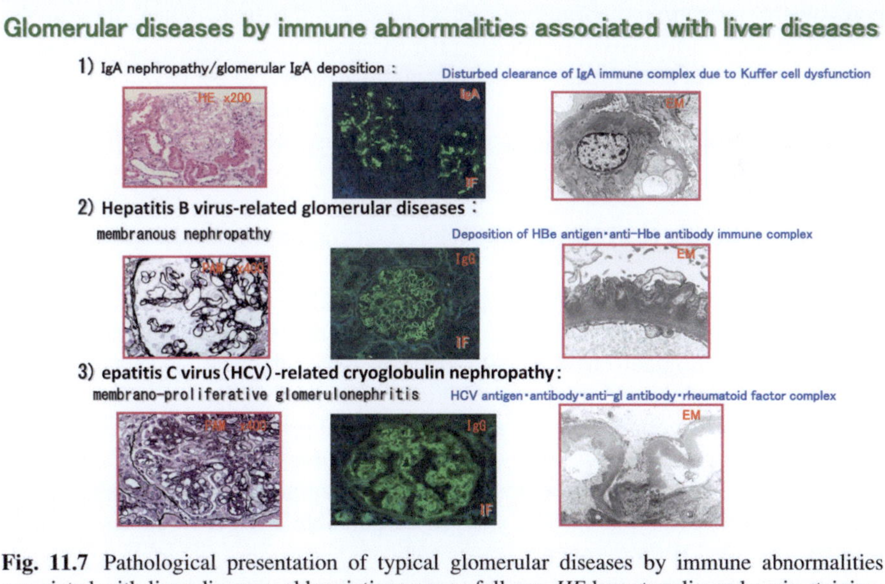

Fig. 11.7 Pathological presentation of typical glomerular diseases by immune abnormalities associated with liver diseases: abbreviations are as follows; *HE* hematoxylin and eosin staining, *PAM* periodic acid methenamine silver staining, *IF* immunofluorescence staining, *EM* electron microscope

hematuria, proteinuria, elevated serum IgA levels, and polyclonal IgA deposition at mesangial area), only small parts of the patients are believed to progress to nephrotic syndrome or renal failure [26]. For pathophysiological mechanisms, experiments using animal model of liver injury suggest that reduced clearance of IgA immune complex due to malfunction of Kupffer cells is suggested as a mechanism contributing to glomerular IgA deposition in liver diseases [27].

11.3.4.2 Hepatitis B Virus (HBV)-Related Glomerular Diseases

Glomerular renal diseases develop mainly in HBs and HBc antigen-positive patients, in which HBe antigen and HBV-DNA are detected, so that HBe antigen-antibody immune complexes are thought to play a role on pathogenesis of its lesion. In these cases, patients often have past histories of acute HBV hepatitis and 80 % of children cases are male. Histologically, children cases predominantly present membranous nephropathy (MN), while adult cases do present MN or membranoproliferative glomerulonephritis (MPGN, which is often complicated with nephrotic syndrome). In laboratory testing, transaminases are not always abnormal, but about 80 % of the patients are positive for immune complex in plasma. Demonstration of histological localization of HBe antigen with lesion of MN or MPGN in renal biopsy specimen of the patients with positive history of HBV infection and abnormality of urinalysis is crucial for definite diagnosis. The principle for treatment is removal of responsible antigens using antiviral drugs such as lamivudine [28, 29] which is recently replaced by entecavir, a drug with less potency for induction of drug-resistant clones, for the first choice drug in the clinical guideline for HBV treatment [10] as mentioned above. Glucocorticoid therapy, which had been thought to be contraindicative due to potency for induction of viral proliferation, was reported to be effective with its short-time use, and effectiveness of interferon (IFN) for infant cases was also reported [30].

11.3.4.3 Hepatitis C Virus (HCV)-Related Cryoglobulin Nephropathy

Some patients with chronic HCV hepatitis/liver cirrhosis develop a typical HCV nephropathy, which is characterized by abnormal urinalysis, cryoglobulinemia, and MPGN-like histological changes with electron dense deposits at subendothelial space proven by electron microscope. Clinically, patients with this disease are often complicated with nephrotic syndrome and poor renal prognosis [31]. Deposition at glomerulus and vascular walls of cryoglobulin (globulin which is precipitated under cold condition) including antibodies against HCV antigen (globulin), antiglobulin antibody, and rheumatoid factors may be responsible for pathogenesis of HCV nephropathy [32]. When patients are complicated with generalized cryoglobulin vasculitis, symptoms characterized for connective tissue diseases such as polyarthritis, purpura, Raynaud phenomena, cold urticaria, and skin ulceration are presented in addition to nonspecific symptoms such as fever and general malaise.

Abnormalities of urinalysis (proteinuria, hematuria, and abnormal urine sediments) in patients with positive for anti-HCV antibody, IgM rheumatoid factors, cryoglobulin, and hypocomplemententemia (about 50 % of the patients) are supportive for diagnosis of this condition, but histological changes typical for MPGN and detection of cryoglobulin in the glomerulus in situ are crucial for its definite diagnosis [33].

Therapeutic principle for HCV-related nephropathy is antigen elimination by antiviral drugs, because effects of interferon (IFN)-α, Peg-IFN-α-2b, and ribavirin were reported, although Peg-IFN-α-2b and ribavirin, half-lives in plasma of which are so long, were not recommended for the patients with impaired renal function (Ccr <50 ml/min) [34, 35]. New direct anti-HCV drugs such as NS3/4A proteinase inhibitors (telaprevir, simeprevir, and asunaprevir) and a NS5A inhibitor (daclatasvir) are developed and will be tested for their effectiveness alone or in combination with other drugs for renal complications in the near future. For patients with progressive nephritic or generalized vasculitis, corticosteroid pulse therapy, uses of immunosuppressants and anti-CD20 monoclonal antibody (rituximab) [36], and plasma exchange therapy, in which sometimes antiviral medication was added during tapering phases of original therapies, were reported to be effectively tried.

11.3.5 Coincidental Involvements in Liver and Kidney by Generalized Systemic Diseases (Fig. 11.8)

11.3.5.1 Congenital Abnormality of Ciliary Functions (Ciliopathy) (Fig. 11.8)

Polycystic kidney disease (PKD) is an inherited disorder characterized by development and growth of numerous abnormal cysts and resultant reduction of functional mass (nephron) in the kidney, which is classified to two types, according to types of genetic inheritance, autosomal dominant form (ADPKD) and autosomal recessive form (ARPKD). Although the kidney is the most severely affected organ, PKD causes frequently cysts and fibrosis in the liver and also pathologic changes elsewhere in the body such as pancreatic cysts, intestinal diverticula, and brain arterial aneurysms.

Individuals with ADPKD, the most prevalent genetic renal disease, may have normal life expectancy, but frequently develop renal dysfunction as growing of renal size due to cyst growth, leading to end-stage renal disease (ESRD) usually by middle ages (the fourth most frequent cause for incidence of ESRD in Japan). Liver cysts are the most common non-kidney complication of ADPKD, which are complicated in more than 90 % of the ADPKD patients, which, however, generally cause no symptoms except for intra-cystic infection, mass effect leading to epigastric discomfort (QOL problems), appetite loss, and malnutrition. Other

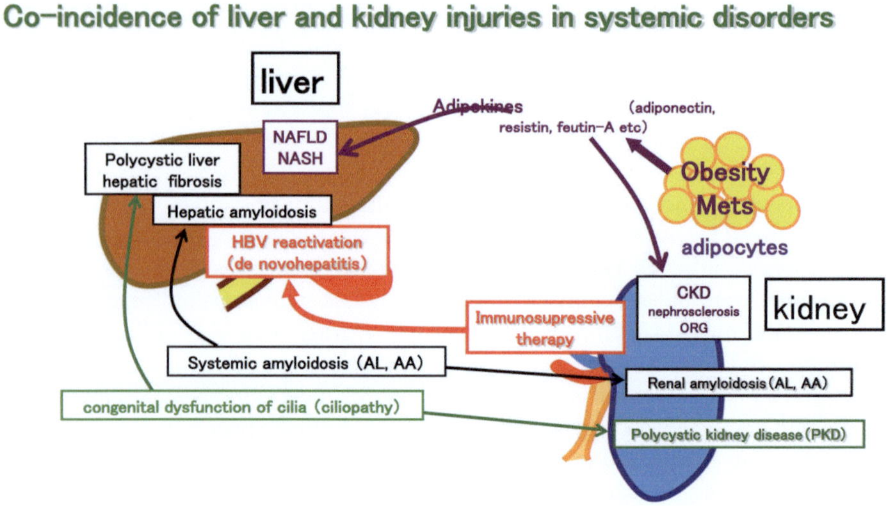

Fig. 11.8 Pathophysiological presentation of typical examples of coincidence of liver and kidney injuries in systemic disorders: abbreviations are shown as in the text

complications of ADPKD include subarachnoid hemorrhage due to aneurysms in the brain and heart failure due to mitral valve prolapse [37].

ARPKD, a rare congenital disorder, is characterized by small renal cysts with diameter of 1–2 mm which are connected to dilated collecting ducts at birth and present a variety of clinical courses, often die by respiratory failure due to hypoplasia of the lung, and sometimes survive to adulthood, or develop ESRD before reaching adulthood. Liver scarring is usually present at birth and then develops in almost all the patients and can lead to portal fibrosis, portal hypertension and dilatation and abnormality of bile duct, and then liver dysfunction as they grow older [38].

PKDs are thought to be one of the genetic defects of functional proteins in primary cilia (ciliopathy); PKD1 gene coded for polycystin-1 (a sensor protein for urinary flow in renal tubule) and PKD2 gene for polycystin-2 (an inward Ca channel in tubular cells) are mutated in patients with ADPKD, and PKHD1 gene for fibrocystin (function unknown and also localized in the centrosome and mitotic spindle of dividing cells) is mutated in ARPKD, which is also proved to be involved in pathogenesis of abnormalities in bile ducts and other epithelial tissues with anatomically and developmentally similar properties to renal tubules [39]. The renal tubular cilium is mechanically sensitive to fluid flow over the renal epithelium, in which polycystin proteins modulate diverse signaling pathways, and may modulate intracellular calcium homoeostasis and other signal transduction pathways. While it is not known how defects in the primary cilium lead to cyst development, it is thought to be possibly related to disruption of one of many signaling pathways regulated by the primary cilium, including intracellular calcium, Hedgehog, Wnt/β-catenin, cyclic adenosine monophosphate (cAMP), or planar cell polarity. Dysfunction of the primary cilium is believed to cause disruption of a number of intracellular signaling cascades that produce dedifferentiation of cystic epithelium, increased cell division, increased apoptosis, and loss of resorptive capacity [40].

For treatment of ADPKD, studies using its animal models implicate that arginine vasopressin, a major stimulant of cAMP production via V2 receptor in the collecting tubule, is shown to be an important promoter of cyst cell proliferation and fluid secretion into cysts. Tolvaptan, a V2 receptor antagonist, dramatically reduces cyst progression in mouse models of ADPKD [41]. Octreotide, a somatostatin analogue, also inhibits cAMP accumulation and produces intriguing results in animal model [42]. Clinically, recent randomized control trials (RCTs) demonstrated that antihypotensive medication mainly with RAS inhibitors, tolvaptan [43] and octreotide [44, 45] (especially in female), was shown to reduce kidney and liver size growth in ADPKD patients. Other drugs with potential actions on cilium-mediated signal transduction such as mTOR inhibitors and statins have been tested [46]. On the other hand, intravascular embolization therapy for liver cysts that are not indicative for surgical removal is shown to improve QOL and nutritional state due to dramatic reduction of liver size in the ADPKD patients with giant liver cysts [47].

11.3.5.2 Acquired Metabolic Disorders Coincidentally Affecting Liver and Kidney

Amyloidosis (Fig. 11.8)

Renal amyloidosis is relatively common etiology for nephrotic syndrome and/or renal failure especially in elderly patients. Amyloidosis is a clinical disorder caused by extracellular and/or intracellular deposition of insoluble abnormal amyloid fibrils with β-sheet structure that alter the normal function of tissues. Amyloidosis is classified to primary and secondary amyloidosis based on the absence or presence of underlying disorders such as chronic infectious, inflammatory diseases and ESRD, respectively. Amyloid protein is amorphously stained slightly eosinophilic with hematoxylin-eosin staining, reddish orange with Congo red staining, and green by birefringence with polarizing microscope. On electron microscope, linear fibril structures with width of 8–15 nm can be detected in the lesion. Systemic amyloidosis is classified to two types according to the protein origin, AL amyloidosis due to denatured protein from immunoglobulin light chain and AA amyloidosis due to that from serum amyloid A protein, an acute phase inflammatory protein secreted from the liver, both of which the kidney, liver, heart, and everywhere in the body are coincidentally affected, among which heart amyloidosis is the most important prognostic factor for life and renal amyloidosis presenting nephrotic syndrome and/or renal failure is also an important prognostic factor. On the other hand, in liver amyloidosis, hepatomegaly and elevation of bile duct-related enzyme titers such as alkaline phosphatase and γGTP are often detected, but transaminases are usually normal or slightly elevated. However, liver amyloidosis complicated with jaundice due to cholestasis (about 8 % incidence) and/or ascites (14–20 %) show poor prognosis for life. On the other hand, β2-microglobulin-derived amyloid protein in dialysis-related amyloidosis and transthyretin-derived one in familial amyloid polyneuropathy are not deposited systematically, but exclusively in connective tissue and bone and in neuronal tissue, respectively (localized amyloidosis).

Definite diagnosis of amyloidosis should be based on histological detection of amyloid proteins in biopsy specimen. However, because biopsy procedure of the liver and kidney for amyloidosis patients is believed to have potential risks for bleeding or rupture of the organ, biopsy specimen from the skin, adipose tissue, or gastrointestinal tracts can be safer substitutes for liver diagnosis and renal amyloidosis.

For treatments of AL amyloidosis, recently, combination therapy of high-dose melphalan and autologous peripheral blood stem cell transplantation [48], bortezomib-based combination chemotherapy, and combination of an immune-modulator such as combination of lenalidomide or pomalidomide and dexamethasone [49, 50] have replaced for a classic combination therapy of melphalan and prednisolone (MP) therapy due to their superiorities in terms of improvements of hematological indicators and renal function. For the treatment of AA amyloidosis, eprodisate, a negatively charged, sulfonated molecule with structural similarities to heparin sulfate, which was shown to interfere with interactions between amyloidogenic proteins and glycosaminoglycans and inhibit development of amyloid deposits in the tissues in mouse models of AA amyloidosis, is shown to slow the decline of renal function in AA amyloidosis [51].

11.3.5.3 Multi-organ Interaction in Obesity and Metabolic Syndrome (Mets) (Fig. 11.9): A Special Attention to Interaction Between Brain, Heart, Kidney, and Liver

Nonalcoholic Fatty Liver Disease (NAFLD)/Nonalcoholic Steatohepatitis (NASH)

NAFLD is a term for hepatic steatosis (fatty liver) in people who drink little or no alcohol (less than 20 g/day of 30 g/day of ethanol for female or male, respectively), and its prevalence is reported to be 15–30 % in general population, more in population with obesity and metabolic syndrome (Mets) and much higher (70–75 %) in patients with type 2 diabetes mellitus. Thus, NAFLD is considered to be a hepatic manifestation of Mets and to be etiologically related to insulin resistance [52, 53]. Although NAFLD is asymptomatic for most of patients, some patients with NAFLD progress to NASH with inflammation and fibrosis in the liver. Recent epidemiological studies on natural histories of NAFLD suggest that 5 % of patients with simple steatosis can develop NASH over a period of 8 years and then 25 % of patients with NASH can progress to advanced fibrosis and cirrhosis [54]. Disease-developing mechanism from simple steatosis to NASH is thought to

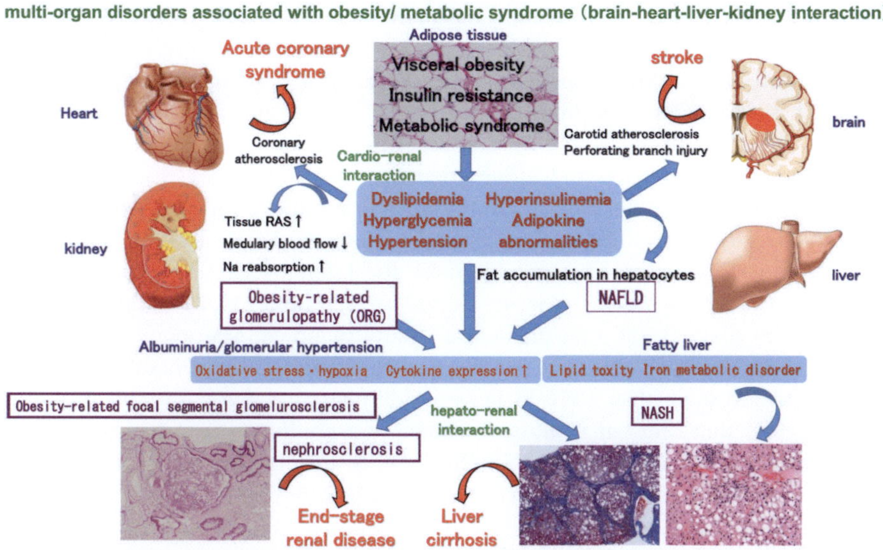

Fig. 11.9 Schematic presentation of multi-organ disorders associated with obesity/metabolic syndrome (brain-heart-liver-kidney interaction): abbreviations are shown as in the text

progress through multiple inflammation and fibrosis steps in the liver, each of which is dependent upon multiple factors such as cytokines, adipokines, fatty acids, oxidized LDL, oxidative stress, apoptosis, and innate immune response via toll-like receptors (multi-hit hypothesis) [55–57]. In addition, incidence of hepatocellular carcinoma (HCC) has been reported to be linked to NAFLD; 15 % of patients with HCC were not related to HBV or HCV infection, but to other factors such as NAFLD even in its non-cirrhotic stage [58]. Elucidation of major systemic and liver-specific molecular mechanisms involved in development of HCC that include insulin resistance and hyperinsulinemia, increased TNF signaling, and abnormalities of lipid metabolism may make pavements to new targets for prevention, early recognition, and effective treatment of HCC associated with NAFLD. So far, both metformin and PPARγ agonists have been proved to be associated with lower risk and improved prognosis of HCC [59].

For definite diagnosis of NAFLD/NASH, histopathological studies on liver biopsy specimen are necessary; hepatic histopathological criteria of NAFLD present broad spectrum ranging from simple steatosis to NASH, which is characterized by large-droplet steatosis, hepatocellular ballooning, Mallory-Denk body, apoptosis, and lobular inflammation with or without fibrosis and cirrhosis [60, 61]. Generally, only 5–20 % of liver specimen from patients with NAFLD is considered to meet criteria for NASH [62]. In contrast, scoring systems for clinical diagnosis of NASH using contribution factors for progression from simple steatosis to NASH such as NAFIC score [63] composed of plasma ferritin (over 200 ng/mL and 300 ng/mL for female and male, respectively), fasting insulin (over 10 μU/mL), and type 4 collagen 7S titer (over 5 ng/mL) are proposed.

Chronic Kidney Disease (CKD) and Obesity-Related Glomerulopathy (ORG)

CKD is defined as kidney damage such as albuminuria > 30 mg/day or glomerular filtration rate (GFR) less than 60 mL/min/1.73 m^2 for 3 months or more, irrespective of cause. GFR can be estimated from serum creatinine (Cr) and estimating equations (eGFR), and kidney damage in many kidney diseases can be ascertained by the presence of albuminuria (>30 mg/day or gCr). Kidney disease severity (stage) is classified according to its cause, the level of GFR, and that of albuminuria (CGA classification) by risks for kidney disease progression and incidence of cardiovascular diseases (CVD) [64] (Table 11.4). Kidney disease treatment by dialysis and transplantation should be noted. Many epidemiological studies show that prevalence of CKD is more than 10 % in general population worldwide and more than 13 % in Japan, which is correlated with BMI (obesity) [65, 66], and that Mets or insulin resistance is a predictive or prognostic factor independent of diabetes mellitus, hypertension, or hyperuricemia for incidence or progression of albuminuria and CKD [67–69], which is similar relation of Mets or insulin resistance to NAFLD.

Moreover, in some patients with massive obesity and Mets, glomerular lesion characterized by enlargement of glomerulus (glomerulomegaly), and glomerular sclerosis similar to glomerular lesion of idiopathic focal, segmental glomerular sclerosis (FSGS) occurs independently of diabetes mellitus or hypertension, for which obesity-related glomerulopathy (ORG) is proposed as an independent disease entity. Renal prognosis of ORG is reported to be better than that of idiopathic FSGS, but not to be necessarily good without successful weight reduction [70, 71]. Experimental studies suggest that glomerular hypertension caused by

Table 11.4 Chronic kidney disease (CKD) classification (2011)

Prognosis of CKD by GFR and Albuminuria Categories: KDIGO 2012				Persistent albuminuria categories Description and range		
				A1	A2	A3
				Normal to mildly increased	Moderately increased	Severely increased
				<30 mg/g <3 mg/mmol	30-300 mg/g 3-30 mg/mmol	>300 mg/g >30 mg/mmol
GFR categories (ml/min/1.73 m^2) Description and range	G1	Normal or high	≥90	Green	Yellow	Orange
	G2	Mildly decreased	60-89	Green	Yellow	Orange
	G3a	Mildly to moderately decreased	45-59	Yellow	Orange	Red
	G3b	Moderately to severely decreased	30-44	Orange	Red	Red
	G4	Severely decreased	15-29	Red	Red	Red
	G5	Kidney failure	<15	Red	Red	Red

Green: low risk (if no other markers of kidney disease, no CKD); Yellow: moderately increased risk; Orange: high risk; Red, very high risk.

activation of sympathetic nerve and RAS systems, intra-glomerular oxidative stress, and inflammation are involved in pathogenesis of ORG [72, 73].

Multi-organ (Brain-Heart-Kidney-Liver) Interactions in Obesity and Mets (Fig. 11.9)

Recent epidemiological studies suggest significant association of NAFLD with prevalence and incidence of CKD in diabetic [74] or nondiabetic and non-hypertensive population [75]. A meta-analysis also proves that the presence of NAFLD exhibits significant predictive values for prevalence and incidence of CKD, which become more significant as inflammation and fibrosis progress in NAFLD (NASH) [76]. Albuminuria and insulin resistance are crossly related in patients with biopsy-proven NAFLD [77]. It is also reported that this pathophysiological interaction between the liver (NAFLD) and kidney (CKD) is proposed to be mediated through dysfunction of AMP kinase signals both in glomerular podocytes and in hepatocytes by disturbed regulation of soluble factors such as fetuin-A and adiponectin secreted from the liver and adipocytes, respectively [78]. Clinically, indicators for insulin resistance (abdominal circumstance, HOMA-IR), noninvasive inflammation/fibrosis markers (increased levels of hsCRP, TNF-α, ferritin, fibrinogen, and reduced IGF-1 titer), and hyperuricemia are predictive biomarkers for fibrosis in the liver, incidence of CKD [79], and cerebrovascular and cardiovascular atherothrombotic events [80] among patients with NAFLD and Mets, suggesting the presence of pathophysiological interactions between multi-organs including the brain, heart, kidney, and liver (Fig. 11.9).

11.3.5.4 Treatment of Multi-organ Interactions in NAFLD and CKD

In experiments using animal models or in clinical studies, weight reduction by lifestyle modification (more than −7 %), antioxidants (vitamin E, pentoxifylline), medication related to lipid metabolism (statin and polyunsaturated fatty acid, eicosapentaenoic acid (EPA), and docosahexaenoic acid (DHA)), and antidiabetic medication to improve insulin resistance (thiazolidine, metformin) are proved to be effective for NAFLD/NASH [81], some of which are also reported to be renoprotective for ORG or CKD with obesity or Mets, and thus are suggested to inhibit vicious multi-organ interactions between the brain, heart, liver, and kidney and to prevent cardiovascular events in patients with CKD and NAFLD.

Weight Reduction

Weight reduction by physical exercise and diet therapy is reported to improve hepatic histological severity in FAFLD [81, 82]. Proteinuria [83, 84] and glomerular hyperfiltration (hypertension) [85] are also corrected by weight reduction with lifestyle modification [83] or by bariatric surgery [84] in ORG and CKD complicated with obesity. However, it is a problem that adherence and persistency of lifestyle modification usually are not good enough.

Anti-oxidative Medication

Vitamin E is proved to improve serum biomarkers and hepatic histopathological severity in nondiabetic adult patients with NASH independently of a marker for insulin resistance in adipocytes (free fatty acids x insulin titer in fasting plasma) according to PIVENS study [86]. The use of vitamin E with or without combination of ursodeoxycholic acid is confirmed to improve serum biochemical markers for hepatic injury solely in patients with NASH according to meta-analyses on recent clinical studies [87–89]. However, vitamin E therapy is reported not to be effective for persistent reduction of serum ALT titer in pediatric patients with NAFLD (TONIC study) [90]. On the other hand, clinical studies on effectiveness of vitamin E single therapy for CKD are scarce, while in a rat model of renal fibrosis (five out of six nephrectomized rats), vitamin E is reported to inhibit renal sclerosis [91].

A nonspecific phosphor-esterase inhibitor with anti-oxidative and anti-inflammatory potency, pentoxifylline, is reported to be effective for reduction of serum transaminases, TNF-α, and various oxidative lipid levels as well as hepatic histopathological improvement of lipid deposition and hepatic inflammation and fibrosis according to various RCTs for NAFLD/NASH [92–95], which is confirmed by a meta-analysis on those studies [96]. Pentoxifylline with or without combination of RAS inhibitors is reported to reduce proteinuria, which is suggested to be associated with reduction of urinary excretion of TNF-α and MCP-1 [97]. Moreover, it is also reported that pentoxifylline significantly slowed GFR decline in a RCT with small number of CKD patients with overt proteinuria [98].

Insulin Sensitizers

Antidiabetic drugs with potency to improve insulin sensitivity, thiazolidine derivatives (pioglitazone, rosiglitazone) [99, 100] and metformin [101–103], are reported to improve biochemical and hepatic histopathological abnormalities accompanied by NAFLD/NASH in diabetic and nondiabetic patients, which is confirmed by meta-analyses [104–106]. However, reported therapeutic effects of metformin on NAFLD/NASH are limited to some part of patients [100, 102], and those of thiazolidine derivatives are not better than those of vitamin E [105–107].

Renoprotective effects of thiazolidine derivatives alone or in combination with RAS inhibitors on renal function and histopathological lesions are reported in ORG model rats caused by high-fat diet [108]; Mets model rats by high-fat, high-salt, and fructose-containing diet [109]; and CKD rodent models by Adriamycin administration [110], adenine administration [111], unilateral ureteral obstruction (UUO) [112], or aging [113]. Clinically, however, the use of a thiazolidine derivative, pioglitazone, is reported to have renoprotective effects additive to the use of a RAS inhibitor, losartan, in patients with type 2 diabetic nephropathy [114].

On the other hand, metformin is reported to inhibit renal function decline and fibrosis via activation of AMP kinase in nondiabetic CKD model rats with five out of six nephrectomies [115]. However, scarce clinical studies are reported on renoprotective effects of metformin, partly because metformin is generally prohibited for advanced CKD patients due to possible risk for lactic acidosis. However, a recent systemic review reveals that incidence of lactic acidosis is not significantly increased in patients with mild to moderate CKD (eGFR, 30–60 mL/min per 1.73 m^2) [116]; thus, clinical studies on renoprotection by metformin had better be tried in patients with mild to moderate CKD.

Medications Related to Lipid Metabolism

HMG-CoA inhibitors (statins) alone or in combination with ezetimibe are reported to reduce transaminases and induce hepatic histopathological improvements, induction of eNOS expression and suppression of iNOS expression, JNK activity, inflammatory factor expression, hepatocyte apoptosis, and fibrosis in NASH models of high-fat-induced Mets model rodents [117, 118]. Clinically, statins reportedly attenuate NASH [119, 120], which is associated with reduction of plasma advanced glycation end-product (AGE) titer in patients with NASH and dyslipidemia [119]. However, therapeutic effects of statin do not reach statistical significance in terms of clinical and hepatic histopathological improvements in patients with NAFLD/NASH at this moment in a recent meta-analysis based on Cochrane Database, due to lack of enough quality and quantity of clinical data on this topic [121].

Statins are reported to reduce albuminuria in that reduction rate by statins is correlated with basal level of albuminuria according to meta-analyses on RCTs in which albuminuria is evaluated by 24 h urine collection for statin effects [122, 123]. On the other hand, beneficial effects of statin to inhibit declining rate of renal function (eGFR) are controversial in each of meta-analyses [123, 124]. Moreover, according to a recent meta-analysis on CKD patients using Cochrane Central Register, the use of statins significantly reduces incidence of cardiovascular events (20 % reduction) except for stroke and also mortality rate in pre-dialysis CKD patients, but not in dialysis or kidney-transplanted patients, while statin use does not significantly inhibit declining rate of eGFR in pre-dialysis CKD patients [125].

Thus, the use of statins can be recommended for patients with NAFLD/NASH, CKD, and dyslipidemia because it should reduce incidence of cardiovascular events and level of proteinuria and may be beneficial for renal function declining rate and histopathological improvements of NAFLD/NASH, even though its beneficial effects for renal function and NAFLD/NASH need to be tested by RCTs in the near future.

ω-3 polyunsaturated fatty acids (PUFA), EPA and DHA, are clinically proved to reduce serum triglyceride (TG) titer via improvement of insulin resistance [126]. There are reports on diet-induced rodent NASH models, presenting that EPA administration inhibits hepatic fibrosis which is associated with reduction in expression of oxidative stress-related factors, but independent of reduction of hepatic TG contents [127]; that DHA is more effective compared to EPA administration in terms of potency to reduce oxidative stress, inflammation, and fibrosis in the liver [128]; and that these beneficial effects of DHA are possibly associated with changes of fatty acid and oxidized fatty acid profiles by metabolome analyses [129].

Clinically, purified EPA administration is reported to reduce serum transaminases, inflammatory cytokines, and oxidative stress markers in patients with biopsy-proven NASH, in some of whom histopathological inflammation and fibrosis are also inhibited in the liver [130]. In comparison of DHA and EPA, DHA administration reportedly is more powerful compared to EPA administration for reduction of hepatic lipid contents estimated by MRI (WELCOME study) [131].

Experimental and clinical beneficial effects of ω-3 PUFA on inflammatory renal diseases such as IgA nephropathy are reported until now [132]. However, there are scarce reports on effects of ω-3 PUFA on obesity- or Mets-related CKD, except that in a Mets model rat, EPA/DHA mix compound is more effective on prevention of renal failure compared to EPA monotherapy, which is supposed to be caused by anti-inflammatory bioactive fatty acids (protectin, resolvin) derived from DHA [133]. Thus, clinical studies on effects of ω-3 PUFA for ORG or obesity-/Mets-related CKD are desired.

11.4 Conclusion

Physiologically, the liver and kidney are two most crucial organs for maintenance of homeostasis and metabolic regulation in the body; although both organs possess their unique functions, the liver and kidney are cooperative and/or compensative for some biological regulations through tight communications through neuronal and humoral mechanisms, such as hepatorenal reflex for volume balance, regulation of glucose metabolism, EPO production, and excretion of drug and toxic substances from the body. Thus, in these contexts, understandings of pathophysiological mechanisms of functional AKI in liver cirrhosis (hepatorenal syndrome), hepatic diabetes, and hypoglycemic tendency in both renal and liver failures and adjustment of medication doses or intervals in both organ dysfunctions are clinically important. Various types of renal diseases are sometimes caused by various types of liver diseases such as HCV- or HBV-related nephritis and hepatic IgA nephropathy; however, usually the opposite relation (liver diseases caused by renal diseases) is not true except for de novo HBV hepatitis by immunosuppression for treatment of immunological renal diseases. Finally, coexistence of diseases in the liver and kidney caused by systemic disorders such as amyloidosis and metabolic syndrome (NAFLD/NASH and CKD/ORG) and their association with cerebrovascular and cardiovascular events (brain-heart-liver-kidney interactions) should be kept in mind for treatment of these complexed disorders, which will become more popular as aging society further progresses in the future. So far, although treatments of some of these complexed pathological conditions mentioned above have been established and proved to be beneficial, evidences for benefits of treatments are generally scarce. Thus, RCTs on treatments of these conditions (brain-heart-liver-kidney interactions) will be needed in the near future.

References

1. Adachi A. Thermosensitive and osmoreceptive afferent fibers in the hepatic branch of the vagus nerve. J Auton Nerve Syst. 1984;10:269–73.
2. Morita H, Matsuda T, Furuya F, et al. Hepatorenal reflex plays an important role in natriuresis after high-NaCl food intake in conscious dogs. Circ Res. 1993;72:552–9.
3. Jimenez-Saenz M, Soria IC, Bernardez JR, et al. Renal sodium retention in portal hypertension and hepatorenal reflex: from practice to science. Hepatology. 2003;37:1494–5.
4. Lubel JS, Herath CB, Burrell LM, et al. Liver disease and the renin-angiotensin system: recent discoveries and clinical implications. J Gastroenterol Hepatol. 2008;23:1327–38.
5. Stanley AJ, Redhead DN, Bouchier IA, et al. Acute effects of transjugular intrahepatic portosystemic stent-shunt (TIPSS) procedure on renal blood flow and cardiopulmonary hemodynamics in cirrhosis. Am J Gastroenterol. 1998;93:2463–8.
6. Jalan R, Forrest EH, Redhead DN, et al. Reduction in renal blood flow following acute increase in the portal pressure: evidence for the existence of a hepatorenal reflex in man? Gut. 1997;40:664–70.
7. Gentilini P, La Villa G. Liver-kidney pathophysiological interrelationships in liver diseases. Dig Liver Dis. 2008;40:909–19.
8. Ming Z, Smyth DD, Lautt WW. Decreases in portal flow trigger a hepatorenal reflex to inhibit renal sodium and water excretion in rats: role of adenosine. Hepatology. 2002;35:167–75.
9. Molino C, Fabbian F, Cozzolino M, et al. The management of viral hepatitis in CKD patients: an unresolved problem. Int J Artif Org. 2008;31:683–96.
10. Clinical guideline for treatment of HBV hepatitis edited by the Japan Society of Hepatology. 2nd ed. 2014.
11. Gentilini P, Laffi G, Buzzelli G, et al. Functional renal alternation in chronic liver disease. Digestion. 1980;20:66–72.
12. Jenq CC, Tsai MH, Tian YC, et al. RIFLE classification can predict short-term prognosis in critically ill cirrhotic patients. Intensiv Care Med. 2007;33:1921–30.
13. Wan ZH, Wang JJ, You SL, et al. Cystatin C is a biomarker for predicting acute kidney injury in patients with acute-on-chronic liver failure. World J Gastroenterol. 2013;19(48):9432–8.
14. Venkat D, Venkat KK. Hepatorenal syndrome. South Med J. 2010;103:654–61.
15. Belcher JM, Sanyal AJ, Peixoto AJ, et al. Kidney biomarkers and differential diagnosis of patients with cirrhosis and acute kidney injury. Hepatology. 2014;60(2):622–32.
16. Davenport A. Management of acute kidney injury in liver disease. Contrib Nephrol. 2010;165:197–205.
17. Salerno F, Gerbes A, Gibes P, et al. Diagnosis, prevention and treatment of the hepato-renal syndrome in cirrhosis. Gut. 2007;56:1310–8.
18. Triantos CK, Samonakis D, Thalheimer U, et al. Terlipressin therapy for renal failure in cirrhosis. Eur J Gastroenterol Hepatol. 2010;22:481–6.
19. Wong F, Pantea L, Sniderman K. Midodrine, octreotide, albumin, and TIPS in selected patients with cirrhosis and type 1 hepato-renal syndrome. Hepatology. 2004;40:55–64.

20. Navasa M, Feu F, Garcia-Pagan JV, et al. Impact of pretransplant renal function on survival after liver transplantation. Transplantation. 1995;59:361–5.
21. Betrosian AP, Agarwal B, Douzinas EE. Acute renal dysfunction in liver diseases. World J Gastroenterol. 2007;13:5552–9.
22. Ahya SN, JoseSoler M, Levitsky J, et al. Acid –base and potassium disorders in liver disease. Semin Nephrol. 2006;26:466–70.
23. Komatsuda A, Wakui H, Ohtani H, et al. Tubulointerstitial nephritis and renal tubular acidosis of different types are rare but important complications of primary biliary cirrhosis. Nephrol Dial Transplant. 2010;25(11):3575–9.
24. Lino M, Binaut R, Noël LH, et al. Tubulointerstitial nephritis and Fanconi syndrome in primary biliary cirrhosis. Am J Kidney Dis. 2005;46(3):e41–6. Steroid therapy can be beneficial in treating PBC patients with these renal complications.
25. Pouria S, Feehally J. Glomerular IgA deposition in liver disease. Nephrol Dial Transplant. 1999;14(10):2279–82.
26. Pouria S, Barratt J. Secondary IgA nephropathy. Semin Nephrol. 2008;28:27–37.
27. Ogata I, Fujiwara K, Nishi T, et al. Contribution of hepatic reticuloendothelial system to glomerular IgA deposition in rat liver injury. Am J Pathol. 1988;131(3):411–7.
28. Tang S, Lai FM, Liu YH, et al. Lamivudine in hepatitis B- associated membranous nephropathy. Kidney Int. 2005;68:1750–8.
29. Wen YK, Chen ML. Remission of hepatitis B virus-associated membranoproliferative glomerulonephritis in a cirrhotic patient after lamivudine therapy. Clin Nephrol. 2006;65:211–5.
30. Farrell GC, Teoh NC. Management of chronic hepatitis B infection: a new era of disease control. Intern Med J. 2006;36:100–13.
31. Johnson RJ, Gretch DR, Yamabe H, et al. Membranoproliferative glomerulonephritis associated with hepatitis C virus infection. N Engl J Med. 1993;328:465–70.
32. Fornasieri A, Armelloni S, Bernasconi P, et al. High binding of immunoglobulin M kappa rheumatoid factor from type II cryoglobulins to cellular fibronectin: a mechanism for induction of in situ immune complex glomerulonephritis? Am J Kidney Dis. 1996;27:476–83.
33. Sansonno D, Gesualdo L, Manno C, et al. Localization of HCV antigens in renal tissue of HCV-infected patients with cryoglobulinemic mesangiocapillary glomerulonephritis (MCGN). J Am Soc Nephrol. 1996;6:431.
34. Sabry AA, Sobh MA, Sheaashaa HA, et al. Effect of combination therapy (ribavirin and interferon) in HCV-related glomerulopathy. Nephrol Dial Transplant. 2007;17:1924–30.
35. Sugiura T, Yamada T, Kimpara Y, et al. Effects of pegylated interferon alpha-2a on hepatitis-C-virus-associated glomerulonephritis. Pediatr Nephrol. 2009;24:199–202.
36. Roccatello D, Baldovino S, Rossi D, et al. Long-term effects of antiCD20 monoclonal antibody treatment of cryoglobunemic glomerulonephritis. Nephrol Dial Transplant. 2004;19:3035–61.
37. Pirson Y. Extrarenal manifestations of autosomal dominant polycystic kidney disease. Adv Chronic Kidney Dis. 2010;17:173–80.
38. Magdalena A, Mounif E-Y, Sandro R, et al. Clinical and molecular characterization defines a broad spectrum of autosomal recessive polycystic kidney disease (ARPKD). Medicine. 2006;85:1–25.
39. Gunay-Aygun M. Liver and kidney disease in ciliopathies. Am J Med Genet Part C Sem Med Genet. 2009;151C:296–306.
40. Hannah CC, Michael JC. The cell biology of polycystic kidney disease. J Cell Biol. 2010;191 (4):701–10. doi:10.1083/jcb.201006173.
41. Torres VE. Vasopressin in chronic kidney disease: an elephant in the room? Kidney Int. 2009;76:925–8.
42. Masyuk TV, Masyuk AI, Torres VE, et al. Octreotide inhibits hepatic cystogenesis in a rodent model of polycystic liver disease by reducing cholangiocyte adenosine 3′,5′-cyclic monophosphate. Gastroenterology. 2007;132:1104–16.

43. Torres VE, Chapman AB, Devuyst O, et al. Tolvaptan in patients with autosomal dominant polycystic kidney disease. N Engl J Med. 2012;367(25):2407–18.
44. Hogan MC, Masyuk TV, Page LJ, et al. Randomized clinical trial of long-acting somatostatin for autosomal dominant polycystic kidney and liver disease. J Am Soc Nephrol. 2010;21:1052–61.
45. Gevers TJ, Inthout J, Caroli A, et al. Young women with polycystic liver disease respond best to somatostatin analogues: a pooled analysis of individual patient data. Gastroenterology. 2013;145(2):357–65.e1–2.
46. Belibi FA, Edelstein CL. Novel targets for the treatment of autosomal dominant polycystic kidney disease. Expert Opin Investig Drugs. 2010;19:315–28.
47. Hoshino J, Ubara Y, Suwabe T, et al. Intravascular embolization therapy in patients with enlarged polycystic liver. Am J Kidney Dis. 2014;63(6):937–44.
48. Hoshino J, Ubara Y, Ohashi K, et al. Pathologic improvement after high-dose melphalan and autologous stem cell transplantation in patients with for primary systemic amyloidosis. Nephro Dial Transplant Plus. 2008;6:414–6.
49. Chaulagain C. New insights and modern treatment of AL amyloidosis. Curr Hematol Malig Rep. 2013;8(4):291–8.
50. Mahmood S, Venner CP, Sachchithanantham S, et al. Lenalidomide and dexamethasone for systemic AL amyloidosis following prior treatment with thalidomide or bortezomib regimens. Br J Haematol. 2014;166(6):842–8.
51. Dember LM, Hawkins PN, Hazenberg BPC, et al. Eprodisate for the treatment of renal disease in AA amyloidosis. N Engl J Med. 2007;356:2349–60.
52. Bedogni G, Miglioli L, Masutti F, et al. Prevalence of and risk factors for non-alcoholic fatty liver disease: the Dionysos Nutrition and Liver Study. Hepatology. 2005;40:1387–95.
53. Marchesini G, Marzocchi R, Agostini F, et al. Nonalcoholic fatty liver disease and metabolic syndrome. Curr Opin Lipidol. 2005;16:421–7.
54. Bhala N, Jouness RI, Bugianesi E. Epidemiology and natural history of patients with NAFLD. Curr Pharm Des. 2013;19:5169–76.
55. Manco M, Marcellini M, Devito R, et al. Metabolic syndrome and liver histology in paediatric non-alcoholic steatohepatitis. Int J Obes (Lond). 2008;32:381–7.
56. Manco M, Bedogni G, Marcellini M, et al. Waist circumference correlates with liver fibrosis in children with nonalcoholic steatohepatitis. Gut. 2008;57:1283–7.
57. Review team: LaBrecque D, Abba Z, Anania F et al. World gastroenterology organisation global guidelines nonalcoholic fatty liver disease and nonalcoholic steatohepatitis. 2012.
58. Nagaoki Y, Hyogo H, Aikata H, et al. Recent trend of clinical features in patients with hepatocellular carcinoma. Hepatol Res. 2012;42:368–75.
59. Baffy G, Brunt EM, Caldwell HJ. Hepatocellular carcinoma in non-alcoholic fatty liver disease: an emerging menace. Hepatology. 2012;56(6):1384–13.
60. Neuschwander-Tetri BA, Clark JM, Bass NM, et al. Clinical, laboratory and histological associations in adults with nonalcoholic fatty liver disease. Hepatology. 2010;52:913–24.
61. Musso G, Gambino R, Cassader M. Non-alcoholic fatty liver disease from pathogenesis to management: an update. Obes Rev. 2010;11:430–45.
62. Torres DM M.D., Stephen A, Harrison MD. Nonalcoholic steatohepatitis and noncirrhotic hepatocellular carcinoma. Semin Liver Dis. 2012;32(1):30–8.
63. Sumida Y, Yoneda M, Hyogo H, et al. A simple clinical scoring system using ferritin, fasting insulin, and type IV collagen 7S for predicting steatohepatitis in nonalcoholic fatty liver disease. J Gastroenterol. 2011;46(2):257–68.
64. Levin A, Stevens PE. Summary of KDIGO 2012 CKD guideline. Behind the scenes, need for guidance, and a framework for moving forward. Kidney Int. 2014;85(1):49–61.
65. Gelber RP, Kurth T, Kausz AT, et al. Association between body mass index and CKD in apparently healthy men. Am J Kidney Dis. 2005;46:871–80.
66. Hsu CY, McCulloch CE, Iribarren C, et al. Body mass index and risk for end-stage renal disease. Ann Intern Med. 2006;144:21–8.

67. Chen J, Muntner P, Hamm LL, et al. The metabolic syndrome and chronic kidney disease in U.S. adults. Ann Intern Med. 2004;140:167–74.
68. Parvanova AI, Trevisan R, Iliev IP, et al. Insulin resistance and microalbuminuria: a cross-sectional, case-control study of 158 patients with type 2 diabetes and different degrees of urinary albumin excretion. Diabetes. 2006;55:1456–62.
69. Kurella M, Lo JC, Chertow GM, et al. Metabolic syndrome and the risk for chronic kidney disease among nondiabetic adults. J Am Soc Nephrol. 2005;16:2134–40.
70. Kambham N, Markowitz GS, Valeri AM, et al. Obesity-related glomerulopathy: an emerging epidemic. Kidney Int. 2001;59(4):1498–509.
71. Praga M, Hernández E, Morales E, et al. Clinical features and long-term outcome of obesity-associated focal segmental glomerulosclerosis. Nephrol Dial Transplant. 2001;16:1790–8.
72. Chen HM, Chen Y, Zhang YD, et al. Evaluation of metabolic risk marker in obesity-related glomerulopathy. J Renal Nutr. 2011;21(4):309–15.
73. Wu Y, Liu Z, Xiang Z, et al. Obesity-related glomerulopathy: insights from gene expression profiles of the glomeruli derived from renal biopsy samples. Endocrinology. 2006;147 (1):44–50.
74. Targher G, Bertolini L, Rodella S, et al. Non-alcoholic fatty liver disease is independently associated with an increased prevalence of chronic kidney disease and proliferative/laser-treated retinopathy in type 2 diabetic patients. Diabetologia. 2008;51:444–50.
75. Chang Y, Ryu S, Sung E, et al. Nonalcoholic fatty liver disease predicts chronic kidney disease in nonhypertensive and nondiabetic Korean men. Metabolism. 2008;57(4):569–76.
76. Musso G, Gambino R, Tabibian JH, et al. Association of non-alcoholic fatty liver disease with chronic kidney disease: a systematic review and meta-analysis. PLoS Med. 2014;11(7): e1001680. PMID:25050550.
77. Manco M, Ciampalini P, DeVito R, et al. Albuminuria and insulin resistance in children with biopsy proven non-alcoholic fatty liver disease. Pediatr Nephrol. 2009;24:1211–7.
78. Ix JH, Sharma K. Mechanisms linking obesity, chronic kidney disease, and fatty liver disease: the roles of fetuin-A, adiponectin, and AMPK. J Am Soc Nephrol. 2010;21:406–12.
79. Sesti G, Fiorentino TV, Arturi F, et al. Association between noninvasive fibrosis markers and chronic kidney disease among adults with nonalcoholic fatty liver disease. PLoS One. 2014;9 (2):e88569. PMID:24520400.
80. Carbone F, Montecucco F, Mach F, et al. The liver and the kidney: two critical organs influencing the atherothrombotic risk in metabolic syndrome. Thromb Haemost. 2013;110 (5):940–58.
81. Musso G, Cassader M, Rosina F, et al. Impact of current treatments on liver disease, glucose metabolism and cardiovascular risk in non-alcoholic fatty liver disease (NAFLD): a systematic review and meta-analysis of randomised trials. Diabetologia. 2012;55(4):885–904.
82. Kistler KD, Brunt EM, Clark JM, et al. Physical activity recommendations, exercise intensity, and histological severity of nonalcoholic fatty liver disease. Am J Gastroenterol. 2011;106 (3):460–8; quiz 469.
83. Shen WW, Chen HM, Chen H, et al. Obesity-related glomerulopathy: body mass index and proteinuria. Clin J Am Soc Nephrol. 2010;5:1401–9.
84. Fowler SM, Kon V, Ma L, et al. Obesity-related focal and segmental glomerulosclerosis: normalization of proteinuria in an adolescent after bariatric surgery. Pediatr Nephrol. 2009;24 (4):851–5.
85. Chagnac A, Weinstein T, Herman M, et al. The effects of weight loss on renal function in patients with severe obesity. J Am Soc Nephrol. 2003;14(6):1480–6.
86. Bell LN, Wang J, Muralidharan S, et al. Relationship between adipose tissue insulin resistance and liver histology in nonalcoholic steatohepatitis: a pioglitazone versus vitamin E versus placebo for the treatment of nondiabetic patients with nonalcoholic steatohepatitis trial follow-up study. Hepatology. 2012;56(4):1311–8.

87. Ji HF, Sun Y, Shen L. Effect of vitamin E supplementation on aminotransferase levels in patients with NAFLD, NASH, and CHC: results from a meta-analysis. Nutrition. 2014;30 (9):986–91.
88. Pacana T, Sanyal AJ. Vitamin E and nonalcoholic fatty liver disease. Curr Opin Clin Nutr Metab Care. 2012;15(6):641–8.
89. Pietu F, Guillaud O, Walter T, et al. Ursodeoxycholic acid with vitamin E in patients with nonalcoholic steatohepatitis: long-term results. Clin Res Hepatol Gastroenterol. 2012;36 (2):146–55. PMID:22154224.
90. Lavine JE, Schwimmer JB, Van Natta ML, et al. Effect of vitamin E or metformin for treatment of nonalcoholic fatty liver disease in children and adolescents: the TONIC randomized controlled trial. JAMA. 2011;305(16):1659–68.
91. Tain YL, Freshour G, Dikalova A, et al. Vitamin E reduces glomerulosclerosis, restores renal neuronal NOS, and suppresses oxidative stress in the 5/6 nephrectomized rat. Am J Physiol Renal Physiol. 2007;292(5):F1404–10.
92. Van Wagner LB, Koppe SW, Brunt EM, et al. Pentoxifylline for the treatment of non-alcoholic steatohepatitis: a randomized controlled trial. Ann Hepatol. 2011;10 (3):277–86. PMID:21677329.
93. Satapathy SK, Sakhuja P, Malhotra V, et al. Beneficial effects of pentoxifylline on hepatic steatosis, fibrosis and necroinflammation in patients with non-alcoholic steatohepatitis. J Gastroenterol Hepatol. 2007;22(5):634–8. PMID:17444848.
94. Lin SL, Chen YM, Chiang WC, et al. Effect of pentoxifylline in addition to losartan on proteinuria and GFR in CKD: a 12-month randomized trial. Am J Kidney Dis. 2008;52 (3):464–74.
95. Zein CO, Lopez R, Fu X, et al. Pentoxifylline decreases oxidized lipid products in nonalcoholic steatohepatitis: new evidence on the potential therapeutic mechanism. Hepatology. 2012;56(4):1291–9. PMID:22505276.
96. Du J, Ma YY, Yu CH, et al. Effects of pentoxifylline on nonalcoholic fatty liver disease: a meta-analysis. World J Gastroenterol. 2014;20(2):569–77. PMID:24574727.
97. Badri S, Dashti-Khavidaki S, Lessan-Pezeshki M, et al. A review of the potential benefits of pentoxifylline in diabetic and non-diabetic proteinuria. J Pharm Pharm Sci. 2011;14 (1):128–37.
98. Perkins RM, Aboudara MC, Uy AL, et al. Effect of pentoxifylline on GFR decline in CKD: a pilot, double-blind, randomized, placebo-controlled trial. Am J Kid Dis. 2009;53(4):606–16.
99. Yki-Järvinen H. Thiazolidinediones and the liver in humans. Curr Opin Lipidol. 2009;20 (6):477–83.
100. Torres DM, Jones FJ, Shaw JC, et al. Rosiglitazone versus rosiglitazone and metformin versus rosiglitazone and losartan in the treatment of nonalcoholic steatohepatitis in humans: a 12-month randomized, prospective, open- label trial. Hepatology. 2011;54(5):1631–9.
101. Duseja A, Das A, Dhiman RK, et al. Metformin is effective in achieving biochemical response in patients with nonalcoholic fatty liver disease (NAFLD) not responding to lifestyle interventions. Ann Hepatol. 2007;6(4):222–6.
102. Loomba R, Lutchman G, Kleiner DE, et al. Clinical trial: pilot study of metformin for the treatment of non-alcoholic steatohepatitis. Aliment Pharmacol Ther. 2009;29(2):172–82.
103. Doycheva I, Loomba R. Effect of metformin on ballooning degeneration in nonalcoholic steatohepatitis (NASH): when to use metformin in nonalcoholic fatty liver disease (NAFLD). Adv Ther. 2014;31(1):30–43.
104. Boettcher E, Csako G, Pucino F, et al. Meta-analysis: pioglitazone improves liver histology and fibrosis in patients with non-alcoholic steatohepatitis. Aliment Pharmacol Ther. 2012;35 (1):66–75.
105. Rakoski MO, Singal AG, Rogers MA, et al. Meta-analysis: insulin sensitizers for the treatment of non-alcoholic steatohepatitis. Aliment Pharmacol Ther. 2010;32(10):1211–21.
106. Shyangdan D, Clar C, Ghouri N, et al. Insulin sensitisers in the treatment of non-alcoholic fatty liver disease: a systematic review. Health Technol Assess. 2011;15(38):1–110.

107. Sanyal AJ, Chalasani N, Kowdley KV, et al. Pioglitazone, vitamin E, or placebo for nonalcoholic steatohepatitis. N Engl J Med. 2010;362(18):1675–85.
108. Yan Z, Ni Y, Wang P, et al. Peroxisome proliferator-activated receptor delta protects against obesity-related glomerulopathy through the P38 MAPK pathway. Obesity. 2013;21 (3):538–45.
109. Kong X, Zhang DY, Wu HB, et al. Losartan and pioglitazone ameliorate nephropathy in experimental metabolic syndrome rats. Biol Pharm Bull. 2011;34(5):693–9.
110. Ochodnicky P, Mesarosova L, Cernecka H, et al. Pioglitazone, a PPAR agonist, provides comparable protection to angiotensin converting enzyme inhibitor ramipril against adriamycin nephropathy in rat. Eur J Pharmacol. 2014;730:51–60.
111. Huang Y, Lei Y, Zheng Z, et al. Rosiglitazone alleviates injury in rats with adenine-induced chronic kidney disease. Mol Med Rep. 2013;8(6):1831–5.
112. Higashi K, Oda T, Kushiyama T, et al. Additive antifibrotic effects of pioglitazone and candesartan on experimental renal fibrosis in mice. Nephrology. 2010;15(3):327–35.
113. Yang HC, Deleuze S, Zuo Y, et al. The PPARgamma agonist pioglitazone ameliorates aging-related progressive renal injury. J Am Soc Nephrol. 2009;20(11):2380–8.
114. Jin HM, Pan Y. Renoprotection provided by losartan in combination with pioglitazone is superior to renoprotection provided by losartan alone in patients with type 2 diabetic nephropathy. Kidney Blood Press Res. 2007;30(4):203–11.
115. Satriano J, Sharma K, Blantz RC, et al. Induction of AMPK activity corrects early pathophysiological alterations in the subtotal nephrectomy model of chronic kidney disease. Am J Physiol Renal Physiol. 2013;305(5):F727–33.
116. Inzucchi SE, Lipska KJ, Mayo H, et al. Metformin in patients with type 2 diabetes and kidney disease: a systematic review. JAMA. 2014;312(24):2668–75.
117. Wang W, Zhao C, Zhou J, et al. Simvastatin ameliorates liver fibrosis via mediating nitric oxide synthase in rats with non-alcoholic steatohepatitis-related liver fibrosis. PLoS One. 2013;8(10):e76538. PMID:24098525.
118. Van Rooyen DM, Gan LT, Yeh MM, et al. Pharmacological cholesterol lowering reverses fibrotic NASH in obese, diabetic mice with metabolic syndrome. J Hepatol. 2013;59 (1):144–52.
119. Kimura Y, Hyogo H, Yamagishi S, et al. Atorvastatin decreases serum levels of advanced glycation endproducts (AGEs) in nonalcoholic steatohepatitis (NASH) patients with dyslipidemia: clinical usefulness of AGEs as a biomarker for the attenuation of NASH. J Gastroenterol. 2010;45(7):750–7.
120. Nseir W, Mograbi J, Ghali M. Lipid-lowering agents in nonalcoholic fatty liver disease and steatohepatitis: human studies. Dig Dis Sci. 2012;57(7):1773–81.
121. Eslami L, Merat S, Malekzadeh R, et al. Statins for non-alcoholic fatty liver disease and non-alcoholic steatohepatitis. Cochrane Database Syst Rev. 2013;12:CD008623.
122. Douglas K, O'Malley PG, Jackson JL. Meta-analysis: the effect of statins on albuminuria. Ann Intern Med. 2006;145(2):117–24.
123. Sandhu S, Wiebe N, Fried LF, et al. Statins for improving renal outcomes: a meta-analysis. J Am Soc Nephrol. 2006;17(7):2006–16.
124. Strippoli GF, Navaneethan SD, Johnson DW, et al. Effects of statins in patients with chronic kidney disease: meta-analysis and meta-regression of randomised controlled trials. BMJ. 2008;336(7645):645–51.
125. Palmer SC, Navaneethan SD, Craig JC, et al. HMG CoA reductase inhibitors (statins) for people with chronic kidney disease not requiring dialysis. Cochrane Database Syst Rev. 2014;5:CD007784.
126. Lopez-Huertas E. The effect of EPA and DHA on metabolic syndrome patients: a systematic review of randomised controlled trials. Br J Nutr. 2012;107 Suppl 2:S185–94.
127. Kajikawa S, Imada K, Takeuchi T, et al. Eicosapentaenoic acid attenuates progression of hepatic fibrosis with inhibition of reactive oxygen species production in rats fed methionine- and choline-deficient diet. Dig Dis Sci. 2011;56(4):1065–74.

128. Depner CM, Philbrick KA, Jump DB. Docosahexaenoic acid attenuates hepatic inflammation, oxidative stress, and fibrosis without decreasing hepatosteatosis in a Ldlr (-/-) mouse model of western diet-induced nonalcoholic steatohepatitis. J Nutr. 2013;143(3):315–23.
129. Depner CM, Traber MG, Bobe G, et al. A metabolomic analysis of omega-3 fatty acid-mediated attenuation of western diet-induced nonalcoholic steatohepatitis in LDLR-/- mice. PLoS One. 2013;8(12):e83756. PMID:24358308.
130. Tanaka N, Sano K, Horiuchi A, et al. Highly purified eicosapentaenoic acid treatment improves nonalcoholic steatohepatitis. J Clin Gastroenterol. 2008;42(4):413–8.
131. Scorletti E, Bhatia L, McCormick KG, et al. Effects of purified eicosapentaenoic and docosahexaenoic acids in non-alcoholic fatty liver disease: results from the *WELCOME study. Hepatology. 2014;60:1211–21. PMID:25043514.
132. Sakurai K, et al. Dietary Perilla seed oil supplement increases plasma omega-3 polyunsaturated fatty acids and ameliorates immunoglobulin A nephropathy in high immunoglobulin A strain of ddY mice. Nephron Exp Nephrol. 2011;119:e33–9.
133. Katakura M, Hashimoto M, Inoue T, et al. Omega-3 fatty acids protect renal functions by increasing docosahexaenoic acid-derived metabolite levels in SHR.Cg-Lepr (cp)/NDmcr rats, a metabolic syndrome model. Molecules. 2014;19(3):3247–63.
134. Mehta RL, Kellum JA, Shah SV, Acute Kidney Injury Network, et al. Acute Kidney Injury Network: report of an initiative to improve outcomes in acute kidney injury. Crit Care. 2007;11(2):R31.

Chapter 12
Endocrine Disease and Liver

Masataka Seike

Abstract Liver diseases are closely related to a wide spectrum of endocrine diseases. The liver plays an important role in the metabolism of not only glucose, lipids, and proteins but also of thyroid, adrenal, sex, and growth hormones. Therefore, liver dysfunction including liver cirrhosis can affect other body organs and lead to abnormalities of endocrine systems. In cirrhotic patients, several abnormal alterations of the thyroid gland, adrenal insufficiency, and hypogonadism have been identified.

On the other hand, endocrine diseases can lead to liver disorders. Hypothyroidism and hyperthyroidism can cause liver injury with hepatocellular or cholestatic injury. Additionally, insufficiency and excessive adrenal hormones can induce liver injury and estrogens are associated with various liver disorders, including cholestatic liver injury and vascular and hepatic tumors. Furthermore, endocrine disorders, such as hypogonadism, hypothyroidism, growth hormone deficiency, and hypercortisolemia are associated with nonalcoholic fatty liver disease (NAFLD).

As endocrine disorders and liver disease are both common in the general population, clinicians should pay attention to the presence of liver disease among patients with endocrine disorders.

Keywords Liver disease • Thyroid hormone • Adrenal hormone • Sex hormone • Growth hormone

12.1 Introduction

Liver diseases are often associated with hormonal disorders, such as thyroid diseases, adrenal disease, hypogonadism, and adult growth hormone (GH) deficiency (AGHD). Endocrine disorders and liver diseases are both common in the general population. Additionally, hormonal treatment for cancer, such as tamoxifen, which is a nonsteroidal antiestrogen drug, causes iatrogenic liver disease. As the liver plays a

M. Seike (✉)
Department of Gastroenterology, Faculty of Medicine, Oita University, 1-1 Idaigaoka, Hasama-machi, Yufu-City, Oita 879-5593, Japan
e-mail: seikem@oita-u.ac.jp

H. Ohira (ed.), *The Liver in Systemic Diseases*, DOI 10.1007/978-4-431-55790-6_12

fundamental role in regulating metabolism, these endocrine abnormalities also play a role in the pathogenesis of nonalcoholic fatty liver disease (NAFLD); yet, awareness of this remains low. Accordingly, liver diseases and endocrine disorders have a bidirectional and complex relationship. It is important that primary care physicians, endocrinologists, and hepatologists are aware of the scope of both diseases.

12.2 Thyroid Hormones and Liver Disease

Thyroid hormones are potent mediators of normal organ growth, development, and function. These hormones regulate energy metabolism in all cells, including hepatocytes. The hypothalamic-pituitary-thyroid (HPT) axis is controlled by a classic endocrine feedback loop. Thyrotropin-releasing hormone (TRH) is released from the hypothalamus and stimulates the anterior pituitary to secrete thyroid-stimulating hormone (TSH). TSH drives the thyroid gland to release the thyroid hormone; the prohormone thyroxine (T4) is converted to triiodothyronine (T3) in peripheral tissues. T3 is the most biologically active form of thyroid hormone. Thyroid hormone receptors (TRs) belong to the nuclear receptor superfamily and mediate the biological functions T3 via transcriptional regulation [1].

According to previous studies, the liver performs functions relating to thyroid hormone transport and metabolism, and contributes to the regulation of systemic endocrine effects. The liver has an important role in metabolism of thyroxine-binding globulin and in alteration of thyroid hormones, and provides a large pool of circulating hormone. More than 99 % of throid hormones are bound to thyroxine-binding globulin, thyroxine-binding prealbumin, and albumin in plasma. Thyroid function is dependent on a normally functioning liver axis. Accordingly, thyroid hormone levels are closely correlated with liver-associated diseases, ranging from hepatic steatosis to hepatocellular carcinoma (HCC). The liver is involved with the synthesis of carrier proteins and metabolism of various hormones; therefore, liver diseases may be associated with various endocrine disturbances [2].

Although further studies are warranted to elucidate the complex mechanism of action of thyroid hormones in the liver, thyroid hormone-based therapeutic strategies for various liver diseases may be used to improve therapeutic outcomes [3, 4].

12.3 Thyroid Dysfunction in Liver Disease

In acute hepatitis of mild to moderate severity, there are elavated serum levels of T4 due to increased thyroid-binding globulin, which is synthesized as an acute-phase reactant; however, there are normal levels of free T4. In more severe cases with impending liver failure, the data is variable, and low T4 levels may reflect reduced hepatocellular synthesis of thyroid-binding globulin. Serum T3 levels are extremely variable, but the free T3:T4 ratio correlates negatively with severity of liver disease and has prognostic value [5]. In a previous study, more than 50 % of patients with acute liver failure presented with abnormal thyroid function. These patients had greater risk for adverse outcomes than euthyroid patients. Patients who recovered without liver transplantation had higher TSH total T4 and T3 concentrations, whereas there were no differences in free hormone concentrations. TSH and total thyroid hormone may serve as additional indicators of disease severity [6]. In patients with hepatitis B related to acute-on-chronic liver failure, serum TSH levels may be a useful indicator for assessing severity and prognosis [7].

Cirrhosis is the common end stage of liver disease. Nonalcoholic steatohepatitis (NASH), viral hepatitis, alcoholic liver disease, autoimmune hepatitis (AIH), and primary biliary choleangitis (PBC) are known causes of liver cirrhosis. Regardless of etiology, liver cirrhosis and its various complications affect other body organs, including endocrine organs.

The liver is a major site of peripheral conversion, degradation, and excretion of thyroid hormones. Therefore, abnormal thyroid function at all levels of hypothalamic-pituitary-peripheral axis is expected in patients with liver cirrhosis [8].

Several abnormal alterations in the thyroid gland have been identified in patients with liver cirrhosis; these range from alterations in thyroid size, morphology, and architectural pattern to alterations in thyroid hormone metabolism and regulation.

The volume of the thyroid gland is reported to increase by up to 17 % in cirrhosis patients compared with non-cirrhotic controls, as measured using ultrasonography [9], the prevalence of thyroid hormone abnormalities ranged from 13 % to 61 %. In patients with cirrhosis, hypothyroidism was more frequently seen, and hyperthyroidism has been also reported [10]. The most consistent thyroid hormone profile in patients with cirrhosis is low total and free T3 and elevated rT3 levels, similar to changes in patients with euthyroid sick syndrome. This results in an increase in conversion of T4 to T3 and an increase in the rT3:T3 ratio. T3:rT3 ratio binds to the same plasma proteins; the T3:rT3 ratio provides a parameter of liver function. Table 12.1 presents a systematic review of dysfunctions of thyroid hormones [11, 12, 37–41].

Regarding the association between severity of cirrhosis and thyroid function, low T4 levels may be related with decreased short- and long-term survival of patients with liver cirrhosis [12]. Low T3 levels are a good indicator of disease severity in cirrhosis [13]. A negative correlation was found between Child-Pugh scores and total serum T3 levels [14].

Low total and free T3 levels may be considered an adaptive hypothyroid condition that contributes to reducing the basal metabolic rate within hepatocytes to preserve liver function. Indeed, recent study showed a significant improvement of liver function, including alanine aminotransferase, alkaline phosphatase, albumin, bilirubin, and prothrombin time in patients with increased TSH [15]. Hypothyroidism is also associated with lesser degrees of decompensation in cirrhosis [16]. Accordingly, euthyroid patients with liver cirrhosis may benefit from a controlled hypothyroidism. However, further studies are required to test this

Table 12.1 Thyroid dysfunction (TD) in liver cirrhosis [8]

Article	Number of patients	Underlying disease	Prevalence of TD	Pattern of TD
Corpechot [38]	205	PBC	26(13 %)	AITD
Caregaro [12]	75	Alc/V	23(30.6 %)	T4↓
Moustafa [39]	59	HCV	NA	T3↓, TSH↑
Tas [40]	106	V/AIH/PBC/Crypt/Alc	65(61.3 %)	SUS
El-Kabbny [37]	40	V/Metabolic/AIH/BA/ Buddchiari/Wilson	NA	FT3↓
Seehofer [41]	22	V/PBC/Alc/Crypt	NA	T3↓, FT3↓
Silveira [10]	67	PBC	9(13.4 %)	Hypo & hyperthyroid

PBC primary biliary cholangitis, *AITD* autoimmune thyroid disease, *Alc* alcoholic, *HCV* Hepatitis C Virus, *AIH* autoimmune hepatitis, *Crypt* cryptogenic, *BA* biliary atresia, *SUS* sick euthyroid syndrome

hypothesis. As thyroid hormone disorders are prevalent in liver cirrhosis, awareness of thyroid function in liver disease is necessary.

12.4 Nonthyroidal Illness Syndrome (NTIS)

Alterations in thyroid hormone metabolism during illness is known as nonthyroidal illness syndrome (NTIS), euthyroid sick syndrome, or low T3 syndrome [4]. In humans, non-thyroidal systemic illness can decrease serum levels of thyroid hormone without a concomitant rise in serum TSH; if negative feedback controls were functional, serum TSH would be substantially increased. This condition is characterized by normal total T4, normal-high freeT4, low free T3, and elevated rT3 levels. Serum T3 further decrease as the severity of disease progresses. Therefore, the scale of the decrease in thyroid hormone plasma levels is associated with the severity and prognosis of disease. NTIS is regarded as a survival advantage in chronically ill patients, as it reduce their basal metabolic rate. In chronic liver disease, a similar process may occur [17]; however, until now, no evidence-based consensus or guidelines have advocated for the use of thyroid hormones to treat NTIS.

12.5 NAFLD and Thyroid

Nonalcoholic fatty liver disease (NAFLD) is recognized as the most common liver disease ranging from simple steatosis to NASH, cirrhosis, and HCC [18]. NAFLD is considered the hepatic manifestation of metabolic syndrome; the mechanisms underlying NAFLD development are closely related to insulin resistance and metabolic syndrome. Thyroid hormones play a fundamental role in lipid metabolism. Hypothyroidism may cause hypercholesterolemia and play an essential role in the pathogenesis of NAFLD. Therefore, thyroid dysfunction, including subclinical hypothyroidism, has been reported to accompany metabolic syndrome.

A recent study demonstrated that the prevalence of NAFLD is negatively correlated with free T4 levels, and decreased free T4 levels contribute to the risk of NAFLD [19]. Furthermore, even subclinical hypothyroidism was suggested to be related to NAFLD in a cross-sectional study with a large general population [19].

Hypothyroidism decreases hepatic uptake of triglyceride-derived free fatty acids [20]. Lipolysis in abdominal subcutaneous adipose tissue is modulated by thyroid function [21].

Thyroid hormone receptor-α knockout mice were protected against high-fat diet-induced hepatic steatosis and insulin resistance [22].

Moreover, a recent study has shown the importance of thyroid hormones for the intrahepatic metabolism via autophagy, including fatty acid β-oxidation and delivery of fatty acids to the mitochondria [23].

Conversely, hyperthyroidism promotes adipose tissue lipolysis and hepatic lipogenesis [24, 25]. A recent systematic review regarding the association between NAFLD and thyroid function has highlighted inconsistent; thus, further studies elucidating this issue are warranted [11].

12.6 AIH PBC and Thyroid Function

Primary biliary cholangitis (PBC) is a chronic inflammatory autoimmune disease frequently associated with extrahepatic autoimmune diseases, such as Sjogren's syndrome, rheumatoid arthritis, Hashimoto's thyroiditis, and Graves's disease. Despite the clear evidence of an association between thyroid disease and PBC, it is uncertain whether this association is stronger than that with other diseases of the liver [26]. Several autoimmune disorders are associated with the diagnoses of primary sclerosing cholangitis (PSC) and autoimmune hepatitis; however, data on the development of thyroid dysfunction in these disorders are limited. A recent report suggested that thyroid dysfunction was as common in patients with PBC as it was in patients with both PSC and NAFLD [10].

12.7 Liver Dysfunction in Thyroid Disease

Hypothyroidism is common in patients with autoimmune liver diseases and its prevalence has recently increased in those with hepatitis C and NAFLD. Patients with hypothyroidism may have myalgia, fatigue, muscle cramps in the presence of elevated muscle aspartate aminotransferase levels, myxedema coma, and myxedema ascites with a high protein concentration. Myxedema ascites was previously considered a consequence of heart failuer or enhance permeability of the vascular endothelium; liver biopsy findings usually show normal or central congestive fibrosis [27, 28]. Hypothyroidism is associated with cholestatic jaundice due to bilirubin and bile excretion. In rat, hypothyroidism resulted in enhanced hepatic bilirubin UDP-glucuronosyltransferase activity and in decreased p-nitrophenol transferase activity, it led to a cholestatic condition with a 50 % decrease in bile flow and bile salt excretion and an increased proportion of conjugated bilirubin in serum [29]. Hypothyroidism should be considered in patients with portal hypertension with refractory ascites, and hormone replacement therapy can make them sensitivve to diuretics. Hepatic abnormalities associated with hypothyroidism can be reversible over a matter of weeks with hormone replacement therapy without residual liver damage [1]. Recently, it has been shown that overt hypothyroidism is more prevalent in patients with NAFLD and in those with HCC of unknown etiology [30, 31].

Such findings may be biologically plausible as overt hypothyroidism can lead to visceral obesity, metabolic syndrome, insulin resistance, and lipid peroxidation, all of which are closely associated with NAFLD [32] and are potential risk factors for liver carcinogenesis. However, further studies are needed to demonstrate an association between NAFLD and hypothyroidism.

Liver injury caused by thyrotoxicosis is relatively common and is classified as hepatic or cholesteric injury. The mechanism of injury is relative hypoxia in the perivenular regions due to an increase in hepatic oxygen demand owing to the presence of thyrotoxicosis [33]. Bile acid production and oxidative stress may lead to a cholestatic pattern of injury. A 10-year retrospective review of patients with acute thyrotoxicosis (90.9 % Graves' disease), excluding iatrogenic causes, who were admitted to a single institution found that 81.8 % of patients had some degree of hepatic abnormality. In patients with hyperthyroidism, these abnormalities were variable in character and magnitude but appeared to have a hepatic predominance [34]. In mild cases, liver histology shows non-specific changes that, on light microscopy, consist of a mild lobular inflammatory infiltrate invoving polymorphic neutrophils, eosinophils, and lymphocytes, associated with nuclear changes and Kupffer cell hyperplasia. Electron microscopy may reveal hyperplasia of the smooth endoplasmic reticulum, a paucity of cytoplasmic glycogen, and an increased number and size of mitochondria, which may contain more cristae [1], whereas liver histology may reveal mild liver injury, with centrilobular cholestasis. Evidence of thyroid dysfunction should be sought in cases of unexpected hepatic abnormalities.

12.8 Therapy for Hyperthyroidism and Liver Damage

Therpies for hyperthyroidism may result in alterations of liver function. Hepatotoxicity is observed more frequently with propylthiouracil than with methimazole treatment (27 % vs 7 %) [35]. In the United States, propylthiouracil is the second leading cause of non-acetaminophen-associated drug-induced liver injury requiring liver transplant [36]. Moreover, therapy may itself cause hepatic complications. Increased serum levels of aspartate aminotransferase and alanine aminotransferase occur in approximately 30 % of patients treated with propylthiouracil. The rise in aspartate aminotransferase appears to be dose-related, resulting in aspartate aminotransferase and alanine aminotransferase levels that are highest during the first few weeks of treatment.

12.9 Liver and Thyroid Dysfunction Owing to Systemic Condition

Malignancies, amyloidosis, and secondary hemochromatosis with diffuse iron deposition cause concomitant liver and thyroid dysfunction. Furthermore, medications such as amiodarone, mefloquine, carbamazepine, and antineoplastic can also result in concomitant liver and thyroid dysfunction.

12.10 Adrenal Hormones and Liver Disease

The relationship between the adrenal gland and liver is complex and bidirectional; in other words, dysfunction in one organ tends to cause functional abnormalities in other organs as well [42].

12.11 Adrenal Insufficiency and Liver Disease

Addison's disease described by Thomas Addison in 1855, which have the cardinal symptoms of adrenal insufficiency (AI), including weakness, fatigue, anorexia, abdominal pain, orthostatic hypotension, salt cravings, and hyperpigmentation of the skin, can cause slightly elevated liver enzymes [43]. Although the mechanisms of interaction remain unclear, chronic hypoperfusion, weight changes, ischemic hepatic injury, and apoptosis induced by cytokines might underlie hepatic injury. The levels of aminotransaminase normalizes after adequate replacement of glucocorticoid. Hepatologists should consider subclinical Addison's disease as a cause of persistently increased transaminase levels with constitutional symptoms in the absence of fatty liver or viral and autoimmune markers [43, 44].

Recent studies have shown that there may be a higher prevalence of AI in patients with liver failure and cirrhosis. The prevalence of AI may range from 33 % in acute liver failure to 69 % in acute-on-chronic liver failure [45, 46]. Relative adrenal dysfunction is frequent in patients with advanced cirrhosis and sepsis, as well as in stable and decompensated cirrhosis without sepsis, such as variceal bleeding and ascites. AI has also documented early and late after liver transplantation. There are discrepancies in the prevalence of AI among studies due to different diffinitions; thus, a consensus is needed on the appropriate tests and criteria used to define AI.

The mechanisms of AI in liver disease remain unclear, but several hypotheses have been suggested (Fig. 12.1). First, total cholesterol, high-density lipoprotein (HDL) cholesterol, and low-density lipoprotein (LDL) cholesterol which are essential precursors for steroid synthesis in adrenal gland decrease in cirrhosis. Second, serum endotoxin levels were increased in patients with cirrhosis. Accordingly, pro-inflammatory cytokines, such as TNF-α, and other peptides derived from blood cells induce the impairment of the HPA axis. Particularly, TNF-α has been shown to inhibit the secretion of adrenocorticotropic hormone (ACTH) from the pituitary gland to suppress the response of corticotropes. Patients with cirrhosis have an increased susceptibility to bacterial infection, which may be partly due to AI. AI results in hemodynamic instability and a reduced response to vasoactive drugs; both of these abnormalities could lead to a higher incidence of hemodynamic dysfunction in patients with cirrhosis and AI.

The effect of corticosteroid therapy on critically ill patients with liver disease has been evaluated in some studies, but the results remain controversial. The use of corticosteroids in liver disease should be reserved for patients with sepsis requiring vasopressors. Further randomized clinical trial should be conducted to determine their use in other patients with liver failure. The mechanism by which liver disease leads to dysfunction of the HPA axis has yet to be clarified; several hypotheses have been suggested (Fig. 12.1) [47].

Corticosteroid replacement may lead to shock resolution and a high survival rate [48]; however, in a recent randomized controlled trial, low-dose hydrocortisone did not reduce mortality [49].

The prevalence of AI in patients with liver cirrhosis who are not critically ill ranged from 7.2 to 60 % in different studies. These studies showed the prognosis of patients with liver cirrhosis with AI was poor [8].

The degree of adrenal dysfunction correlates with severity of liver disease. Although the mechanisms of HPA dysfunction are not clear in liver disease, Marik et al. have used the term “hepatoadrenal syndrome” to describe these findings [50].

Hepatoadrenal syndrome has also been characterized in children with end-stage liver disease [51].

Regarding the risk factors for the development of AI, the serum level of high-density lipoprotein (HDL) was inversely correlated with the degree of RAL, and

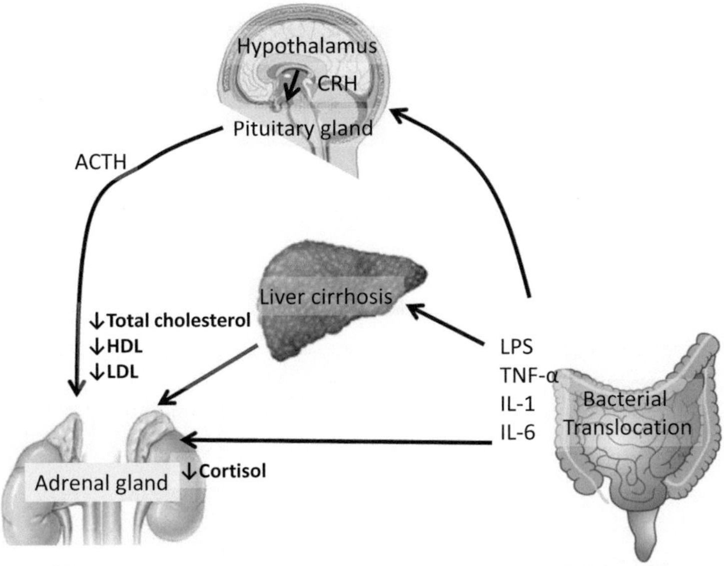

Fig. 12.1 Possible causes of adrenal dysfunction in liver disease [47]. *LPS*; lipopolysaccharide. *CRH*; corticotropin releasing hormone. *TNF-α*; r tumor necrotizing factor-α

it has been proposed that low HDL levels could be used as a surrogate marker for the development of AI [52]. Because AI is extremely common in patients with advanced liver cirrhosis, free cortisol measurements may also be useful. However, there is controversy concerning the effect of corticosteroid therapy on cirrhotic patients with AI. Further research on adrenal function in patients with cirrhosis is needed to confirm the relationship between AI and its outcome in cirrhotic patients.

12.12 Adrenal Excess and the Liver

Cushing's syndrome is associated with features of metabolic syndrome, including NAFLD and insulin resistance. NAFLD is also observed in patients with excess because of exogenous corticosteroid administration. Emerging data suggest that patients with metabolic syndrome show hyperactivity of the HPA axis, which leads to a state of "functional hypercortisolism." The increased exposure to cortisol contributes to increased fat accumulation in visceral depots. However, cortisol metabolism is not only centrally regulated; the action of 11β-hydroxysteroid dehydrogenase-type 1 at the tissue level also modulates cortisol metabolism. Increased 11β-hydroxysteroid dehydrogenase-type 1 activity in adipose tissue and liver might contribute to the development of several features of the metabolic syndrome. Metabolic syndrome shares many characteristics of Cushing's syndrome, and the cortisol might play a role, at both a central and a peripheral level in the development of metabolic syndrome [53, 54].

12.13 Adrenocortical Dysfunction in Liver Disease

In patients with cirrhosis, AI during critical illnesses, such as of sepsis and septic shock, is associated with increased mortality.

Some studies have investigated the prevalence of AI in patients with stable cirrhosis, as well as in those with decompensated cirrhosis other than sepsis, such as bleeding (30–48 %) and ascites (26–64 %). Moreover, other studies showed a high prevalence in liver transplant recipients immediately or after liver transplantation.

12.14 Sex Hormones and Liver Disease

Estrogens considered to play a role in the development of liver damage involving the biliary duct. The prevalence of PBC is more frequent in females than it is in males [55, 56]. Chronic hepatic rejection leading to ductopenia occurs more frequent with male donors and female recipients [57].

Endocrine disorders are frequent in PBC, including a high prevalence of osteoporosis, which is a sign of estrogen deficiency [58, 59].

Bile duct pathology is frequent in Turner syndrome, and estrogen replacement therapy is an effective treatment, which suggests a strong association between estrogens and cholangiopathy [60].

Furthermore, it is well known that oral contraceptives are associated with cholestasis. The incidence of hepatic disorders has steadily declined over the years and may be related to the use of lower doses of estrogen and progesterone in currently available contraceptive preparations [61]. Estrogen can induce intrahepatic cholestasis and jaundice. Oral contraceptives with concomitant progestin, genetic susceptibility, prior history of pregnancy-associated cholestasis [62], subclinical PBC, Dubin-Johnson syndrome, and familial intrahepatic cholestasis are thought to increase the risk of cholestasis [63, 64].

Moreover, jaundice usually presents within the first 6 months of oral contraceptive use and is not associated with elevations of aminotransferase or alkaline phosphatase levels. It resolves with discontinuation of the drug; full recovery may take weeks to months [65].

A variety of hepatic disorders associated with estrogens have been reported (Table 12.2). The long-term use of oral contraceptives can cause both benign tumors, including hemangioma, adenoma, and focal nodular hyperplasia (FNH), as well as

Table 12.2 Liver disease associated with sex hormones [42]

	Estrogens	Androgens
Disorder of hepatic metabolism	Cholestatic jaundice	Abnormal liver function test cholestatic jaundice secondary biliary cirrhosis
Vascular disorder	Budd-Chiari syndrome	Peliosis hepatis
	Portal vein thrombosis	
	Peliosis hepatis	
Hepatic tumors	Hepatic adenoma	Hepatic adenoma hepatocellular carcinoma
	Focal nodular hyperplasia	
	Hemagioma	
	Hepatocellular carcinoma	

malignant hepatocellular tumors [66]. Hepatic vein or portal vein and peliosis hepatis are recognized as hepatic vascular disorders related to estrogen use [67].

Peliosis hepatis is a rare complication of estrogen use that has characteristics of hepatomegaly and elevations of aminotransferase levels. The pathogenesis of peliosis remains uncertain; however, the lesion resolves with cessation of estrogen use [68]. As previously stated, benign hepatic tumors, such as adenoma, FNH, and hemangiomas are associated with oral contraceptive use. Hepatic adenomas are rare benign tumors that usually occur in young women; their development and complications are related to the strength of and duration of use of oral contraceptives. Hepatic adenoma incidence has decreased since the introduction of oral contraceptive pills containing smaller amounts of estrogen. FNH is a benign local hyperplasia. Due to the female predominance and the young age of onset, estrogen may play a role in the development of tumor. Furthermore, 50–75 % of women with FNH use oral contraceptives [66]. Liver hemangioma is the most common benign tumor and is usually seen in young adult female. This female predilection and clinical observations of liver hemangioma growth under estrogenic exposure suggest a possible role for estrogen in its pathogenesis. However, evidence of the role of oral contraceptives in causing either lesion is lacking. HCC, one of the most frequent primary liver cancers, is the third most common cause of cancer mortality worldwide [70]. Animal models of experimental liver carcinogenesis and epidemiological studies in humans suggest a relationship between exposure to sex hormones and HCC growth. These hormones may play a role as inducers and promoters in the hepatic carcinogenesis. Androgens are considered to promote carcinogenesis, whereas estrogens has diverse roles in the development of HCC. Regardless of etiology, chronic liver disease progresses at unequal rates in women and men. These epidemiological data have prompted researchers to investigate the relationship between sex hormone and liver tumors [71].

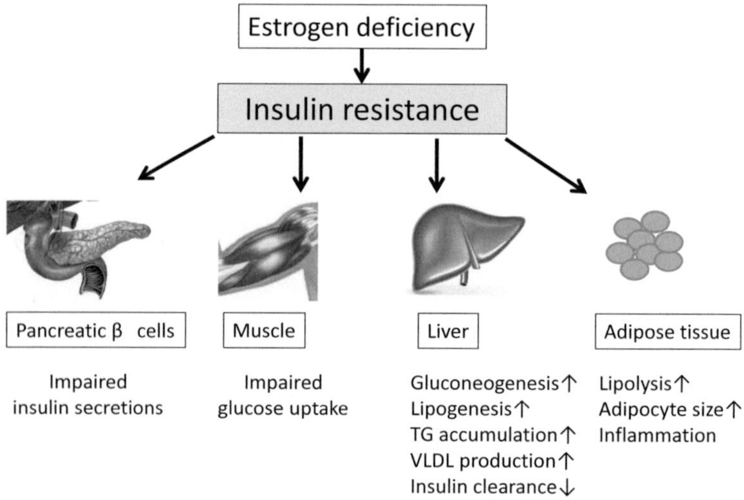

Fig. 12.2 The relationship between estrogen and insulin resistance [72]

Furthermore, estrogen and estrogen receptors (ERs) are known regulators of several aspects of metabolism, including glucose and lipid metabolism, and impaired estrogen signaling is associated with the development of metabolic disease. Metabolic syndrome is a complex condition characterized by obesity, insulin resistance, decreased HDL cholesterol, and hypertension; it is associated with a high risk of developing type 2 diabetes and cardiovascular disease. A major increase in the incidence of metabolic syndrome and its related disease has been observed worldwide in association with a transition to a less active lifestyle and increased food consumption. Humans and rodents studies have linked estrogen to the regulation of glucose homeostasis. Estrogen deficiency is strongly associated with the development of insulin resitance and subsequent manifestations in various metabolic tissues [72] (Fig. 12.2).

12.15 PCOS and Liver Disease

Polycystic ovary syndrome (PCOS) is the most common endocrinopathy in women of reproductive-age. Women with PCOS are at increased risk for metabolic disorder, such as insulin resistance, diabetes mellitus, hypertension, and dyslipidemia. Recently, PCOS has been considered a significant risk factor for the development of NAFLD in women. Conversely, NAFLD may also be a risk factor for PCOS [73]. PCOS is clinically characterized by clinical features including anovulatory infertility, hirsutism, menstrual dysfunction, acne, and alopecia, as well as by increases in serum androgen and luteinizing hormone. Moreover, the ovarian follicles develop poorly, giving rise to multiple cysts. PCOS is diagnosed with oligo-anovulation, clinical, and/or biochemical hyperandrogenism, and polycystic ovaries. The prevalence of PCOS ranges from 5 % to 16 % in the normal population and varies across studies according to the diagnostic criteria used and the characteristics of the participants [74–77]. Obesity is more frequent in women with PCOS. Even in lean patients, PCOS is often accompanied by abnormalities in insulin secretion [78, 79].

Insulin resitance and androgen excess in PCOS patients may contribute to NAFLD. The prevalence of NAFLD in the PCOS population is estimated to be between 15 and 55 %. As the prevalence of NAFLD is higher in women with PCOS compared with the general population, early recognition is important. PCOS and NAFLD share a common attribute with regard to the pathogenesis of insulin resistance. Multiple factors, including environmental and genetic variables, steroid biosynthesis, and androgen excess, contribute to the development of insulin resistance. Both PCOS and NAFLD are frequently accompanied by metabolic syndrome, and these two diseases can coexist and may respond to similar therapeutic strategies.

12.16 Growth Hormone and Liver Disease

Growth hormone (GH) is secreted in peaks shortly after the onset of sleep and a few hours. GH excess leads to both hepatic and peripheral insulin resistance, and GH also promotes lipolysis and fat oxidation. Insulin-like growth factor-1 (IGF-1) has insulin-sensitizing effects and is considered a the second messenger of GH as it mediates important anabolic effect. Moreover, it has been used as a first-line marker for the diagnosis and therapeutic monitoring of patients with acromegaly. Acromegaly is usually caused by a GH-secreting pituitary adenoma, and prolonged excess GH/IGF-1 exposure leads to somatic and metabolic effects [80]. Acromegaly is a rare condition with an annual incidence of 3 patients per million [81]. Patients with acromegaly develop insulin resistance and hyperinsulinemia, and a previous study found that approximately 28–53 % of patients with acromegaly who underwent an oral glucose tolerance test were diagnosed with diabetes mellitus [82].

GH hypersecretion can result in excess linear bone growth and gigantism. Long-term complications include arthropathy, cardiomyopathy, hypertension, and impaired glucose tolerance [83].

Neurosurgery in acromegaly leads to increase in insulin sensitivity and serum adiponectin levels and decreases in serum alanine aminotransferase activity. The modest increase in adiponectin in acromegaly patients undergoing pituitary surgery was associated with improved insulin resistance, as well as a decrease in alanine aminotransferase activity [84].

The main causes of reduced life expectancy in acromegaly are cardiovascular and respiratory diseases. GH and IGF-1 play essential roles in linear growth in childhood, and have important metabolic actions throughout life.

The metabolic syndrome is a cluster of cardiovascular risk factors including central obesity, dyslipidemia, hypertension, insulin resistance, and type 2 diabetes.

GH plays an important role in the regulation of hepatic LDL receptors and may be of important in the control of plasma LDL cholesterol levels. Moreover, GH is involved in complex actions related to carbohydrate metabolism, and GH excess is associated with both hepatic and peripheral insulin resistance.

12.17 Adult GH Deficiency (AGHD)

AGHD has with various symptoms, such as increased visceral fat, decreased muscle mass, osteoporosis, and hyperlipidemia. Adult patients with hypothalamic-pituitary masses either before or after therapy (neurosurgery, radiotherapy, and/or medical therapy) are at risk for severe AGHD. The large majority of patients with childhood-onset multiple hypopituitarism show persistent severe GH deficiency (GHD) [85]. Traumatic and vascular brain injuries also cause AGHD; some degree of hypopituitarism is found in 35–40 % of patients with traumatic brain injury (TBI). In previous studies, 10–15 % of patients presented with severe GHD and 15 % presented with partial GHD. In Italy, the prevalence of AGHD is 300 patients per year of 1,000,000 people [86, 87].

The Growth Hormone Research Society (GRS) arranged a workshop in 1997, to formulate consensus guidelines for the diagnosis and treatment of AGHD.

AGHD symptoms improve with GH replacement; however, AGHD can lead to impairments in body composition and function, as well as disrupted lipoprotein and carbohydrate metabolism and increased cardiovascular disease [88]. AGHD has similarities with metabolic syndrome [88], and AGHD patients have a metabolic syndrome-like phenotype that is also associated with the development of NASH [89]. The metabolic changes that accompany hypopituitarism are central obesity, hyperlipidemia, and insulin resistance, which are thought to be caused primarily by GH deficiency [90]. Moreover, adult patients with anterior pituitary deficiency and associated GH deficiency experience fatty infiltration of the liver more frequently than patients with anterior pituitary hormone deficiency than in those without GH deficiency [91].

The liver is one of the important target tissues of GH. IGF-1 is a single-chain peptide, which has structural homology with proinsulin, and the majority of circulating IGF-1 is derived from the liver [92]. Recently, physiological significance of the hepatic GH/IGF-1 axis has been recognized [93].

GH promotes lipid metabolism by enhancing lipolysis and oxidation and activates hormone-sensitive lipase through β-adrenergic stimulation. It also enhances the clearance of LDL cholesterol by activating the expression of its hepatic receptors [94].

GH regulates glucose metabolism both directly and by antagonizing the acrions of insulin. Furthermore, it suppresses glucose oxidation and utilization while enhancing hepatic glucose production. In protein metabolism, GH reduces urea synthesis, blood urea concentration, urinary urea excretion, and protein oxidation and stimulates protein synthesis. Although these effects are mainly mediated by

IGF-1, a direct effect of GH has also been proposed. Conversely, IGF-1 improves glucose sensitivity due to its direct and indirect actions to reduce GH secretion. IGF-1 strongly stimulates protein synthesis and inhibits protein breakdown. GH and IGF-1 cooperatively exert their effects in various tissues with the exception of the insulin-like action of IGF-1 [95].

A case report published in 1997 noted improvements in fatty liver associated with panhypopituitarism after GH administration, suggesting that fatty liver is at least partly attributable to GH deficiency. Few reports have demonstrated that GH replacement therapy reversed nonalcoholic steatohepatitis (NASH) in AGHD. On the other hand, Grader et al. reported that NAFLD is equally common in patients with GHD and matched controls. GHR is associated with a hierarchical reduction in fat deposition (as follows: visceral > subcutaneous > liver) [96]. Several factors may explain this discrepancy, including race, age, gender, and BMI. Further studies investigating GHD in patients with NAFLD are required to determine the role of GH replacement in treating NAFLD.

Recently, Lonardo et al. demonstrated that low GH levels are independent predictors of NAFLD in males, and other reports suggest that hypothalamic and/or pituitary disease involves a rapid progressive NAFLD [90, 97]. Furthermore, patients with more advanced NAFLD have low circulating levels of IGF-1 [91, 98], suggesting that GH, IGF-1, and IGFBP-3 are associated with fibrosis and steatosis in NAFLD. These data suggest that in addition to conventional therapies, such as Vitec and pioglitazone, GH replacement and IGF-1 supplementation may be candidate treatments of NAFLD. Further investigation is necessary to clarify the precise mechanisms by which GH and IGF-1 exert their effects in the liver. Hepatologists should recognize the similarities and mechanisms of association between AGHD and NAFLD, and collaboration with endocrinologists is recommended to perform clinical screening for AGHD.

References

1. Huang MJ, Liaw YF. Clinical associations between thyroid and liver diseases. J Gastroenterol Hepatol. 1995;10(3):344–50.
2. Kharb S, Garg MK, Puri P, Brar KS, Pandit A, Srivastava S. Assessment of thyroid and gonadal function in liver diseases. Indian J Endocrinol Metab. 2015;19(1):89–94.
3. Cable EE, Finn PD, Stebbins JW, Hou J, Ito BR, van Poelje PD, Linemeyer DL, Erion MD. Reduction of hepatic steatosis in rats and mice after treatment with a liver-targeted thyroid hormone receptor agonist. Hepatology. 2009;49(2):407–17.
4. Fliers E, Bianco AC, Langouche L, Boelen A. Thyroid function in critically ill patients. Lancet Diabetes Endocrinol. 2015;3(10):816–25. Pii: S2213-8587(15)00225-9.
5. Kano T, Kojima T, Takahashi T, Muto Y. Serum thyroid hormone levels in patients with fulminant hepatitis: usefulness of rT3 and the rT3/T3 ratio as prognostic indices. Gastroenterol Jpn. 1987;22(3):344–53.
6. Anastasiou O, Sydor S, Sowa JP, Manka P, Katsounas A, Syn WK, Führer D, Gieseler RK, Bechmann LP, Gerken G, Moeller LC, Canbay A. Higher thyroid-stimulating hormone,

triiodothyronine and thyroxine values are associated with better outcome in acute liver failure. PLoS One. 2015;10(7):e0132189.
7. Wu Y, You S, Zang H, Liu H, Mao Y, Mao P, Zhu B, Xu J, Xie G, Guo J, Li D, Xin S, Wan Z. Usefulness of serum thyroid-stimulation hormone (TSH) as a prognostic indicator for acute-on-chronic liver failure. Ann Hepatol. 2015;14(2):218–24.
8. Eshraghian A, Taghavi SA. Systematic review: endocrine abnormalities in patients with liver cirrhosis. Arch Iran Med. 2014;17(10):713–21.
9. Bianchi GP, Zoli M, Marchesini G, Volta U, Vecchi F, Iervese T, Bonazzi C, Pisi E. Thyroid gland size and function in patients with cirrhosis of the liver. Liver. 1991;11(2):71–7.
10. Silveira MG, Mendes FD, Diehl NN, Enders FT, Lindor KD. Thyroid dysfunction in primary biliary cirrhosis, primary sclerosing cholangitis and non-alcoholic fatty liver disease. Liver Int. 2009;29(7):1094–100.
11. Eshraghian A, Hamidian JA. Non-alcoholic fatty liver disease and thyroid dysfunction: a systematic review. World J Gastroenterol. 2014;20(25):8102–9.
12. Caregaro L, Alberino F, Amodio P, Merkel C, Angeli P, Plebani M, Gatta A. Nutritional and prognostic significance of serum hypothyroxinemia in hospitalized patients with liver cirrhosis. J Hepatol. 1998;28(1):115–21.
13. Rodríguez-Torres M, Ríos-Bedoya CF, Ortiz-Lasanta G, Marxuach-Cuétara AM, Jiménez-Rivera J. Thyroid dysfunction (TD) among chronic hepatitis C patients with mild and severe hepatic fibrosis. Ann Hepatol. 2008;7(1):72–7.
14. Mansour-Ghanaei F, Mehrdad M, Mortazavi S, Joukar F, Khak M, Atrkar-Roushan Z. Decreased serum total T3 level in hepatitis B and C related cirrhosis by severity of liver damage. Ann Hepatol. 2012;11(5):667–71.
15. Oren R, Sikuler E, Wong F, Blendis LM, Halpern Z. The effects of hypothyroidism on liver status of cirrhotic patients. J Clin Gastroenterol. 2000;31(2):162–3.
16. Oren R, Brill S, Dotan I, Halpern Z. Liver function in cirrhotic patients in the euthyroid versus the hypothyroid state. J Clin Gastroenterol. 1998;27(4):339–41.
17. Boelen A, Kwakkel J, Fliers E. Beyond low plasma T3: local thyroid hormone metabolism during inflammation and infection. Endocr Rev. 2011;32(5):670–93.
18. Farrell GC, Larter CZ. Nonalcoholic fatty liver disease: from steatosis to cirrhosis. Hepatology. 2006;43(2 Suppl 1):S99–112.
19. Chung GE, Kim D, Kim W, Yim JY, Park MJ, Kim YJ, Yoon JH, Lee HS. Non-alcoholic fatty liver disease across the spectrum of hypothyroidism. J Hepatol. 2012;57(1):150–6.
20. Klieverik LP, Coomans CP, Endert E, Sauerwein HP, Havekes LM, Voshol PJ, Rensen PC, Romijn JA, Kalsbeek A, Fliers E. Thyroid hormone effects on whole-body energy homeostasis and tissue-specific fatty acid uptake in vivo. Endocrinology. 2009;150(12):5639–48.
21. Nedvidkova J, Haluzik M, Bartak V, Dostalova I, Vlcek P, Racek P, Taus M, Behanova M, Svacina S, Alesci S, Pacak K. Changes of noradrenergic activity and lipolysis in the subcutaneous abdominal adipose tissue of hypo- and hyperthyroid patients: an in vivo microdialysis study. Ann N Y Acad Sci. 2004;1018:541–9.
22. Jornayvaz FR, Lee HY, Jurczak MJ, Alves TC, Guebre-Egziabher F, Guigni BA, Zhang D, Samuel VT, Silva JE, Shulman GI. Thyroid hormone receptor-α gene knockout mice are protected from diet-induced hepatic insulin resistance. Endocrinology. 2012;153(2):583–91.
23. Sinha RA, You SH, Zhou J, Siddique MM, Bay BH, Zhu X, Privalsky ML, Cheng SY, Stevens RD, Summers SA, Newgard CB, Lazar MA, Yen PM. Thyroid hormone stimulates hepatic lipid catabolism via activation of autophagy. J Clin Invest. 2012;122(7):2428–38.
24. Riis AL, Gravholt CH, Djurhuus CB, Nørrelund H, Jørgensen JO, Weeke J, Møller N. Elevated regional lipolysis in hyperthyroidism. J Clin Endocrinol Metab. 2002;87 (10):4747–53.
25. Cachefo A, Boucher P, Vidon C, Dusserre E, Diraison F, Beylot M. Hepatic lipogenesis and cholesterol synthesis in hyperthyroid patients. J Clin Endocrinol Metab. 2001;86(11):5353–7.

26. Borzio M, Borzio M, Caldara R, Borzio F, Piepoli V, Rampini P, Ferrari C. Thyroid function tests in chronic liver disease: evidence for multiple abnormalities despite clinical euthyroidism. Gut. 1983;24(7):631–6.
27. Baker A, Kaplan M, Wolfe H. Central congestive fibrosis of the liver in myxedema ascites. Ann Intern Med. 1972;77(6):927–9.
28. Kinney EL, Wright RJ, Caldwell JW. Value of clinical features for distinguishing myxedema ascites from other forms of ascites. Comput Biol Med. 1989;19(1):55–9.
29. Van Steenbergen W, Fevery J, De Vos R, Leyten R, Heirwegh KP, De Groote J. Thyroid hormones and the hepatic handling of bilirubin. I. Effects of hypothyroidism and hyperthyroidism on the hepatic transport of bilirubin mono- and diconjugates in the Wistar rat. Hepatology. 1989;9(2):314–21.
30. Liangpunsakul S, Chalasani N. Is hypothyroidism a risk factor for non-alcoholic steatohepatitis? J Clin Gastroenterol. 2003;37(4):340–3.
31. Reddy A, Dash C, Leerapun A, Mettler TA, Stadheim LM, Lazaridis KN, Roberts RO, Roberts LR. Hypothyroidism: a possible risk factor for liver cancer in patients with no known underlying cause of liver Disease. Clin Gastroenterol Hepatol. 2007;5(1):118–23.
32. Uzunlulu M, Yorulmaz E, Oguz A. Prevalence of subclinical hypothyroidism in patients with metabolic syndrome. Endocr J. 2007;54(1):71–6.
33. Malik R, Hodgson H. The relationship between the thyroid gland and the liver. QJM. 2002;95 (9):559–69.
34. Elias RM, Dean DS, Barsness GW. Hepatic dysfunction in hospitalized patients with acute thyrotoxicosis: a decade of experience. Endocrinology. 2012;2012:325092.
35. Nakamura H, Noh JY, Itoh K, Fukata S, Miyauchi A, Hamada N. Comparison of methimazole and propylthiouracil in patients with hyperthyroidism caused by Graves' disease. J Clin Endocrinol Metab. 2007;92(6):2157–62.
36. Russo MW, Galanko JA, Shrestha R, Fried MW, Watkins P. Liver transplantation for acute liver failure from drug induced liver injury in the United States. Liver Transpl. 2004;10 (8):1018–23.
37. El-Kabbany ZA, Hamza RT, Abd El Hakim AS, Tawfik LM. Thyroid and hepatic haemodynamic alterations among Egyptian children with liver cirrhosis. ISRN Gastroenterol. 2012;2012:595734.
38. Corpechot C, Chrétien Y, Chazouillères O, Poupon R. Demographic, lifestyle, medical and familial factors associated with primary biliary cirrhosis. J Hepatol. 2010;53(1):162–9.
39. Moustafa AH, Ali EM, Mohamed TM, Abdou HI. Oxidative stress and thyroid hormones in patients with liver diseases. Eur J Intern Med. 2009;20(7):703–8.
40. Taş A, Köklü S, Beyazit Y, Kurt M, Sayilir A, Yeşil Y, Çelik H. Thyroid hormone levels predict mortality in intensive care patients with cirrhosis. Am J Med Sci. 2012;344(3):175–9.
41. Seehofer D, Steinmueller T, Graef KJ, Rayes N, Wiegand W, Tullius SG, Settmacher U, Neuhaus P. Pituitary function test and endocrine status in patient with cirrhosis of the liver before and after hepatic transplantation. Ann Transplant. 2002;7(2):32–7.
42. Maheshwari A, Thuluvath PJ. Endocrine diseases and the liver. Clin Liver Dis. 2011;15 (1):55–67.
43. Boulton R, Hamilton MI, Dhillon AP, Kinloch JD, Burroughs AK. Subclinical Addison's disease: a cause of persistent abnormalities in transaminase values. Gastroenterology. 1995;109:1324–7.
44. Ersan O, Demirezer B. Addison's disease: a rare cause of hypertransaminasaemia. Dig Dis Sci. 2008;53(12):3269–71.
45. Harry R, Auzinger G, Wendon J. The clinical importance of adrenal insufficiency in acute hepatic dysfunction. Hepatology. 2002;36(2):395–402.
46. Tsai MH, Peng YS, Chen YC, Liu NJ, Ho YP, Fang JT, Lien JM, Yang C, Chen PC, Wu CS. Adrenal insufficiency in patients with cirrhosis, severe sepsis and septic shock. Hepatology. 2006;43(4):673–81.

47. Fede G, Spadaro L, Tomaselli T, Privitera G, Germani G, Tsochatzis E, Thomas M, Bouloux PM, Burroughs AK, Purrello F. Adrenocortical dysfunction in liver disease: a systematic review. Hepatology. 2012;55(4):1282–91.
48. Fernández J, Escorsell A, Zabalza M, Felipe V, Navasa M, Mas A, Lacy AM, Ginès P, Arroyo V. Adrenal insufficiency in patients with cirrhosis and septic shock: Effect of treatment with hydrocortisone on survival. Hepatology. 2006;44(5):1288–95.
49. Arabi YM, Aljumah A, Dabbagh O, Tamim HM, Rishu AH, Al-Abdulkareem A, Knawy BA, Hajeer AH, Tamimi W, Cherfan A. Low-dose hydrocortisone in patients with cirrhosis and septic shock: a randomized controlled trial. CMAJ. 2010;182(18):1971–7.
50. Marik PE, Gayowski T, Starzl TE, Hepatic Cortisol Research and Adrenal Pathophysiology Study Group. The hepatoadrenal syndrome: a common yet unrecognized clinical condition. Crit Care Med. 2005;33(6):1254–9.
51. Hauser GJ, Brotzman HM, Kaufman SS. Hepatoadrenal syndrome in pediatric patients with end-stage liver disease. Pediatr Crit Care Med. 2012;13(3):e145–9.
52. Marik PE. Adrenal-exhaustion syndrome in patients with liver disease. Intensive Care Med. 2006;32(2):275–80.
53. Tarantino G, Finelli C. Pathogenesis of hepatic steatosis: the link between hypercortisolism and non-alcoholic fatty liver disease. World J Gastroenterol. 2013;19(40):6735–43.
54. Anagnostis P, Athyros VG, Tziomalos K, Karagiannis A, Mikhailidis DP. Clinical review: the pathogenetic role of cortisol in the metabolic syndrome: a hypothesis. J Clin Endocrinol Metab. 2009;94(8):2692–701.
55. Ahlqvist J. Can endocrine factors influence pathogenetic mechanisms in chronic active hepatitis (CAH) and primary biliary cirrhosis (PBC)? A hypothesis. Hepatogastroenterology. 1980;27(1):64–7. Review.
56. Floreani A, Titta M, Plebani M, Faggian D, Chiaramonte M, Naccarato R. Sex hormone changes in post-menopausal women with primary biliary cirrhosis (PBC) and with cryptogenic chronic liver disease. Clin Exp Obstet Gynecol. 1991;18(4):229–34.
57. Wiesner RH, Batts KP, Krom RA. Evolving concepts in the diagnosis, pathogenesis, and treatment of chronic hepatic allograft rejection. Liver Transpl Surg. 1999;5(5):388–400.
58. Hodgson SF, Dickson ER, Wahner HW, Johnson KA, Mann KG, Riggs BL. Bone loss and reduced osteoblast function in primary biliary cirrhosis. Ann Intern Med. 1985;103 (6 (Pt 1)):855–60.
59. Stellon AJ, Webb A, Compston J, Williams R. Low bone turnover state in primary biliary cirrhosis. Hepatology. 1987;7(1):137–42.
60. Elsheikh M, Hodgson HJ, Wass JA, Conway GS. Hormone replacement therapy may improve hepatic function in women with Turner's syndrome. Clin Endocrinol (Oxf). 2001;55 (2):227–31.
61. Lindgren A, Olsson R. Liver damage from low-dose oral contraceptives. J Intern Med. 1993;234(3):287–92.
62. Reyes H, Gonzalez MC, Ribalta J, Aburto H, Matus C, Schramm G, Katz R, Medina E. Prevalence of intrahepatic cholestasis of pregnancy in Chile. Ann Intern Med. 1978;88 (4):487–93.
63. Kreek MJ. Female sex steroids and cholestasis. Semin Liver Dis. 1987;7(1):8–23.
64. Metreau JM, Dhumeaux D, Berthelot P. Oral contraceptives and the liver. Digestion. 1972;7 (5):318–35. Dourakis SP, Tolis G. Sex hormonal preparations and the liver. Eur J Contracept Reprod Health Care. 1998;3(1):7–16. Sex hormonal preparations and the liver.
65. Dourakis SP, Tolis G. Eur J Contracept Reprod Health Care. 1998;3(1):7–16.
66. Giannitrapani L, Soresi M, La Spada E, Cervello M, D'Alessandro N, Montalto G. Sex hormones and risk of liver tumor. Ann N Y Acad Sci. 2006;1089:228–36.
67. Maddrey WC. Hepatic vein thrombosis (Budd Chiari syndrome): possible association with the use of oral contraceptives. Semin Liver Dis. 1987;7(1):32–9.
68. Weinberger M, Garty M, Cohen M, Russo Y, Rosenfeld JB. Ultrasonography in the diagnosis and follow-up of hepatic sinusoidal dilatation. Arch Intern Med. 1985;145(5):927–9.

69. Llovet JM, Burroughs A, Bruix J. Hepatocellular carcinoma. Lancet. 2003;362:1907–17.
70. Parkin DM. Global cancer statistics in the year 2000. Lancet Oncol. 2001;2:533–43.
71. Di Maio M, De Maio E, Morabito A, D'Aniello R, De Feo G, Gallo C, Perrone F. Hormonal treatment of human hepatocellular carcinoma. Ann N Y Acad Sci. 2006;1089:252–61.
72. Faulds MH, Zhao C, Dahlman-Wright K, Gustafsson JÅ. The diversity of sex steroid action: regulation of metabolism by estrogen signaling. J Endocrinol. 2012;212(1):3–12.
73. Kelley CE, Brown AJ, Diehl AM, Setji TL. Review of nonalcoholic fatty liver disease in women with polycystic ovary syndrome. World J Gastroenterol. 2014;20(39):14172–84.
74. Lauritsen MP, Bentzen JG, Pinborg A, Loft A, Forman JL, Thuesen LL, Cohen A, Hougaard DM, Nyboe Andersen A. The prevalence of polycystic ovary syndrome in a normal population according to the Rotterdam criteria versus revised criteria including anti-Mullerian hormone. Hum Reprod. 2014;29(4):791–801.
75. Azziz R, Woods KS, Reyna R, Key TJ, Knochenhauer ES, Yildiz BO. The prevalence and features of the polycystic ovary syndrome in an unselected population. J Clin Endocrinol Metab. 2004;89(6):2745–9.
76. Vassilatou E. Nonalcoholic fatty liver disease and polycystic ovary syndrome. World J Gastroenterol. 2014;20(26):8351–63.
77. Baranova A, Tran TP, Birerdinc A, Younossi ZM. Systematic review: association of polycystic ovary syndrome with metabolic syndrome and non-alcoholic fatty liver disease. Aliment Pharmacol Ther. 2011;33(7):801–14.
78. Kulshreshtha B, Ganie MA, Praveen EP, Gupta N, Lal Khurana M, Seith A, Dwivedi SN, Kumar G, Ammini AC. Insulin response to oral glucose in healthy, lean young women and patients with polycystic ovary syndrome. Gynecol Endocrinol. 2008;24(11):637–43. やせと PCO.
79. Diamanti-Kandarakis E, Katsikis I, Piperi C, Kandaraki E, Piouka A, Papavassiliou AG, Panidis D. Increased serum advanced glycation end-products is a distinct finding in lean women with polycystic ovary syndrome (PCOS). Clin Endocrinol (Oxf). 2008;69(4):634–41.
80. Melmed S. Acromegaly. N Engl J Med. 1990;322(14):966–77.
81. Holdaway IM, Rajasoorya C. Epidemiology of acromegaly. Pituitary. 1999;2(1):29–41. Prevalence of diabetes mellitus in patients with acromegaly.
82. Dreval AV, Trigolosova IV, Misnikova IV, Kovalyova YA, Tishenina RS, Barsukov IA, Vinogradova AV, Wolffenbuttel BH. Prevalence of diabetes mellitus in patients with acromegaly. Endocrinol Connect. 2014;3(2):93–8.
83. Colao A, Ferone D, Marzullo P, Lombardi G. Systemic complications of acromegaly: epidemiology, pathogenesis, and management. Endocr Rev. 2004;25(1):102–52.
84. Wiesli P, Bernays R, Brändle M, Zwimpfer C, Seiler H, Zapf J, A Spinas G, Schmid C. Effect of pituitary surgery in patients with acromegaly on adiponectin serum concentrations and alanine aminotransferase activity. Clin Chim Acta. 2005;352(1–2):175–81.
85. Molitch ME, Clemmons DR, Malozowski S, Merriam GR, Vance ML, Endocrine Society. Evaluation and treatment of adult growth hormone deficiency: an Endocrine Society clinical practice guideline. J Clin Endocrinol Metab. 2011;96(6):1587–609.
86. Ghigo E, Aimaretti G, Corneli G. Diagnosis of adult GH deficiency. Growth Horm IGF Res. 2008;18(1):1–16.
87. Tagliaferri F, Compagnone C, Korsic M, Servadei F, Kraus J. A systematic review of brain injury epidemiology in Europe. Acta Neurochir (Wien). 2006;148(3):255–68.
88. Johannsson G, Bengtsson BA. Growth hormone and the metabolic syndrome. J Endocrinol Invest. 1999;22(5 Suppl):41–6.
89. Loria P, Carulli L, Bertolotti M, Lonardo A. Endocrine and liver interaction: the role of endocrine pathways in NASH. Nat Rev Gastroenterol Hepatol. 2009;6(4):236–47.
90. Adams LA, Feldstein A, Lindor KD, Angulo P. Nonalcoholic fatty liver disease among patients with hypothalamic and pituitary dysfunction. Hepatology. 2004;39(4):909–14.

91. Ichikawa T, Nakao K, Hamasaki K, Furukawa R, Tsuruta S, Ueda Y, Taura N, Shibata H, Fujimoto M, Toriyama K, Eguchi K. Role of growth hormone, insulin-like growth factor 1 and insulin-like growth factor-binding protein 3 in development of non-alcoholic fatty liver disease. Hepatol Int. 2007;1(2):287–94.
92. Yakar S, Liu JL, Stannard B, Butler A, Accili D, Sauer B, LeRoith D. Normal growth and development in the absence of hepatic insulin-like growth factor I. Proc Natl Acad Sci U S A. 1999;96(13):7324–9.
93. Holt RI, Simpson HL, Sönksen PH. The role of the growth hormone-insulin-like growth factor axis in glucose homeostasis. Diabet Med. 2003;20(1):3–15.
94. Rudling M, Norstedt G, Olivecrona H, Reihnér E, Gustafsson JA, Angelin B. Importance of growth hormone for the induction of hepatic low density lipoprotein receptors. Proc Natl Acad Sci U S A. 1992;89(15):6983–7.
95. Takahashi Y. Essential roles of growth hormone (GH) and insulin-like growth factor-I (IGF-I) in the liver. Endocr J. 2012;59(11):955–62.
96. Gardner CJ, Irwin AJ, Daousi C, McFarlane IA, Joseph F, Bell JD, Thomas EL, Adams VL, Kemp GJ, Cuthbertson DJ. Hepatic steatosis, GH deficiency and the effects of GH replacement: a Liverpool magnetic resonance spectroscopy study. Eur J Endocrinol. 2012;166 (6):993–1002.
97. Gasco V, Prodam F, Grottoli S, Marzullo P, Longobardi S, Ghigo E, Aimaretti G. GH therapy in adult GH deficiency: a review of treatment schedules and the evidence for low starting doses. Eur J Endocrinol. 2013;168(3):R55–66.
98. Sumida Y, Yonei Y, Tanaka S, Mori K, Kanemasa K, Imai S, Taketani H, Hara T, Seko Y, Ishiba H, Okajima A, Yamaguchi K, Moriguchi M, Mitsuyoshi H, Yasui K, Minami M, Itoh Y. Lower levels of insulin-like growth factor-1 standard deviation score are associated with histological severity of non-alcoholic fatty liver disease. Hepatol Res. 2015;45(7):771–81.

Chapter 13
Rheumatic Diseases and the Liver

Atsushi Takahashi, Kazumichi Abe, Hiroshi Watanabe, and Hiromasa Ohira

Abstract Rheumatic diseases affect multiple organs, including the liver. Liver dysfunction is not rare in patients with rheumatic diseases. Not only rheumatic disease itself, but also other factors such as drug toxicity, virus, fatty infiltration and overlapping autoimmune liver disease can cause liver dysfunction. Therefore, liver dysfunction in patients with collagen diseases needs to be considered separately from the rheumatic disease itself and other causes. Liver dysfunction in patients with rheumatic disease is tended to be mild and temporary, so the causes are often overlooked. However, acute liver failure occurs infrequently by some causes such as de novo hepatitis B or adult-onset Still's disease. Liver dysfunction in patients with rheumatic disease shows relatively specific tendencies for each collagen disease. On the other hand, liver dysfunction caused by systemic lupus erythematosus (SLE) itself is difficult to distinguish from autoimmune hepatitis (AIH) because of the laboratory findings are similar. Histological examination of the liver is useful for differentially diagnosing AIH and SLE-associated hepatitis. The feature of liver dysfunction and its causes need to be elucidated and considered when treating rheumatic diseases.

13.1 Introduction

Rheumatic diseases develop primarily on the basis of immunological disorders, but the detailed causes and mechanisms remain unknown. Rheumatic diseases often have target organs, but most diseases show systemic involvement, including the liver, and other forms of liver dysfunction are induced by many causes, such as viruses, drugs, alcohol, obesity, and overlapping autoimmune liver diseases [1–7]. Liver dysfunction in patients with rheumatic diseases thus comprises a broad spectrum of liver diseases. Consequently, liver dysfunction in patients with

A. Takahashi (✉) • K. Abe • H. Watanabe • H. Ohira
Department of Gastroenterology and Rheumatology, Fukushima Medical School of Medicine, Fukushima, Japan
e-mail: junior@fmu.ac.jp

H. Ohira (ed.), *The Liver in Systemic Diseases*, DOI 10.1007/978-4-431-55790-6_13

collagen diseases needs to be considered separately from the rheumatic disease itself and other causes. Moreover, the liver dysfunction caused by rheumatic diseases themselves differs by disease. In this chapter, we first describe the characteristics of liver dysfunction in rheumatic diseases as a whole and then review them by each disease, including systemic lupus erythematosus (SLE), rheumatoid arthritis (RA), Sjögren's syndrome (SjS), systemic sclerosis (SSc), vasculitis, and adult-onset Still's disease (AOSD).

13.2 Laboratory Findings in Patients with Liver Dysfunction Caused by Rheumatic Diseases Themselves

Liver dysfunction is generally classified into two patterns: predominantly hepatocellular (with elevated alanine aminotransferase [ALT] and aspartate aminotransferase [AST] levels) and cholestatic damage (with elevated alkaline phosphatase [ALP] and gamma-glutamyl transferase [γ-GTP] levels). Liver dysfunction in patients with rheumatic diseases has been defined as the elevation of liver and biliary enzyme levels [2–7]. These elevations of liver and biliary enzyme levels are, on the whole, mild in rheumatic disease patients with liver dysfunction. However, liver dysfunction shows different tendencies by disease. ALT levels are higher in AOSD than in other collagen diseases [5]. Conversely, ALP or γ-GTP levels are higher in vasculitis syndrome than in other collagen diseases [2, 5]. Aminotransferase and bilirubin levels are generally normal in RA, though ALP is increased in 18–46 % of patients with RA [8–10]. Moreover, γ-GTP is elevated in 23–77 % of patients and correlates with disease activity [9–11]. The degree of liver and biliary enzyme elevation is generally associated with disease activity.

13.3 Liver Histological Findings in Patients with Liver Dysfunction by Rheumatic Disease

The histological abnormalities in most rheumatic disease patients are generally nonspecific and nonprogressive. A wide variation has been described in each rheumatic disease [1–3]. The spectrum of histomorphological findings in rheumatic disease is commonly categorized into portal changes, lobular changes, and vascular changes. The various alterations seen in the portal areas include portal inflammation, interface hepatitis, chronic active hepatitis, nonspecific reactive hepatitis, abnormal vessels, and portal tract fibrosis. Portal tract inflammation is a relatively common histopathologic finding in SLE patients with liver dysfunction [2, 12, 13]. Lobular changes are not as frequent as portal changes, but lobular inflammation, steatosis, and focal necrosis have been reported [2, 12, 13]. Many reports have described vascular changes, such as arteritis, abnormal vessels in portal tracts, hemangioma, peliosis hepatis, and infarcts due to arthritis in rheumatic diseases with liver dysfunction [1–3].

13.4 Systemic Lupus Erythematosus

13.4.1 Prevalence of Liver Dysfunction

SLE affects multiple organs including the liver. Not only SLE itself but other factors such as drug toxicity, fatty infiltration, and overlapping autoimmune diseases can also cause liver dysfunction [2, 14–18]. The reported incidence of liver dysfunction in SLE patients ranges from 8.6 to 59.7 % [2, 13–21] (Table 13.1). This wide range of prevalences may result from different definitions of liver dysfunction.

13.4.2 Liver Dysfunction Caused by SLE Itself (Lupus Hepatitis)

'Lupus hepatitis' has traditionally been used to describe the liver dysfunction caused by SLE itself [15, 22]. However, older reports may have used 'lupus hepatitis' without ruling out other causes. Therefore, it is important to strictly exclude other liver diseases, including drug-induced liver injury, viral hepatitis, alcoholic liver disease, nonalcoholic fatty liver disease (NAFLD), and autoimmune liver diseases. The prevalence of liver dysfunction caused by SLE itself reported in the literature is rather variable. Our previous reports based on lenient discrimination criteria reported a prevalence of 59.7 % among 206 SLE patients [18], while Zheng et al., using much stricter discrimination criteria, reported a prevalence of 9.3 % among 504 SLE patients [13].

This liver dysfunction mostly presents as mild to moderate elevation of serum aminotransferase levels, while ALP and γ-GTP elevations are less frequent [2, 13]. The diagnosis of liver dysfunction caused by SLE itself is achieved by ruling out other causes, such as drugs, viral hepatitis, fatty infiltration, and overlapping autoimmune diseases. Moreover, the activity of SLE is often helpful in making the diagnosis [13]. The incidence of nervous system involvement is higher in patients with liver dysfunction caused by SLE itself [18].

The anti-ribosomal P protein antibody has been described as a marker of central nervous system (CNS) lupus or lupus hepatitis, and the antibody is used in the differentiating between lupus hepatitis and overlapping SLE-autoimmune hepatitis (AIH) [23–26]. Anti-ribosomal P protein antibody is also detected in patients with SLE-AIH overlap or AIH alone [18]. In a recent study of 93 AIH patients without clinical or laboratory evidence of SLE, 9 patients (9.7 %) had moderate to high

Table 13.1 The prevalence of liver dysfunction in patients with rheumatic disease

Rheumatic disease	Prevalence of liver dysfunction	Reference
Systemic erythematosus (SLE)		
	46/106 (43.4 %)	Kojima [2]
	47/504 (9.3 %)	Zheng [13]
	84/260 (32.3 %)	Miller [14]
	40/192 (20.8 %)	Chowdhary [15]
	45/242 (18.6 %)	Piga [16]
	134/1553 (8.6 %)	Huang [17]
	123/206 (59.7 %)	Takahashi [18]
	124/238 (52.1 %)	Runyon [19]
	80/225 (35.6 %)	Luangjaru [20]
	46/141 (32.6 %)	Her [21]
Rheumatoid arthritis (RA)		
	24/59 (40.7 %)	Kojima [2]
	79/220 (35.9 %)	Takahashi [5]
	45/100 (45.0 %)	Fernandes [8]
	45/98 (45.9 %)	Spooner [9]
	48/62 (77.4 %)	Lowe [11]
	86/183 (47.0 %)	Akesson [68]
Sjögren's syndromes (SjS)		
	37/71 (52.1 %)	Kojima [2]
	20/44 (45.5 %)	Takahashi [5]
	21/300 (7.0 %)	Skopouli [88]
	12/45 (26.7 %)	Lindgren [89]
	42/95 (44.2 %)	Montano-Loza [90]
Systemic sclerosis (SSc)		
	10/27 (37.0 %)	Kojima [2]
	21/47 (44.7 %)	Takahashi [5]
	8/727 (1.1 %)	Chen [98]
Vasculitis syndrome		
	7/13 (53.8 %)	Kojima [2]
	12/25 (48.0 %)	Takahashi [5]
Adult-onset Still's disease (AOSD)		
	13/16 (81.3 %)	Takahashi [5]
	47/62 (75.8 %)	Pouchot [107]
	53/72 (73.6 %)	Fautrel [108]
	59/95 (62.1 %)	Pay [109]
	30/84 (35.7 %)	Cagatary [110]
	48/77 (62.3 %)	Zhu [111]
	65/104 (62.5 %)	Kong [112]
	57/76 (75.0 %)	Colina [113]
	43/61 (70.5 %)	Chen [114]
	27/50 (54.0 %)	Gerfaud-Valentin [115]
	25/28 (89.3 %)	Mehrpoor [116]

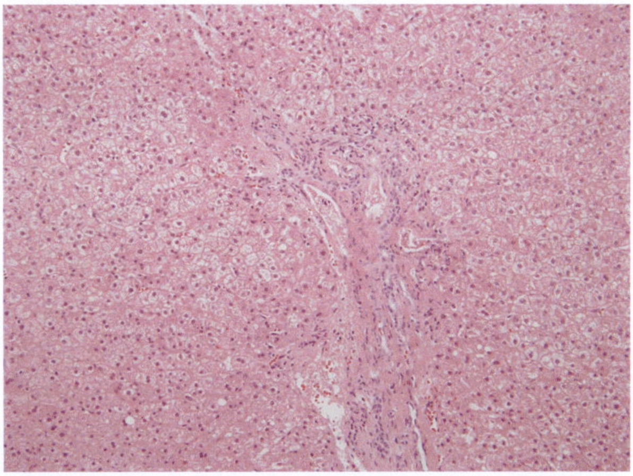

Fig. 13.1 Nonspecific reactive hepatitis in patients with SLE

titers of anti-ribosomal P protein antibody [27]. The diagnosis of liver dysfunction caused by SLE itself therefore requires histological examination.

The histological findings of the liver in SLE patients show a broad morphological spectrum of liver dysfunction when caused by SLE itself. Common histopathologic findings in SLE include fatty liver, portal inflammation, nonspecific reactive hepatitis, arthritis, congestion, nodular regenerative hyperplasia (NRH), abnormal vessels in portal tracts, and vascular changes such as hemangioma [1, 12, 18, 28] (Fig. 13.1).

Survival rates do not differ between SLE patients with and without liver dysfunction [18]. Liver dysfunction caused by SLE itself is generally subclinical with a fluctuating course and responds well to moderate to high doses of prednisone without progression to end-stage liver disease [16].

13.4.3 Liver Dysfunction Caused by Drugs

SLE is treated using many drugs for various symptoms; as a result, drug-induced liver injury (DILI) is not rare. In fact, we reported DILI as the most frequent cause (31 %) of liver dysfunction among 123 SLE patients with liver dysfunction [18]. Huang et al. also reported 35 cases of DILI among 1553 SLE patients [17] (Table 13.2).

The causative drugs vary. About 80 % of SLE cases are treated by nonsteroidal anti-inflammatory drugs (NSAIDs) and analgesics for major symptoms such as arthralgia, serositis, and headache [29]. Liver injury caused by NSAIDs is common and appears dose independent [30]. Patients with SLE usually present with a higher rate of NSAID-related complications than SLE-negative patients. Common complications include increased aminotransferase levels, skin rashes, retention of body fluids, gastric ulcers, and aseptic meningitis [28].

Table 13.2 Numbers of cause of liver dysfunction in systemic lupus erythematosus and rheumatoid arthritis

Ref	Number/ total	Disease-related	Drug	Fatty liver	Viral hepatitis	AIH/ PBC	Alcohol	Others
Systemic erythematosus (SLE)								
Kojima [2]	46/106	22	8	6	5	0	0	5
Miller [14]	67/260	0	28	0	2	0	8	29
Chowdaharay [15]	40/192	0	4	8	8	6/3	0	11
Piga [16]	45/283	14	18	3	3	1/0	2	4
Huang [17]	134/1553	10*	35	31	3	10*/0	0	55
Takahashi [18]	123/206	35	38	22	1	6/3	2	16
Rheumatoid arthritis (RA)								
Kojima [2]	24/59	7	8	2	3	0/1	0	3
Takahashi [5]	79/220	2	32	5	1	1/3	0	35

AIH autoimmune hepatitis, *PBC* primary biliary cholangitis, *NA* not available
*Either SLE related or AIH

Aspirin is the most common drug associated with DILI in SLE patients, and the liver toxicity of aspirin is considered dose-dependent. Hypoalbuminemia in SLE patients is one risk factor for increased susceptibility to liver injury [31]. The clinical presentation of liver toxicity is often non-icteric with markedly elevated aminotransferase levels. Aspirin can injure the mitochondria, leading to free fatty acid accumulation in the liver and hepatic steatosis [30].

Azathioprine (AZA) is an immunosuppressive drug used to achieve or maintain remission in SLE [32]. Liver injury caused by AZA generally presents as elevated serum aminotransferase levels [28]. It is not generally severe and responds to dose reduction. NRH can arise as a rare but severe complication of thiopurine-based therapies [28].

Methotrexate (MTX) is associated with significant reductions in the SLE disease activity index and the average dose of corticosteroid in SLE patients [33]. In a study involving 18 SLE patients who received MTX, 10 (55.5 %) showed elevated AST levels [34].

13.4.4 Liver Dysfunction Caused by Viruses

The etiology of SLE is suspected to result from an interaction between a genetic predisposition and an environmental trigger, including infection [35]. Many viral infections have been documented in SLE at presentation and during the course of the disease. The prevalence of anti-hepatitis C virus (HCV) antibodies among SLE patients is 13 %, compared to 0.5–2 % among voluntary blood donors [35]. Chronic HCV infection can induce clinical and serological changes and mimic SLE. For example, about 20 % of hepatitis C patients are antinuclear antibody (ANA)-positive [36], and chronic hepatitis C can occur with cryoglobulinemia, which can lead to an erroneous diagnosis of SLE. Therefore, previous reports have suggested that a positive result for HCV antibody could reflect various conditions in SLE patients. First, it could show a true association between SLE and hepatitis C. Second, it may represent a false-positive finding of HCV antibody, because of the high levels of autoantibodies present in SLE patients. Third, HCV can trigger the occurrence of ANA or cryoglobulinemia without typical skin changes. Steroid therapy for SLE patients does not alter the course of HCV [23].

The prevalence of hepatitis B is lower than that of hepatitis C in SLE patients [16, 19, 20]. Although the prevalence of hepatitis B virus (HBV) infection in SLE patients has a wide range across countries, the rate of the presence of hepatitis B surface antigen (HBsAg) is 0.8 % in SLE patients, while that of hepatitis B surface antibody (HBsAb) and/or hepatitis B core antibody (HBcAb) is 16.5 % in Japan [37]. These prevalences are generally comparable to those in healthy individuals. Recently, de novo hepatitis B has become a serious problem in patients undergoing chemotherapy or immunosuppressive therapies [38]. Since acute liver failure due to de novo HBV is lethal, some guidelines now recommend serological screening for HBV prior to starting immunosuppressive therapy for patients with rheumatic disease [39–42]. The guideline proposed by the Japanese College of Rheumatology recommends that antiviral drugs be started if positive results are obtained for HBsAg or HBV DNA [41]. Other immunosuppressive therapies affect the markers of HBV infection. In a study of 248 SLE patients, anti-HBcAb and anti-HBsAb levels became undetectable during immunosuppressive treatment in 2 of 16 patients with anti-HBcAb (16.7 %) and 2 of 10 patients with anti-HBs (20 %), respectively [37]. These results suggest that careful monitoring is essential during immunosuppressive therapy, even if results for all HBV-related markers are negative.

Immunosuppressive therapy in SLE patients increases the risk of bacterial and viral infections. Ramos-Casals et al. reported a high prevalence of aminotransferase elevation (56 %) in SLE patients presenting with acute viral infection [42]. CMV infection is closely associated with the occurrence and development of SLE and also correlates with disease activity and mortality in SLE [43]. In a study of 105 SLE patients with active CMV infection, hematocytopenia (81 %), fever (73.3 %), and liver dysfunction (54.3 %) were the three most common clinical manifestations [44].

13.4.5 Hemophagocytic Syndrome

Reactive hemophagocytic syndrome (HPS) is a potentially fatal condition associated with neoplasms, viral infections, and autoimmune diseases, including SLE [45–47]. HPS is usually characterized by high fever, lymphadenopathy, hepatosplenomegaly, pancytopenia, elevated liver enzymes, hyperferritinemia, and hypercoagulopathy. Reactive HPS in SLE patients was first reported by

Wong et al. in 1991 [45], and five cases of HPS were reported among 88 SLE patients with acute viral infections [42]. The precise mechanisms underlying the development of reactive HPS in SLE are unclear, but sustained activation of macrophages following production of inflammatory cytokines such as interleukin (IL)-6 and tumor necrosis factor (TNF)-α leads to the clinical findings, including fever, liver dysfunction, and coagulopathy [47–49].

13.4.6 Liver Dysfunction Caused by Obesity

Fatty liver is one of the major causes of liver dysfunction in SLE patients. The prevalence of fatty liver is 13–23.1 % among SLE patients with liver dysfunction [2, 20, 21]. Moreover, steatosis is one of the major liver histological findings in SLE patients with liver dysfunction [1, 28]. Corticosteroids are standard and first-line therapy for SLE, but they can also cause secondary nonalcoholic steatohepatitis [50]. We previously confirmed that fatty liver usually develops during the course of SLE [18].

13.4.7 AIH Overlap

AIH is an autoimmune liver disease characterized by the presence of ANA and hypergammaglobulinemia. The histopathological features of AIH in the liver include interface hepatitis, rosette formation of hepatocytes, emperipolesis, and progression to inflammation and fibrosis [51]. Patients with AIH occasionally suffer from other autoimmune diseases [52]. Overlap of AIH and SLE is considered to be a rare condition, because only a few case reports have been published to date [53]. Moreover, it is not clear whether such damage is caused by a primary liver disease such as AIH or a hepatic manifestation of SLE. The elevated immunoglobulin (Ig)G and ANA levels are characteristic of both AIH and SLE [54]. Anti-double-stranded DNA (anti-dsDNA) and anti-ribosomal P protein antibodies are associated with SLE but are also found in patients with AIH [21, 27]. In fact, 30 (57 %) of 53 AIH patients were found to have anti-dsDNA antibody according to enzyme immunosorbent assay and indirect immunofluorescence [54]. Oka reported that 5 (3 %) of 162 patients with AIH satisfied the American College of Rheumatology criteria for SLE [55]. Similarly, Onder et al. reported that 7 of 30 patients with AIH satisfied the criteria [56] (Table 13.3). Specific markers such as anti-smooth muscle antibody (ASMA) and liver-kidney microsomal (LKM) antibody for AIH may help to differentiate AIH from SLE serologically. However, the positive rate for serum ASMA is 42.5 % [52]; moreover, positivity for LKM antibody alone, seen with type 2 AIH, is extremely rare in Japan. Therefore, histological assessment of the liver is essential for differentially diagnosing AIH and SLE-associated hepatitis [57].

Table 13.3 The prevalence of rheumatic disease in autoimmune liver disease

Overlap	Prevalence	References
Primary biliary cholangitis (PBC)		
PBC+SLE	24/7926 (0.3 %)	Hirohara [60]
	12/322 (3.7 %)	Wang [61]
	2/160 (1.3 %)	Watt [62]
	3/170 (1.8 %)	Marasini [63]
PBC+RA	285/7926 (3.6 %)	Hirohara [60]
	9/322 (2.8 %)	Wang [61]
	27/160 (16.9 %)	Watt [62]
	3/170 (1.8 %)	Marasini [63]
PBC+SjS	947/7926 (11.9 %)	Hirohara [60]
	121/322 (37.6 %)	Wang [61]
	40/160 (25.0 %)	Watt [62]
	6/170 (3.5 %)	Marasini [63]
PBC+SSc (CREST)	214/7926 (2.7 %)	Hirohara [60]
	9/322 (2.8 %)	Wang [61]
	12/160 (7.5 %)	Watt [62]
	21/170 (12.4 %)	Marasini [63]
Autoimmune hepatitis (AIH)		
AIH+SLE	27/1056 (2.6 %)	Abe [52]
	5/162 (3.1 %)	Oka [55]
	7/30 (23.3 %)	Onder [56]
	2/278 (0.7 %)	Teufel [93]
AIH+RA	30/1056 (2.8 %)	Abe [52]
	5/278 (1.8 %)	Teufel [93]
AIH+SjS	76/1056 (7.2 %)	Abe [52]
	4/278 (1.4 %)	Teufel [93]

SLE systemic erythematosus, *RA* rheumatoid arthritis, *SjS* Sjögren's syndromes, *SSc* systemic sclerosis, *CREST* calcinosis, Raynaud's phenomenon, esophageal dysmotility, sclerodactyly, and telangiectasia

13.4.8 Primary Biliary Cholangitis Overlap

Primary biliary cholangitis (PBC) is a chronic cholestatic disease of unknown cause characterized by progressive destruction of intrahepatic bile ducts [58]. PBC is often accompanied by other autoimmune diseases, indicating the involvement of autoimmune mechanisms in its pathogenesis [59]. An epidemiological study from Japan showed that 1965 (23.8 %) of 7926 patients with PBC were affected by another autoimmune disease at the time of PBC diagnosis [60]. The autoimmune diseases in PBC are wide ranging, including SjS (11.9 %), Hashimoto disease (6.5 %), RA (3.6 %), and SSc (2.7 %) [60]. SLE-PBC overlap is relatively rare. The prevalence of SLE in PBC patients has been reported to be 0.3–3.7 % [60–63] (Table 13.3), while the prevalence of PBC in SLE patients is 1.5–1.6 % [15, 21]. In

15 SLE-PBC overlap cases, PBC developed before SLE (73.3 %) [64]. SLE-PBC overlap patients had lower white blood cell counts and higher frequencies of renal involvement than patients with PBC alone [61]. SLE-PBC patients appeared to have much less extensive liver damage, suggesting that SLE may protect against progression of PBC [65]. Although SLE-PBC overlap may involve a genetic abnormality, e.g., STAT 4, which is associated with disease activity in both SLE and PBC [66, 67], the detailed roles of genetic factors remain to be established.

13.5 Rheumatoid Arthritis

13.5.1 Prevalence of Liver Dysfunction

RA is a systemic disease characterized by joint involvement but also affects other organs, including the liver. The prevalence of liver dysfunction is 36–77 % [2, 5, 8, 9, 11, 68] (Table 13.1). The causes of liver dysfunction in patients with RA vary, as in SLE (Table 13.2). Liver dysfunction in patients with RA is mostly the cholestatic pattern; serum ALP or γ-GTP levels are elevated, while serum aminotransferase levels are usually normal [69].

13.5.2 Liver Dysfunction Caused by RA Itself

The prevalence of liver dysfunction caused by RA itself is 2.5–29.2 % [2, 5] (Table 13.2). In general, the degree of liver dysfunction reflects the activity of the underlying disease, including in RA [10]. The ALP elevations in RA require attention, because increased ALP levels reflect not only liver damage but also bone lesions. Examination of ALP isozymes is therefore needed to evaluate the liver dysfunction caused by RA in patients showing ALP elevation alone. The histology of the liver with dysfunction caused by RA itself does not show any consistent structural abnormalities. A previous paper reported nonspecific findings, such as nonspecific reactive hepatitis, hepatic arthritis, and fatty liver [1]. Moreover, NRH is also associated with RA and has been seen in Felty's syndrome, a subtype of RA characterized by leucopenia and splenomegaly [4].

13.5.3 Liver Dysfunction Caused by Drugs

DILI is the main cause of liver dysfunction in RA patients, with a prevalence of 33–40.5 % [2, 5] (Table 13.2). MTX is a disease-modifying antirheumatic drug (DMARD) and has been used to treat RA since the 1950s. A systematic review reported that the incidence of elevated liver enzymes in the first 3 years of MTX use was 13/100 patient-years, and the cumulative incidence was 31 % [70]. The liver dysfunction caused by MTX in patients with RA is rather broad, ranging from mild elevation of transaminases to liver failure [71, 72]. NAFLD has also been associated with MTX therapy. A recent study showed that the prevalence of MTX-associated NAFLD with transaminitis was 4.7 % among 987 RA patients on MTX therapy [71]. Moreover, the cumulative MTX dose was an independent predictor of MTX-associated NAFLD transaminitis, although the mechanisms remain unclear.

Biologics are the first-line therapy for RA and are effective at reducing RA activity, achieving remission, and preventing joint destruction. Infliximab is a TNF-α antagonist that is used for the treatment of inflammatory diseases, including RA. A large study showed that 154 (3.1 %) of 5000 RA patients treated with infliximab had a hepatic disorder [73].

13.5.4 Liver Dysfunction Caused by Viruses

Chronic HCV infection has extrahepatic manifestations including arthropathy. The prevalence of arthropathy is 40–70 % in patients with HCV infection [74]. In a large prospective study, 23 % of 1614 patients with chronic HCV infection had arthralgia and arthritis [75]. A nationwide population-based study in Taiwan recently showed that chronic HCV infection was associated with the development of RA [76]. TNF-α antagonists have usually been safe in HCV-positive RA patients [77].

About 350 million individuals have chronic HBV infection, and more than one-third of the global population has been considered to be infected with HBV [78]. Previous reports have shown that more than one-quarter of patients with RA in Japan may be infected with HBV [79, 80]. Reactivation of HBV represents a serious problem among patients undergoing immunosuppressive therapy. Urata et al. reported that HBV DNA became positive in 7 of 135 RA patients with resolved hepatitis B (HBsAg-negative, HBcAb/HBsAb-positive) during 12 months of treatment [80]. Moreover, use of biologic agents was significantly more frequent in patients who developed reactivation of DNA replication (87.5 %) than in patients who did not (36 %). Immunosuppressive therapy for RA has the potential to induce HBV reactivation and de novo hepatitis, so HBV screening before treatment should always be performed.

13.5.5 AIH Overlap

AIH and RA overlap is a rare condition. Abe et al. diagnosed RA in 2.8 % of 1056 patients with AIH [53]. We diagnosed AIH in 1.3 % of 79 RA patients [5]. A study of RA patients on long-term low-dose MTX therapy reported that 13 (52.5 %) of

25 RA patients with elevated liver enzymes showed AIH-like lesions in liver biopsy specimens [81].

13.5.6 *PBC Overlap*

In a large-scale nationwide study in Japan, 285 (3.6 %) of 7926 patients with PBC had RA [60]. Some articles reported a similar prevalence (1.8–2.8 %) [61, 63], and one report described 27 (17 %) of 160 PBC patients as having RA [63]. This wide spectrum of prevalence may be explained by differences in ethnicity and environment. Some reports have indicated that the rate of RA is higher in PBC [61–63], as in a large Japanese cohort study, which may suggest a common background for the pathogenesis of both diseases.

Antimitochondrial antibodies (AMA) are a disease-specific maker for PBC. Several studies have estimated that 10–18 % of RA patients have AMA, while about half of PBC patients become rheumatoid factor-positive during the clinical course of PBC [82–84]. Moreover, Koga et al. indicated that 2 (2.7 %) of 73 PBC patients showed positive results for anti-cyclic citrullinated peptide antibodies [85]. Genome-wide association studies (GWAS) have indicated several common genes, such as CTLA4, STAT4, IRF5, and CXCR5, in RA and PBC [86]. These common serum and genetic profiles may explain PBC-RA overlap.

A study by Siegel et al. found that RA was diagnosed before PBC in 17 (68 %) of 25 patients with both RA and PBC [87]. Laboratory findings from patients with PBC-RA overlap have shown higher levels of hemoglobin, ALP, and IgG and increased erythrocyte sedimentation rate and rheumatoid factor-positivity than in PBC patients without RA.

13.6 Sjögren's Syndrome

SjS is a chronic autoimmune disorder that is clinically characterized by keratoconjunctivitis sicca, xerostomia, and swollen salivary glands. The prevalence of liver dysfunction is seen in 7–52 % of SjS patients [2, 5, 88–90]. Liver dysfunction is usually mild and predominantly a cholestatic biochemical profile. The clonality of B cells infiltrating the hepatic tissues of SjS patients with liver dysfunction suggests the contribution of a specific autoimmune abnormality to SjS-associated liver dysfunction [91].

PBC is the main cause (27–70 %) of liver dysfunction in SjS patients [2, 5]. In previous studies, 47–73 % of PBC patients had sicca symptoms [92], whereas SjS is found in 4–38 % of PBC patients [60–63] (Table 13.3). AMA is detected in 7 % of patients with SjS. Among AMA-positive SjS patients, 60 % have an elevated ALP and 82 % have histological findings of PBC [88]. Bile duct and salivary gland epithelia are common major targets of both SjS and PBC. In addition, SjS and PBC have a common histological characteristic, showing a predominance of CD4-positive T-cell infiltrates, around the bile duct in PBC and around the salivary duct in SjS. Although the prevalence of liver dysfunction caused by SjS itself has been reported as 30 % [2], some patients may be affected by PBC, including subclinical PBC.

SjS is present in 1.4–7.2 % of patients with AIH [52, 93]. Although only a small number of studies have been conducted, AIH was found in 4 % of patients with SjS [89]. Histological findings of SjS patients with AIH have been reported as a predominance of CD3-positive T-cell infiltrates in both the salivary glands and liver [94].

HCV infection has long been suspected to play a pathogenetic role in the development of SjS. HCV RNA is present in the salivary glands of SjS patients with HCV infection [95]. SjS patients with HCV infection have a higher prevalence of liver involvement than those without [96].

13.7 Systemic Sclerosis

SSc is a chronic autoimmune disease characterized by fibrosis and vascular endothelial damage in multiple internal organs. D'Angelo et al. identified cirrhosis in 5 (9 %) of 57 patients with SSc [97]. Matsumoto et al. also reported that 1 (8.3 %) of 12 autopsy patients with SSc had hepatic arteritis [1].

Liver dysfunction was reported in 1.1–44.7 % of patients with SSc [2, 5, 98]. PBC often overlaps with SSc and is the main cause of liver dysfunction in these patients [2, 5]. About 3–12 % of PBC patients have been reported to have scleroderma [60–63] (Table 13.3). In a large-scale nationwide study in Japan, 214 (2.7 %) of 7926 patients with PBC were reported to show overlap with SSc [60]. SSc is classified into two types: diffuse type (diffuse cutaneous SSc), characterized by generalized dermal sclerosis, and limited type (limited cutaneous SSc (lcSSc)), affecting only the hands and fingers. Furthermore, lcSSc includes a subtype referred to as CREST (calcinosis, Raynaud's phenomenon, esophageal dysmotility, sclerodactyly, and telangiectasia) syndrome. Assassi et al. reported that PBC was detected in 16 (2 %) of 817 patients with SSc, of whom 13 (81 %) displayed CREST syndrome [99].

Anticentromere antibody (ACA), a hallmark antibody of SSc, has also been detected in 10 % of PBC patients [100]. In a study of PBC patients with ACA, 10 (63 %) of 16 patients showed features of lcSSc [101]. Raynaud's phenomenon is also more commonly seen in PBC patients with ACA than in those without. Rigamonti et al. showed a higher prevalence of ACA in patients with PBC-SSc overlap than in patients with PBC alone [102]. Moreover, patients with PBC-CREST overlap syndrome also showed a higher prevalence of ACA compared to patients with PBC alone, with asymptomatic PBC accounting for about 80 % of all PBC cases, and characterized by a high prevalence of HLA-DR9 [103]. At the same time, about 60 % of PBC-CREST overlap syndrome patients are known to have incomplete types of CREST syndrome, such as CRST (calcinosis, Raynaud's phenomenon, sclerodactyly, and telangiectasia) and RST (Raynaud's phenomenon, sclerodactyly, and telangiectasia). Outcomes of PBC-SSc overlap are significantly better than those of PBC alone in terms of 10-year survival, but not in terms of overall survival. Moreover, rates of progressive jaundice and liver transplantation are significantly lower in patients with PBC-SSc overlap than in those with PBC alone [102]. AIH-SSc overlap has been reported only occasionally, and most cases had lcSSc.

13.8 Vasculitis

A new system that classifies vasculitis according to the size of the affected blood vessels was proposed in 2012 [104]. Vasculitides affecting large blood vessels include Takayasu arteritis and giant cell arteritis; vasculitides affecting medium-sized vessels include polyarteritis nodosa (PN) and Kawasaki disease; and vasculitides affecting small vessels include microscopic polyangiitis, granulomatosis with polyangiitis (Wegener's granulomatosis), eosinophilic granulomatosis with polyangiitis (Churg-Strauss syndrome), anti-glomerular basement membrane disease, cryoglobulinemic vasculitis, IgA vasculitis (Henoch-Schonlein purpura), and hypocomplementemic urticarial vasculitis.

Liver dysfunction is rare in patients with vasculitis syndrome, but liver arteritis is a frequent finding, especially in patients with PN [1]. Kojima et al. identified liver dysfunction in 54 % of PN patients and determined that the hepatopathy was caused by PN itself in 71 % [2]. The severity of liver injury correlates with the activity of vasculitis, and liver dysfunction associated with PN is characterized by higher ALP levels than liver dysfunction caused by other collagen diseases [5].

Wegener's granulomatosis and Churg-Strauss syndrome are classified as small vessel vasculitides and newly named as granulomatosis with polyangiitis and eosinophilic granulomatosis with polyangiitis, respectively, by the recent classification system. In Wegener's granulomatosis, liver injury is extremely rare, but a few reports have described hepatic granuloma [105, 106]. Liver dysfunction is also rare in patients with Churg-Strauss syndrome. Although a recent study showed eosinophilic infiltrates in vessels in the portal area of the liver in patients with Churg-Strauss syndrome, direct pathological demonstration of vasculitis in the liver is very rare.

13.9 Adult-Onset Still's Disease

AOSD is a rare systemic autoinflammatory disorder of unknown etiology. Liver dysfunction is common, as 36–89 % of patients display elevated levels of liver enzymes [5, 107–116] (Table 13.1). The presence of abnormal liver function tests is therefore one of the diagnostic items in the classification criteria of Yamaguchi et al. [117]. Liver dysfunction can be caused by drugs, such as antipyretic analgesics and antibiotics, and by viral infections, or can be directly associated with AOSD, making differential diagnosis important.

Serum levels of IL-18, which induces the production of Th1 cytokines, are higher in AOSD patients [118]. Moreover, Priori et al. reported markedly increased IL-18 liver expression in AOSD-related hepatitis [119]. Liver dysfunction in AOSD is mainly asymptomatic, with mild to moderate elevations of transaminase levels. Histologically, nonspecific interstitial inflammation is the most common finding in organs including the liver. Acute liver failure occurs infrequently at the time of AOSD diagnosis, during tapering of immunosuppressive therapy, or long after diagnosis when other symptoms are well controlled by therapy. In patients with severe AOSD, submassive hepatic necrosis in the centrilobular area and piecemeal necrosis have been described [120]. The severity of liver dysfunction directly associated with AOSD usually correlates with the intensity of the underlying disease, as reflected in ferritin and ALT levels [121, 122].

13.10 Conclusion

The liver is involved in rheumatic disease with a wide spectrum of clinical findings and severities. Moreover, treatment for rheumatic disease or following viral infections could induce liver dysfunction. Liver dysfunction in patients with rheumatic disease shows relatively specific tendencies for each collagen disease. An adequate understanding of the characteristics of liver dysfunction is necessary when treating rheumatic disease. Consideration should also be given to the possibility of concomitant autoimmune hepatic diseases, such as AIH and PBC.

References

1. Matsumoto T, Kobayashi S, Shimizu H, Nakajima M, Watanabe S, Kitami N, et al. The liver in collagen diseases: pathologic study of 160 cases with particular reference to hepatic arteritis, primary biliary cirrhosis, autoimmune hepatitis and nodular regenerative hyperplasia of the liver. Liver. 2000;20:366–73.
2. Kojima H, Uemura M, Sakurai S, Ann T, Ishii Y, Imazu H, et al. Clinical features of liver disturbance in rheumatoid diseases: clinicopathological study with special reference to the cause of liver disturbance. J Gastroenterol. 2002;37:617–25.
3. Abraham S, Begum S, Isenberg D. Hepatic manifestations of autoimmune rheumatic diseases. Ann Rheum Dis. 2004;63:123–9.
4. Malnick S, Melzer E, Sokolowski N, Basevitz A. The involvement of the liver in systemic diseases. J Clin Gastroenterol. 2008;42:69–80.
5. Takahashi A, Abe K, Yokokawa J, Iwadate H, Kobayashi H, Watanabe H, et al. Clinical features of liver dysfunction in collagen diseases. Hepatol Res. 2010;40:1092–7. doi:10.1111/j.1872-034X.2010.00707.x.

6. Schlenker C, Halterman T, Kowdley KV. Rheumatologic disease and the liver. Clin Liver Dis. 2011;15:153–64. doi:10.1016/j.cld.2010.09.006.
7. Ohira H, Abe K, Takahashi A. Involvement of the liver in rheumatic disease. Clin J Gastroenterol. 2012;5:9–14. doi:10.1007/s12328-011-0271-4.
8. Fernandes L, Sullivan S, McFarlane IG, Wojcicka BM, Warnes TW, Eddleston AL, et al. Studies on the frequency and pathogenesis of liver involvement in rheumatoid arthritis. Ann Rheum Dis. 1979;38:501–6.
9. Spooner RJ, Smith DH, Bedford D, Beck PR. Serum gamma-glutamyltransferase and alkaline phosphatase in rheumatoid arthritis. J Clin Pathol. 1982;35:638–41.
10. Aida S. Alkaline phosphatase isoenzyme activities in rheumatoid arthritis: hepatobiliary enzyme dissociation and relation to disease activity. Ann Rheum Dis. 1993;52:511–6.
11. Lowe JR, Pickup ME, Dixon JS, Leatham PA, Rhind VM, Wright V, et al. Gamma glutamyl transpeptidase levels in arthritis: a correlation with clinical and laboratory indices of disease activity. Ann Rheum Dis. 1978;37:428–31.
12. Grover S, Rastogi A, Singh J, Rajbongshi A, Bihari C. Spectrum of histomorphologic findings in liver in patients with SLE: a review. Hepat Res Treat. 2014;2014:562979. doi:10.1155/2014/562979.
13. Zheng RH, Wang JH, Wang SB, Chen J, Guan WM, Chen MH. Clinical and immunopathological features of patients with lupus hepatitis. Chin Med J (Engl). 2013;126:260–6.
14. Miller MH, Urowitz MB, Gladman DD, Blendis LM. The liver in systemic lupus erythematosus. Q J Med. 1984;53:401–9.
15. Chowdhary VR, Crowson CS, Poterucha JJ, Moder KG. Liver involvement in systemic lupus erythematosus: case review of 40 patients. J Rheumatol. 2008;35:2159–64.
16. Piga M, Vacca A, Porru G, Cauli A, Mathieu A. Liver involvement in systemic lupus erythematosus: incidence, clinical course and outcome of lupus hepatitis. Clin Exp Rheumatol. 2010;28:504–10.
17. Huang D, Aghdassi E, Su J, Mosko J, Hirschfield GM, Gladman DD, et al. Prevalence and risk factors for liver biochemical abnormalities in Canadian patients with systemic lupus erythematosus. J Rheumatol. 2012;39:254–61. doi:10.3899/jrheum.110310.
18. Takahashi A, Abe K, Saito R, Iwadate H, Okai K, Katsushima F, et al. Liver dysfunction in patients with systemic lupus erythematosus. Intern Med. 2013;52:1461–5.
19. Runyon BA, LaBrecque DR, Anuras S. The spectrum of liver disease in systemic lupus erythematosus. Report of 33 histologically-proved cases and review of the literature. Am J Med. 1980;69:187–94.
20. Luangjaru S, Kullavanijaya P. Gastrointestinal and hepatobiliary manifestations in systemic lupus erythematosus. J Med Assoc Thai. 2005;88:71–5.
21. Her M, Lee Y, Jung E, Kim T, Kim D. Liver enzyme abnormalities in systemic lupus erythematosus: a focus on toxic hepatitis. Rheumatol Int. 2011;31:79–84. doi:10.1007/s00296-009-1237-4.
22. Gibson T, Myers AR. Subclinical liver disease in systemic lupus erythematosus. J Rheumatol. 1981;8:752–9.
23. Arnett FC, Reichlin M. Lupus hepatitis: an under-recognized disease feature associated with autoantibodies to ribosomal P. Am J Med. 1995;99:465–72.
24. Hulsey M, Goldstein R, Scully L, Surbeck W, Reichlin M. Anti-ribosomal P antibodies in systemic lupus erythematosus: a case-control study correlating hepatic and renal disease. Clin Immunol Immunopathol. 1995;74:252–6.
25. Yoshio T, Masuyama JI, Minota S, Kaneko N, Iwamoto M, Okazaki H, et al. A close temporal relationship of liver disease to antiribosomal P0 protein antibodies and central nervous system disease in patients with systemic lupus erythematosus. J Rheumatol. 1998;25:681–8.
26. Ohira H, Takiguchi J, Rai T, Abe K, Yokokawa J, Sato Y, et al. High frequency of anti-ribosomal P antibody in patients with systemic lupus erythematosus-associated hepatitis. Hepatol Res. 2004;28:137–9.

27. Calich AL, Viana VS, Cancado E, Tustumi F, Terrabuio DR, Leon EP, et al. Anti-ribosomal P protein: a novel antibody in autoimmune hepatitis. Liver Int. 2013;33:909–13. doi:10.1111/liv.12155.
28. Bessone F, Poles N, Roma MG. Challenge of liver disease in systemic lupus erythematosus: clues for diagnosis and hints for pathogenesis. World J Hepatol. 2014;6(6):394–409. doi:10.4254/wjh.v6.i6.394.
29. Horizon AA, Wallace DJ. Risk:benefit ratio of nonsteroidal anti-inflammatory drugs in systemic lupus erythematosus. Expert Opin Drug Saf. 2004;3:273–8.
30. Bessone F. Non-steroidal anti-inflammatory drugs: what is the actual risk of liver damage? World J Gastroenterol. 2010;16:5651–61.
31. Zimmerman HJ. Editorial: aspirin-induced hepatic injury. Ann Intern Med. 1974;80:103–5.
32. Yildirim-Toruner C, Diamond B. Current and novel therapeutics in the treatment of systemic lupus erythematosus. J Allergy Clin Immunol. 2011;127:303–14. doi:10.1016/j.jaci.2010.12.1087.
33. Sakthiswary R, Suresh E. Methotrexate in systemic lupus erythematosus: a systematic review of its efficacy. Lupus. 2014;23:225–35. doi:10.1177/0961203313519159.
34. Carneiro JR, Sato EI. Double blind, randomized, placebo controlled clinical trial of methotrexate in systemic lupus erythematosus. J Rheumatol. 1999;26:1275–9.
35. Ramos-Casals M, Font J, García-Carrasco M, Cervera R, Jiménez S, Trejo O, et al. Hepatitis C virus infection mimicking systemic lupus erythematosus: study of hepatitis C virus infection in a series of 134 Spanish patients with systemic lupus erythematosus. Arthritis Rheum. 2000;43(12):2801–6.
36. Manns MP, Obermayer-Straub P. Viral induction of autoimmunity: mechanisms and examples in hepatology. J Viral Hepat. 1997;4 Suppl 2:42–7.
37. Watanabe R, Ishii T, Nakamura K, Shirai T, Tajima Y, Fujii H, et al. Prevalence and time course of hepatitis B virus infection in patients with systemic lupus erythematosus under immunosuppressive therapy. Mod Rheumatol. 2013;23:1094–100. doi:10.1007/s10165-012-0797-4.
38. Hoofnagle JH. Reactivation of hepatitis B. Hepatology. 2009;49:S156–65. doi:10.1002/hep.22945.
39. Weinbaum CM, Williams I, Mast EE, Wang SA, Finelli L, Wasley A, et al. Recommendations for identification and public health management of persons with chronic hepatitis B virus infection. MMWR Recomm Rep. 2008;57:1–20.
40. Singh JA, Furst DE, Bharat A, Curtis JR, Kavanaugh AF, Kremer JM, et al. 2012 update of the 2008 American College of Rheumatology recommendations for the use of disease-modifying antirheumatic drugs and biologic agents in the treatment of rheumatoid arthritis. Arthritis Care Res. 2012;64:625–39. doi:10.1002/acr.21641.
41. Harigai M, Mochida S, Mimura T, Koike T, Miyasaka N. A proposal for management of rheumatic disease patients with hepatitis B virus infection receiving immunosuppressive therapy. Mod Rheumatol. 2014;24:1–7. doi:10.3109/14397595.2013.852834.
42. Ramos-Casals M, Cuadrado MJ, Alba P, Sanna G, Brito-Zerón P, Bertolaccini L, et al. Acute viral infections in patients with systemic lupus erythematosus: description of 23 cases and review of the literature. Medicine. 2008;87:311–8. doi:10.1097/MD.0b013e31818ec711.
43. Tsai WP, Chen MH, Lee MH, Yu KH, Wu MW, Liou LB. Cytomegalovirus infection causes morbidity and mortality in patients with autoimmune diseases, particularly systemic lupus: in a Chinese population in Taiwan. Rheumatol Int. 2012;32(9):2901–8. doi:10.1007/s00296-011-2131-4.
44. Zhang J, Dou Y, Zhong Z, Su J, Xu D, Tang F, et al. Clinical characteristics and therapy exploration of active human cytomegalovirus infection in 105 lupus patients. Lupus. 2014;23:889–97.
45. Wong KF, Hui PK, Chan JK, Chan YW, Ha SY. The acute lupus hemophagocytic syndrome. Ann Intern Med. 1991;114:387–90.

46. Dhote R, Simon J, Papo T, Detournay B, Sailler L, Andre MH, et al. Reactive hemophagocytic syndrome in adult systemic disease: report of twenty-six cases and literature review. Arthritis Rheum. 2003;49:633–9.
47. Larroche C, Mouthon L. Pathogenesis of hemophagocytic syndrome (HPS). Autoimmun Rev. 2004;3:69–75.
48. Sekigawa I, Suzuki J, Nawata M, Ikeda K, Koike M, Iida N, et al. Hemophagocytosis in autoimmune disease. Clin Exp Rheumatol. 2001;19:333–8.
49. Kumakura S, Ishikura H, Kondo M, Murakawa Y, Masuda J, et al. Autoimmune-associated hemophagocytic syndrome. Mod Rheumatol. 2004;14:205–15.
50. Reid AE. Nonalcoholic steatohepatitis. Gastroenterology. 2001;121:710–23.
51. Harada K. Autoimmune hepatitis: histological findings of autoimmune hepatitis. In: Ohira H, editor. Autoimmune liver disease. Tokyo: Springer; 2014.
52. Abe M, Mashiba T, Zeniya M, Yamamoto K, Onji M, Tsubouchi H, Autoimmune Hepatitis Study Group-Subgroup of the Intractable Hepato-Biliary Disease Study Group in Japan. Present status of autoimmune hepatitis in Japan: a nationwide survey. J Gastroenterol. 2011;46:1136–41. doi:10.1007/s00535-011-0421-y.
53. Beisel C, Weiler-Normann C, Teufel A, Lohse AW. Association of autoimmune hepatitis and systemic lupus erythematodes: a case series and review of the literature. World J Gastroenterol. 2014;20:12662–7. doi:10.3748/wjg.v20.i35.12662.
54. Czaja AJ, Morshed SA, Parveen S, Nishioka M. Antibodies to single-stranded and double-stranded DNA in antinuclear antibody-positive type 1-autoimmune hepatitis. Hepatology. 1997;26:567–72.
55. Oka H. The survey of autoimmune hepatitis in Japan. Annual report of the Study Group on Severe Hepatitis. Japanese Ministry of Health and Welfare. 1988;235–241 (Japanese).
56. Onder FO, Yürekli OT, Oztaş E, Kalkan IH, Köksal AS, Akdoğan M, et al. Features of systemic lupus erythematosus in patients with autoimmune hepatitis. Rheumatol Int. 2013;33 (6):1581–5. doi:10.1007/s00296-012-2607-x.
57. Iwai M, Harada Y, Ishii M, Tanaka S, Muramatsu A, Mori T. Autoimmune hepatitis in a patient with systemic lupus erythematosus. Clin Rheumatol. 2003;22:234–6.
58. Kaplan MM, Gershwin ME. Primary biliary cirrhosis. N Engl J Med. 2005;353:1261–73.
59. Hirschfield GM, Gershwin ME. The immunobiology and pathophysiology of primary biliary cirrhosis. Annu Rev Pathol. 2013;8:303–30. doi:10.1146/annurev-pathol-020712-164014.
60. Hirohara J. National surveys of primary biliary cirrhosis (PBC) in Japan. Annual report of the intractable Liver and Biliary Diseases Study Group of Japan. Japanese Ministry of Health, Labour and Welfare. 2013;63–67 (Japanese).
61. Wang L, Zhang FC, Chen H, Zhang X, Xu D, Li YZ, et al. Connective tissue diseases in primary biliary cirrhosis: a population-based cohort study. World J Gastroenterol. 2013;19:5131–7. doi:10.3748/wjg.v19.i31.5131.
62. Watt FE, James OF, Jones DE. Patterns of autoimmunity in primary biliary cirrhosis patients and their families: a population-based cohort study. QJM. 2004;97:397–406.
63. Marasini B, Gagetta M, Rossi V, Ferrari P. Rheumatic disorders and primary biliary cirrhosis: an appraisal of 170 Italian patients. Ann Rheum Dis. 2001;60:1046–9.
64. Saito H, Takahashi A, Abe K, Monoe K, Kanno Y, Yokokawa J, et al. Two cases of primary biliary cirrhosis associated with systemic lupus erythematosus. Kanzo. 2011;52:169–75 (Japanese).
65. Corpechot C, Abenavoli L, Rabahi N, Chrétien Y, Andréani T, Johanet C, et al. Biochemical response to ursodeoxycholic acid and long-term prognosis in primary biliary cirrhosis. Hepatology. 2008;48:871–7. doi:10.1002/hep.22428.
66. Hirschfield GM, Liu X, Xu C, Lu Y, Xie G, Lu Y, et al. Primary biliary cirrhosis associated with HLA, IL12A, and IL12RB2 variants. N Engl J Med. 2009;360(24):2544–55. doi:10.1056/NEJMoa0810440.
67. Han JW, Zheng HF, Cui Y, Sun LD, Ye DQ, Hu Z, et al. Genome-wide association study in a Chinese Han population identifies nine new susceptibility loci for systemic lupus erythematosus. Nat Genet. 2009;41:1234–7. doi:10.1038/ng.472.

68. Akesson A, Berglund K, Karlsson M. Liver function in some common rheumatic disorders. Scand J Rheumatol. 1980;9:81–8.
69. Rau R, Pfenninger K, Boni A. Proceedings: liver function tests and liver biopsies in patients with rheumatoid arthritis. Ann Rheum Dis. 1975;34:198–9.
70. Visser K, van der Heijde DM. Risk and management of liver toxicity during methotrexate treatment in rheumatoid and psoriatic arthritis: a systematic review of the literature. Clin Exp Rheumatol. 2009;27(6):1017–25.
71. Sakthiswary R, Chan GY, Koh ET, Leong KP, Thong BY. Methotrexate-associated nonalcoholic fatty liver disease with transaminitis in rheumatoid arthritis. Sci World J. 2014;2014:823763. doi:10.1155/2014/823763.
72. Hakim NS, Kobienia B, Benedetti E, Bloomer J, Payne WD. Methotrexate-induced hepatic necrosis requiring liver transplantation in a patient with rheumatoid arthritis. Int Surg. 1998;83:224–5.
73. Takeuchi T, Tatsuki Y, Nogami Y, Ishiguro N, Tanaka Y, Yamanaka H, et al. Postmarketing surveillance of the safety profile of infliximab in 5000 Japanese patients with rheumatoid arthritis. Ann Rheum Dis. 2008;67:189–94.
74. Antonelli A, Ferri C, Galeazzi M, Giannitti C, Manno D, Mieli-Vergani G, et al. HCV infection: pathogenesis, clinical manifestations and therapy. Clin Exp Rheumatol. 2008;26: S39–47.
75. Cacoub P, Poynard T, Ghillani P, Charlotte F, Olivi M, Piette JC, et al. Extrahepatic manifestations of chronic hepatitis C. MULTIVIRC Group. Multidepartment Virus C. Arthritis Rheum. 1999;42:2204–12.
76. Su FH, Wu CS, Sung FC, Chang SN, Su CT, Shieh YH, et al. Chronic hepatitis C virus infection is associated with the development of rheumatoid arthritis: a nationwide population-based study in Taiwan. PLoS One. 2014;9(11):e113579. doi:10.1371/journal.pone.0113579.
77. Brunasso AM, Puntoni M, Gulia A, Massone C. Safety of anti-tumour necrosis factor agents in patients with chronic hepatitis C infection: a systematic review. Rheumatology. 2011;50:1700–11. doi:10.1093/rheumatology/ker190.
78. Lok AS, McMahon BJ. Chronic hepatitis B: update 2009. Hepatology. 2009;50(3):661–2. doi:10.1002/hep.23190.
79. Mori S. Past hepatitis B virus infection in rheumatoid arthritis patients receiving biological and/or nonbiological disease-modifying antirheumatic drugs. Mod Rheumatol. 2011;21:621–7. doi:10.1007/s10165-011-0458-z.
80. Urata Y, Uesato R, Tanaka D, Kowatari K, Nitobe T, Nakamura Y, et al. Prevalence of reactivation of hepatitis B virus replication in rheumatoid arthritis patients. Mod Rheumatol. 2011;21:16–23. doi:10.1007/s10165-010-0337-z.
81. Quintin E, Scoazec JY, Marotte H, Miossec P. Rare incidence of methotrexate-specific lesions in liver biopsy of patients with arthritis and elevated liver enzymes. Arthritis Res Ther. 2010;12:R143. doi:10.1186/ar3085.
82. Datta A, Deodhar SD, Datta U, Sehgal S. Non-organ specific & organ specific antibodies in rheumatoid arthritis. Indian J Med Res. 1990;92:228–32.
83. Zurgil N, Bakimer R, Moutsopoulos HM, Tzioufas AG, Youinou P, Isenberg DA, et al. Antimitochondrial (pyruvate dehydrogenase) autoantibodies in autoimmune rheumatic diseases. J Clin Immunol. 1992;12:201–9.
84. Mouritsen S, Demant E, Permin H, Wiik A. High prevalence of anti-mitochondrial antibodies among patients with some well-defined connective tissue diseases. Clin Exp Immunol. 1986;66:68–76.
85. Koga T, Migita K, Miyashita T, Maeda Y, Nakamura M, Abiru S, et al. Determination of anti-cyclic citrullinated peptide antibodies in the sera of patients with liver diseases. Clin Exp Rheumatol. 2008;26:121–4.
86. Smyk DS, Bogdanos DP, Mytilinaiou MG, Burroughs AK, Rigopoulou EI. Rheumatoid arthritis and primary biliary cirrhosis: cause, consequence, or coincidence? Arthritis. 2012;2012:391567. doi:10.1155/2012/391567.

87. Siegel JL, Luthra H, Donlinger J, Angulo P, Lindor K. Association of primary biliary cirrhosis and rheumatoid arthritis. J Clin Rheumatol. 2003;9:340–3.
88. Skopouli FN, Barbatis C, Moutsopoulos HM. Liver involvement in primary Sjögren's syndrome. Br J Rheumatol. 1994;33:745–8.
89. Lindgren S, Manthorpe R, Eriksson S. Autoimmune liver disease in patients with primary Sjögren's syndrome. J Hepatol. 1994;20:354–8.
90. Montaño-Loza AJ, Crispín-Acuña JC, Remes-Troche JM, Uribe M. Abnormal hepatic biochemistries and clinical liver disease in patients with primary Sjögren's syndrome. Ann Hepatol. 2007;6:150–5.
91. Tokuno T, Takahashi H, Suzuki C, Yamamoto M, Naishiro Y, Sugaya A, et al. Analysis of B-cell clonality in the hepatic tissue of patients with Sjögren's syndrome. Scand J Rheumatol. 2003;32:268–72.
92. De Santis M, Crotti C, Selmi C. Liver abnormalities in connective tissue diseases. Clin Gastroenterol. 2013;27:543–51. doi:10.1016/j.bpg.2013.06.016.
93. Teufel A, Weinmann A, Kahaly GJ, Centner C, Piendl A, Wörns M, et al. Concurrent autoimmune diseases in patients with autoimmune hepatitis. J Clin Gastroenterol. 2010;44 (3):208–13. doi:10.1097/MCG.0b013e3181c74e0d.
94. Matsumoto T, Morizane T, Aoki Y, Yamasaki S, Nakajima M, Enomoto N, et al. Autoimmune hepatitis in primary Sjogren's syndrome: pathological study of the livers and labial salivary glands in 17 patients with primary Sjogren's syndrome. Pathol Int. 2005;55:70–6.
95. Toussirot E, Le Huédé G, Mougin C, Balblanc JC, Bettinger D, Wendling D. Presence of hepatitis C virus RNA in the salivary glands of patients with Sjögren's syndrome and hepatitis C virus infection. J Rheumatol. 2002;29:2382–5.
96. Esteban JI, Esteban R, Viladomiu L, López-Talavera JC, González A, Hernández JM, et al. Hepatitis C virus antibodies among risk groups in Spain. Lancet. 1989;2:294–7.
97. D'Angelo WA, Fries JF, Masi AT, Shulman LE. Pathologic observations in systemic sclerosis (scleroderma). A study of fifty-eight autopsy cases and fifty-eight matched controls. Am J Med. 1969;46:428–40.
98. Chen J. Liver, gall and pancreas. In: Liu TH, Liu TH, Li WH, editors. Diagnostic pathology. Beijing: People Health Press; 1995. p. 242.
99. Assassi S, Fritzler MJ, Arnett FC, Norman GL, Shah KR, Gourh P, et al. Primary biliary cirrhosis (PBC), PBC autoantibodies, and hepatic parameter abnormalities in a large population of systemic sclerosis patients. J Rheumatol. 2009;36:2250–6. doi:10.3899/jrheum.090340.
100. Hansen BU, Eriksson S, Lindgren S. High prevalence of autoimmune liver disease in patients with multiple nuclear dot, anti-centromere, and mitotic spindle antibodies. Scand J Gastroenterol. 1991;26:707–13.
101. Shoji I, Takagi T, Kasukawa R. Anti-centromere antibody and CREST syndrome in patients with primary biliary cirrhosis. Intern Med. 1992;31:1348–55.
102. Rigamonti C, Shand LM, Feudjo M, Bunn CC, Black CM, Denton CP, et al. Clinical features and prognosis of primary biliary cirrhosis associated with systemic sclerosis. Gut. 2006;55:388–94.
103. Tojo J, Ohira H, Suzuki T, Takeda I, Shoji I, Kojima T, et al. Clinicolaboratory characteristics of patients with primary biliary cirrhosis associated with CREST symptoms. Hepatol Res. 2002;22:187–95.
104. Jennette JC, Falk RJ, Bacon PA, Basu N, Cid MC, Ferrario F, et al. 2012 revised International Chapel Hill Consensus Conference Nomenclature of Vasculitides. Arthritis Rheum. 2013;65 (1):1–11. doi:10.1002/art.37715.
105. Shah IA, Holstege A, Riede UN. Bioptic diagnosis of Wegener's granulomatosis in the absence of vasculitis and granulomas. Pathol Res Pract. 1984;178:407–15.
106. Boissy C, Bernard E, Chazal M, Fuzibet JG, Michiels JF, Saint-Paul MC. Wegener's granulomatosis disclosed by hepato-splenic involvement. Gastroenterol Clin Biol. 1997;21:633–5 (in French).

107. Pouchot J, Sampalis JS, Beaudet F, Carette S, Décary F, Salusinsky-Sternbach M, et al. Adult Still's disease: manifestations, disease course, and outcome in 62 patients. Medicine. 1991;70:118–36.
108. Fautrel B, Zing E, Golmard JL, Le Moel G, Bissery A, Rioux C, et al. Proposal for a new set of classification criteria for adult-onset still disease. Medicine. 2002;81:194–200.
109. Pay S, Türkçapar N, Kalyoncu M, Simşek I, Beyan E, Ertenli I, et al. A multicenter study of patients with adult-onset Still's disease compared with systemic juvenile idiopathic arthritis. Clin Rheumatol. 2006;25:639–44.
110. Cagatay Y, Gul A, Cagatay A, Kamali S, Karadeniz A, Inanc M, et al. Adult-onset Still's disease. Int J Clin Pract. 2009;63:1050–5.
111. Zhu G, Liu G, Liu Y, Xie Q, Shi G. Liver abnormalities in adult onset Still's disease: a retrospective study of 77 Chinese patients. J Clin Rheumatol. 2009;15:284–8. doi:10.1097/RHU.0b013e3181b57199.
112. Kong XD, Xu D, Zhang W, Zhao Y, Zeng X, Zhang F. Clinical features and prognosis in adult-onset Still's disease: a study of 104 cases. Clin Rheumatol. 2010;29:1015–9. doi:10.1007/s10067-010-1516-1.
113. Colina M, Zucchini W, Ciancio G, Orzincolo C, Trotta F, Govoni M. The evolution of adult-onset Still disease: an observational and comparative study in a cohort of 76 Italian patients. Semin Arthritis Rheum. 2011;41:279–85. doi:10.1016/j.semarthrit.2010.12.006.
114. Chen PD, Yu SL, Chen S, Weng XH. Retrospective study of 61 patients with adult-onset Still's disease admitted with fever of unknown origin in China. Clin Rheumatol. 2012;31:175–81. doi:10.1007/s10067-011-1798-y.
115. Gerfaud-Valentin M, Maucort-Boulch D, Hot A, Iwaz J, Ninet J, et al. Adult-onset still disease: manifestations, treatment, outcome, and prognostic factors in 57 patients. Medicine (Baltimore). 2014;93(2):91–9. doi:10.1097/MD.0000000000000021.
116. Mehrpoor G, Owlia MB, Soleimani H, Ayatollahi J. Adult-onset Still's disease: a report of 28 cases and review of the literature. Mod Rheumatol. 2008;18:480–5. doi:10.1007/s10165-008-0104-6.
117. Yamaguchi M, Ohta A, Tsunematsu T, Kasukawa R, Mizushima Y, Kashiwagi H, et al. Preliminary criteria for classification of adult Still's disease. J Rheumatol. 1992;19:424–30.
118. Fujii T, Nojima T, Yasuoka H, Satoh S, Nakamura K, Kuwana M, et al. Cytokine and immunogenetic profiles in Japanese patients with adult Still's disease. Association with chronic articular disease. Rheumatology. 2001;40:1398–404.
119. Priori R, Barone F, Alessandri C, Colafrancesco S, McInnes IB, Pitzalis C, et al. Markedly increased IL-18 liver expression in adult-onset Still's disease-related hepatitis. Rheumatology. 2011;50:776–80. doi:10.1093/rheumatology/keq397.
120. Takami A, Nakao S, Miyamori H, Ooi M, Machi T, Chujo T, et al. Adult-onset Still's disease with submassive hepatic necrosis. Intern Med. 1995;34:89–91.
121. Motoo Y, Ohta H, Okai T, Sawabu N. Adult-onset Still's disease: hepatic involvement and various serum markers relating to the disease activity. Jpn J Med. 1991;30:247–50.
122. Andrès E, Kurtz JE, Perrin AE, Pflumio F, Ruellan A, Goichot B, et al. Retrospective monocentric study of 17 patients with adult Still's disease, with special focus on liver abnormalities. Hepatogastroenterology. 2003;50:192–5.

Chapter 14
Hematologic Diseases and Liver

Nobuhiko Nakamura, Hisashi Tsurumi, and Masahito Shimizu

Abstract Liver involvement is often observed in several hematologic diseases, as shown by abnormal liver function tests, abnormalities in liver imaging studies, or clinical symptoms presenting with hepatic manifestations. In hematologic malignancies, malignant cells often infiltrate into the liver and produce abnormal liver function test results accompanied by hepatosplenomegaly or formation of multiple nodules in the liver. These cases may further evolve into fulminant hepatic failure. The treatment for hematologic diseases can cause liver problems. Iron overload is a major concern in patients with congenital and acquired anemias for whom regular transfusions are needed. Hepatitis B virus reactivation is a potentially fatal but preventable complication of chemotherapy or immunosuppressive therapy for hematologic diseases. Hepatic diseases such as veno-occlusive disease are common complications of hematopoietic cell transplantation. The types of liver complications occurring with hematologic diseases are many and varied, and acute and chronic liver disease contributes significantly to morbidity and mortality. Pre-transplant evaluation and prevention of liver injury are often more useful than treatment of deeply jaundiced patients in improving transplant outcomes.

Keywords Hematologic diseases • Iron overload • Hepatitis B virus reactivation • Hematopoietic cell transplantation

14.1 Introduction

Liver abnormalities are frequently seen in patients with hematologic diseases. The liver is a major component of the reticuloendothelial system, and malignant tumor cell infiltration of the liver commonly occurs in hematological malignancies. Occasionally, clinical evidence of liver disease may be the first manifestation of a primary hematological condition. This chapter summarizes the hepatic

N. Nakamura • H. Tsurumi • M. Shimizu (✉)
First Department of Internal Medicine, Gifu University Graduate School of Medicine, 1-1 Yanagido, Gifu 501-1194, Japan
e-mail: shimim-gif@umin.ac.jp

H. Ohira (ed.), *The Liver in Systemic Diseases*, DOI 10.1007/978-4-431-55790-6_14

Table 14.1 Involvement of the liver in patients with hematological malignancies

Diseases	Frequency of liver involvement	
	Clinical evaluation	Post mortem
Acute lymphocytic leukemia	–	>95 %
Acute myelogenous leukemia	–	75 %
Chronic lymphocytic leukemia	–	98 %
Hodgkin lymphoma	8–14 %	55 %
Non-Hodgkin lymphoma	16–57 %	52 %
Multiple myeloma	30–40 %	40–50 %

abnormalities found in the different hematological diseases and the treatment for hematologic diseases.

14.2 Malignant Hematologic Diseases

Liver involvement in hematologic malignancies is rarely life threatening or a source of great morbidity. The frequency of malignant infiltration varies from less than 10 % to nearly 100 % depending on the nature of the underlying hematologic malignancy (Table 14.1) [1].

14.2.1 Acute Leukemia

Acute leukemia is a rapidly progressing cancer that starts in the blood-forming tissue, such as the bone marrow, and causes large numbers of white blood cells to be produced and enter the blood stream. Although hepatic involvement is usually silent at the time of diagnosis, greater than 95 % of patients with acute lymphocytic leukemia (ALL) and 75 % of patients with acute myeloid leukemia (AML) have hepatic infiltration at autopsy [2]. In ALL, the infiltration is in the portal tracts, while in AML, it is in both the portal tracts and sinusoids [3]. A slight elevation in serum alkaline phosphatase activity and mild to moderate liver enlargement may be noted. Massive leukemic cell infiltration of the liver may present as fulminant hepatic failure (FHF) [4, 5]. The hemorrhagic complications of these acute leukemias rarely permit histological evaluation of the liver in patients with early, active disease. Therefore, it is difficult to discern the relative contributions of leukemic infiltration, extramedullary hematopoiesis, and infectious or toxic complications of the underlying leukemia (or the therapies employed) to the development of hepatomegaly and liver test abnormalities.

ALL is a common acute leukemia in the pediatric population, and FHF caused by ALL has sometimes been described in children. The pathogenesis is not clear but may be related to comorbid viral infections, sepsis, or ischemic hepatopathy with submassive necrosis resulting from the obstruction of hepatic blood flow by infiltrating leukemic cells [4]. In any child who presents with FHF, acute leukemia should be considered in the differential diagnosis, especially if there is hepatosplenomegaly, pancytopenia, and increased lactate dehydrogenase [5]. There is a report of obstructive jaundice as a rare presentation of ALL in an adult [6].

AML does not usually cause liver injury as a presenting feature; however, there have been reported cases of obstructive jaundice and cholestatic hepatitis secondary to sinusoidal infiltration, which improved with chemotherapy [7]. Acute megakaryoblastic leukemia is a rare type of AML that occurs in 3–5 % of AML cases and may present with thrombocytopenia, hepatic failure, and ascites secondary to massive infiltration of hepatic sinusoids by leukemia cells [8]. An important condition is veno-occlusive disease of the liver or sinusoidal obstruction syndrome. This is an established complication of high-dose chemotherapy before hematopoietic stem cell transplantation, which is often the treatment chosen for the aforementioned leukemias. Although it is not common, significant veno-occlusive disease may also occur with less intense induction therapy for ALL [9].

14.2.2 Chronic Lymphocytic Leukemia

Chronic lymphocytic leukemia (CLL) is one of the B-cell chronic lymphoproliferative disorders. According to the WHO classification, B-cell chronic lymphocytic leukemia is considered to be identical to the mature B-cell neoplasm small lymphocytic lymphoma. Patients with CLL often show mild to moderate liver enlargement at the time of initial diagnosis, in 15–25 % of cases [10]. In an autopsy series, 98 % of patients with CLL were found to have leukemic infiltration, which consisted predominantly of portal infiltrates that usually left the hepatic limiting plates intact [11]. However, in some cases, leukemic infiltration was observed to bridge adjacent portal tracts and to be associated with hepatocellular necrosis, bridging necrosis, and occasionally pseudolobule formation.

The development of portal hypertension is uncommon. However, there is a case report in the literature describing the feasibility of developing splenomegaly, portal hypertension, and bleeding esophageal varices in the absence of regenerative nodular hyperplasia or significant liver infiltration, favoring the role of increased splenic/portal blood flow [12]. This is a mechanism of portal hypertension similar to that described earlier in idiopathic portal hypertension.

CLL is generally indolent, and most patients are symptom-free for years. However, in 2–9 % of patients with CLL, Richter's transformation can occur, in which a highly aggressive non-Hodgkin lymphoma develops. This situation may be triggered by a viral infection such as Epstein-Barr virus (EBV) and/or be related to chromosomal abnormalities [13]. Most of these patients experience weight loss, fever, increasing lymphadenopathy, and hepatosplenomegaly; acute hepatic failure has been described as well. The prognosis is poor; the median survival after this condition occurs can be approximately 6 months [14]. The key to treating acute hepatic failure as a result of Richter's transformation is making the appropriate tissue diagnosis and initiating chemotherapy rapidly; success has been reported in treating patients in this manner.

14.2.3 Hodgkin Lymphoma

Hodgkin lymphoma (HL, formerly called Hodgkin's disease) is a group of cancers characterized by Reed-Sternberg cells in an appropriately reactive cellular background. HL has a bimodal age distribution with one peak in the 20s and 30s and a second peak over the age of 50 years. Presentation is variable, and liver involvement is possible [15]. Liver infiltration of malignant cells has been reported in 14 % of patients with HL, and hepatomegaly has been reported in 9 % of patients with stage I–II and in 45 % of patients with stage III–IV disease [16]. Acute hepatic failure can be caused by ischemia secondary to compression of the hepatic sinusoids by infiltrating lymphoma cells [17]. Cholestasis can be caused by direct infiltration of lymphoma cells, extrahepatic biliary obstruction, hemolysis, viral hepatitis, drug hepatotoxicity, or vanishing bile duct syndrome [18]. Cholestasis in zone 3 has been described as the result of vanishing bile duct syndrome associated with HL, a syndrome that causes irreversible destruction of the small intrahepatic bile ducts and leads to significant liver damage [18]. The mechanism by which this syndrome occurs is poorly understood but may be a paraneoplastic effect, a defect in liver microsomal function, or a toxic effect of cytokines produced from lymphoma cells [19]. Other causes of vanishing bile duct syndrome should be considered in the differential diagnosis before attributing it to HL [20]. Even with adequate treatment of lymphoma, most of these patients die of hepatic failure. These patients also often experience lymphoma progression because of the difficulty in administering potentially hepatotoxic agents to them [21].

14.2.4 Non-Hodgkin Lymphoma

Non-Hodgkin lymphoma (NHL) is a large and diffuse group of malignancies involving mutations of B and T cells that essentially include all lymphomas other than HL. Compared with HL, this type of lymphoma is more common, it spreads in a less contiguous fashion, and it usually affects patients over the age of 60 years. Treatment, survival, and presenting symptoms differ between NHL and HL.

The frequency of liver involvement in initial clinical staging is significantly higher in patients with NHL than in those with HL. When evaluated by percutaneous liver biopsy, 16–26 % of patients with NHL are found to have liver infiltration [22, 23]; higher percentages of patients are found to have hepatic involvement when evaluated at staging laparotomy (56 %) [24] or at autopsy (52 %) [25].

As described earlier with HL, acute hepatic failure can also occur in NHL. The mechanism by which this occurs is likely similar to that in HL, with sudden ischemia related to massive infiltration of the sinusoids or replacement of liver parenchyma by malignant cells [26]. Submassive necrosis has been described in patients with the cytotoxic phenotype of peripheral T-cell lymphoma and is often fatal [27]. Although the prognosis is poor, there have been reports of successful treatment with immediate initiation of chemotherapy [26].

Primary NHL of the liver is a rare condition, accounting for less than 1 % of all extranodal lymphomas. Two thirds of cases occur in men aged approximately 50 years. Although the cause is unclear, some hypothesize the involvement of viral hepatitis or EBV. Patients typically present with right upper quadrant or epigastric pain, fever, anorexia, nausea, hepatomegaly, and abnormal liver tests with a greater increase in lactate dehydrogenase than alanine aminotransferase [28, 29]. The most common type of primary hepatic NHL is diffuse large B-cell lymphoma, comprising 80–90 % of cases. This disease may present with nodules in the liver or diffuse portal infiltration and sinusoidal spread [30]. Rapid identification of this lymphoma is critical so that appropriate chemotherapy can be initiated in a timely manner. Because this condition is uniformly fatal, patients with FHF from primary hepatic lymphoma have been treated with liver transplantation and subsequent chemotherapy [31]. The long-term success of this approach has not been substantiated and is probably poor.

14.2.5 Multiple Myeloma and Amyloidosis

Multiple myeloma (MM) is a malignancy of clonal plasma cells that predominantly affects bone marrow and the bones. Hepatomegaly and abnormalities of liver biochemical tests are commonly observed in patients with MM [32]. In up to one half of patients who undergo a hepatic histological evaluation, either diffuse sinusoidal or portal infiltration or, less commonly, nodule formation by malignant plasma cells has been observed [25]. The frequency of jaundice has ranged from 0 to 30 % in series of patients with hepatic infiltration by MM [33]. Ascites has been reported to complicate the course of disease in 10–35 % of patients with massive hepatic infiltration [32, 34]; esophageal varices occur more rarely. Portal hypertension secondary to tumor infiltration appears to be a cause of ascites in most affected patients; other potential causes include congestive heart failure, dissemination of myeloma cells into the peritoneal cavity, and tuberculous peritonitis. Extramedullary hematopoiesis may also contribute to hepatomegaly or liver test abnormalities in these patients [32]. The clinical significance of liver involvement in MM is uncertain. Treatment of MM with hepatic involvement requires systemic treatment. A number of reports have described successful treatment with combination chemotherapy or steroids alone [35, 36]. Amyloidosis, another plasma cell dyscrasia manifested as tissue deposition of clonal light-chain fibrils, can be seen as a concomitant finding in approximately 15 % of patients with MM. Liver involvement has been reported in patients with MM as well as in primary systemic amyloidosis [37].

14.2.6 Myeloproliferative Neoplasms

Chronic myeloproliferative neoplasms (MPN) include chronic myeloid leukemia (CML), polycythemia vera (PV), essential thrombocythemia (ET), and primary myelofibrosis (PMF).

CML is a specific type of MPN characterized by dysregulated production and uncontrolled proliferation of mature and immature granulocytes with normal morphology. The tumor cells are derived from a pluripotent hematopoietic stem cell having acquired the *BCR-ABL1* fusion gene, usually through translocation between chromosomes 9 and 22, t(9;22)(q34;q11), referred to as the Philadelphia (Ph) chromosome. In the chronic phase, approximately 50 % of patients with CML show mild to moderate hepatomegaly at presentation, with no liver function abnormalities [38]. At the time of blast crisis, however, liver sinusoidal infiltration by immature cells may lead to liver enlargement and elevated serum alkaline phosphatase activity [39].

PV, ET, and PMF are classified as Ph-negative MPN and are characterized by an overproduction of certain cell types: PV is caused by overproduction of red blood cells; ET is caused by overproduction of platelets; and PMF is caused by red blood cells and granulocytes that do not mature properly. The hepatic manifestations in this group of hematologic disorders are similar.

The hepatic circulatory system is most affected by MPN, causing Budd-Chiari syndrome (BCS), portal vein thrombosis, and/or nodular regenerative hyperplasia [40]. Patients may present with acute or chronic BCS as a result of the prothrombotic and hyperviscous state seen in PV [41]. When BSC occurs, the liver becomes acutely hypoxic, causing injury and necrosis. It is possible that the surge in erythropoietin (Epo) levels that occurs in this setting is related to spillage from necrotic liver tissue, because small amounts of Epo are produced in the adult liver. This situation may confuse the diagnosis of PV in a patient with BCS, which is usually associated with a low Epo level, but other diagnostic tools, such as the analysis of the V617F point mutation of the Janus 2 tyrosine kinase (JAK2), have helped to make the diagnosis easier [41]. Testing for JAK2 secures a diagnosis of occult MPN in patients who were previously believed to have BCS of unclear cause. After PV, ET is also commonly associated with BCS [40, 42].

Portal vein thrombosis may also occur in MPN, more commonly in PV and ET [43]. After the thrombosis occurs, collaterals often develop, resulting in cavernous transformation of the portal vein. Patients usually present with variceal hemorrhage but may be seen with abdominal pain related to mesenteric ischemia [40]. Many of these patients can also have the JAK2 mutation. Screening for this mutation in patients with portal vein thrombosis may provide useful information to recognize patients with occult MPN or those at risk of developing MPN [43].

14.3 Nonmalignant Hematologic Diseases

14.3.1 Aplastic Anemia

Aplastic anemia is characterized by diminished or absent hematopoietic precursors in the bone marrow, most often due to injury to the pluripotent stem cells. The most typical form of aplastic anemia is an immune-mediated bone marrow aplasia. In addition, the major causes of acquired aplastic anemia are exposure to a wide variety of drugs and chemicals, ionizing radiation, and some viruses including hepatitis viruses [44]. The mechanism may involve T-cell activation with release of cytokines [45] or activation of a cytotoxic T-cell clone which recognizes similar target antigens on both liver and bone marrow cells [46]. Hepatitis-associated aplastic anemia most often affects boys and young men, with aplasia developing 2–3 months after an episode of acute hepatitis [47]. The responsible virus has not been identified; neither hepatitis A, B, C, nor G appears to be involved [44].

14.3.2 Paroxysmal Nocturnal Hemoglobinuria

Paroxysmal nocturnal hemoglobinuria (PNH) is caused by an acquired defect of glycosylphosphatidylinositol-anchored protein in the erythrocyte membrane that results in complement-mediated hemolysis. The disease usually occurs in middle-aged adults and affects men and women equally. Patients usually present with complaints of red or dark brown urine, often seen in the mornings. Mild hepatosplenomegaly and jaundice can occur, as it does in other hemolytic anemias [48, 49]. One of the more serious complications of PNH is the development of a hypercoagulable state and the formation of thrombosis as a result of thrombogenic material released into the bloodstream after hemolysis [48]. Thromboses in PNH typically occur in the intracranial, hepatic, or portal vessels and thus may have devastating effects. PNH is one of the more common types of de novo presentation of portal vein thrombosis and a rare cause of BCS [48]. The diagnosis is suggested by the sucrose lysis test and confirmed with the acid Ham test [48]. To identify the absence of CD55 and CD59 in erythrocytes and/or granulocytes is important. Recently, eculizumab became available for the inhibition of terminal complement and is the treatment of choice for severe manifestations of PNH. Supportive care, treatment of the underlying process, and prevention of thrombotic events with anticoagulants are the mainstays of management.

14.3.3 Thrombotic Thrombocytopenic Purpura-Hemolytic Uremic Syndromes

Thrombotic thrombocytopenic purpura (TTP) and hemolytic uremic syndrome (HUS) result from platelet aggregation in the microvasculature, either systemically or in the renal circulation, respectively. In pregnancy, it can be difficult to distinguish preeclampsia and HELLP from TTP and HUS, because all of those conditions can be associated with microangiopathic hemolytic anemia. It is important to make the appropriate diagnosis in pregnancy because there have been reports of TTP-HUS being associated with BCS [50]. Although this hemolytic disorder is associated with thrombosis in the microvasculature, there may be a common pathway by which thrombosis of the hepatic vein can occur, resulting in worsening jaundice, hepatosplenomegaly, and liver dysfunction. Diagnosis is made by imaging the hepatic vasculature, and treatment may include plasma exchange therapy for TTP and anticoagulation for BCS [50].

14.4 Liver Diseases Associated with Treatment for Hematologic Diseases

14.4.1 Transfusional Iron Overload

Red blood cell transfusions are increasingly used in the management of various anemias. Iron overload is inevitable in both children and adults who require lifelong transfusion support [51]. Each unit of transfused red cells introduces 200–250 mg of elemental iron into the body. Since iron cannot be actively excreted and is utilized poorly in patients with ineffective erythropoiesis, the excess iron is deposited in macrophages of the reticuloendothelial system. When this iron burden overwhelms the ability of reticuloendothelial cells to sequester the iron, parenchymal iron overload develops, leading to end-organ dysfunction, especially in the liver, myocardium, pancreas, and endocrine organs. If patients with transfusional iron overload achieve remission and no longer require transfusion, phlebotomy treatment is the safest and most efficient method to remove the excessive iron burden [52]. For subjects still requiring transfusion, iron chelation is the only available treatment. This treatment has been shown to significantly reduce tissue iron overload and prolong overall survival in such patients [53].

14.4.2 Hepatitis B Virus Reactivation

Hepatitis B virus (HBV) reactivation is a potentially fatal but preventable complication of chemotherapy or immunosuppressive therapy for hematologic diseases. It can develop not only in patients seropositive for hepatitis B surface antigen (HBsAg) but also in those with resolved HBV infection who are seronegative for HBsAg but seropositive for antibodies against hepatitis B core antigen (anti-HBc) and/or antibodies against HBsAg (anti-HBs) [54]. The risk of HBV reactivation depends on the balance between replication of the virus and the immune response of the host. The risk of HBV reactivation with each of the drug classes administrated to HBsAg-positive or HBsAg-negative/anti-HBc positive patients has been estimated by the American Gastroenterological Association (AGA) based on a thorough systematic review of the existing literature (Table 14.2) [55]. All patients should be screened to identify if they belong to any of the risk groups for HBV reactivation before initiating chemotherapy or immunosuppressive therapy for hematologic diseases. Screening is accomplished by measuring serum HBV markers including HBsAg, anti-HBc, and anti-HBs. To prevent the development of hepatitis due to HBV reactivation, antiviral prophylaxis is recommended for HBsAg-positive patients and/or patients in whom HBV DNA is detectable at the baseline. In patients with resolved HBV infection, regular monitoring of HBV DNA-guided preemptive antiviral therapy is a reasonable and useful approach [56].

Table 14.2 Immunosuppressive drug classes and corresponding risk estimates of hepatitis B virus reactivation (HBVr)

Drug class	Drug	Risk estimate of HBVr for HBsAg-positive patients	Risk estimate of HBVr for HBsAg-negative/anti-HBc-positive patients
B-cell depleting agents	Rituximab	High (30 %–60 %)	High (>10 %)
	Ofatumumab		
Anthracycline derivatives	Doxorubicin	High (15 %–30 %)	High (>10 %)
	Epirubicin		
Tyrosine kinase inhibitors	Imatinib	Moderate (1 %–10 %)	Moderate (1 %)
	Nilotinib		
Corticosteroids	High dose	High (>10 %)	NA
	Moderate dose	Moderate (1 %–10 %)	Moderate (1 %–10 %)
	Low dose	Low (<1 %)	Low (<<1 %)
Traditional immunosuppression	Methotrexate	Low (<1 %)	Low (<<1 %)

HBVr hepatitis B virus reactivation, *HBsAg* hepatitis B surface antigen, *NA* not available, *anti-HBc* antibody to hepatitis B core antigen; corticosteroids, prednisone: high dose, >20 mg; moderate dose, 10–20 mg; low dose, <10 mg

14.4.3 Hepatic Complications of Hematopoietic Cell Transplantation

Human hematopoietic cell transplantation (HCT) is now standard procedure for many patients with hematologic malignancy and genetic disorders. The liver may be damaged by drugs used during the transplant process, particularly drugs in high-dose myeloablative regimens that prepare patients for infusion of stem cells. After infusion of stem cells, patients remain profoundly immunosuppressed until engraftment; full recovery of immune function is often delayed for a year or longer, exposing patients to infection with viruses, fungi, and bacteria. Recipients of allogeneic stem cells are also at risk for graft versus host disease (GVHD) involving the liver. Thus, a patient undergoing transplantation is at risk for drug-liver toxicity, infections, and immunologic liver injury (Table 14.3). Development of jaundice following HCT is an ominous prognostic sign, with increased non-relapse mortality in patients whose total serum bilirubin exceeds 4 mg/dL [57]. Because treatment of

Table 14.3 Hepatic complications after hematopoietic cell transplantation

Disease	Frequency	Timing
Sinusoidal obstructive syndrome (SOS)	10–35 % (regimen dependent)	Before day 20
Cholestasis of sepsis	Common in neutropenic patients	Before day 30
Acute GVHD of the liver	10–20 % of allograft recipients	Day 15–50
Acute viral hepatitis	Uncommon when prophylaxis is used against HSV or HBV	HSV, day 20–50
		ADV, day 30–80
		VZV, day 80–250
		HBV and HCV, during immune reconstitution
Fungal abscess	Rare when prophylaxis is used	Day 10–60
Drug liver injury	Common	Day 0–100
Ischemic liver disease	Confined to patients with septic or hemorrhagic shock	Day 0–30
Biliary obstruction	Transient biliary sludge, common	Day 15–60
	Stones or chloromas, rare	
Idiopathic hyperammonemia	Rare	Day 10–50
Chronic hepatitis C	Formerly common	After day 80
Iron overload	Very common	Pre-transplant
		Long-term follow-up after transplantation
Chronic GHVD	Common after allografts	After day 80
Nodular regenerative hyperplasia	Rare complication of toxic liver injury	Years after transplantation

GVHD graft-vs-host disease, *HSV* herpes simplex virus, *ADV* adenovirus, *VZV* varicella zoster virus, *HBV* hepatitis B virus, *HCV* hepatitis C virus

severe liver dysfunction is often futile, it is important to recognize risk factors for hepatobiliary problems before the transplant process starts, implement measures to prevent liver damage, and identify posttransplant disorders that have specific treatments. Over the last decade, this approach has resulted in a marked reduction in the incidence of liver infections and clinical jaundice, due to prevention of hepatic sinusoidal injury, fungal, and viral prophylaxis and the introduction of prophylactic ursodiol for all patients undergoing transplantation [58].

14.5 Conclusion

Hepatologists or general physicians sometimes encounter hepatic manifestations of various hematologic diseases in daily practice, including various abnormalities in liver function tests or imaging studies of the liver. In hematologic malignancies, malignant cells often infiltrate the liver and demonstrate hepatosplenomegaly. It is important to differentiate liver problems occurring as a result of hematologic diseases from liver dysfunction as the primary etiology. Treatment for hematologic diseases often causes several types of liver problems. Hematologists should consult with hepatologists when their patients with hematologic diseases experience liver complications.

References

1. Thiele D. Hepatic manifestations of systemic diseases and other disorders of the liver. In: Feldman M, Friedman LS, Sleisenger MH, editors. Sleisenger & Fordtran's gastrointestinal and liver disease: pathophysiology, diagnosis, management. 7th ed. Philadelphia: Saunders; 2002. p. 1603–19.
2. Singh MM, Pockros PJ. Hematologic and oncologic diseases and the liver. Clin Liver Dis. 2011;15(1):69–87. doi:10.1016/j.cld.2010.09.013.
3. Shimizu Y. Liver in systemic disease. World J Gastroenterol. 2008;14(26):4111–9.
4. Litten JB, Rodriguez MM, Maniaci V. Acute lymphoblastic leukemia presenting in fulminant hepatic failure. Pediatr Blood Cancer. 2006;47(6):842–5. doi:10.1002/pbc.20544.
5. Kader A, Vara R, Egberongbe Y, Height S, Dhawan A. Leukaemia presenting with fulminant hepatic failure in a child. Eur J Pediatr. 2004;163(10):628–9. doi:10.1007/s00431-004-1510-1.
6. Daniel SV, Vani DH, Smith AM, Hill QA, Menon KV. Obstructive jaundice due to a pancreatic mass: a rare presentation of acute lymphoblastic leukaemia in an adult. JOP. 2010;11(1):72–4.
7. Wandroo FA, Murray J, Mutimer D, Hubscher S. Acute myeloid leukaemia presenting as cholestatic hepatitis. J Clin Pathol. 2004;57(5):544–5.
8. Lewis MS, Kaicker S, Strauchen JA, Morotti RA. Hepatic involvement in congenital acute megakaryoblastic leukemia: a case report with emphasis on the liver pathology findings. Pediatr Dev Pathol. 2008;11(1):55–8. doi:10.2350/07-03-0243.1.
9. Papadopoulos A, Ntaios G, Kaiafa G, Girtovitis F, Saouli Z, Kontoninas Z, et al. Veno-occlusive disease of the liver during induction therapy for acute lymphoblastic leukemia. Int J Hematol. 2008;88(4):441–2. doi:10.1007/s12185-008-0172-6.

10. Binet JL, Auquier A, Dighiero G, Chastang C, Piguet H, Goasguen J, et al. A new prognostic classification of chronic lymphocytic leukemia derived from a multivariate survival analysis. Cancer. 1981;48(1):198–206.
11. Schwartz JB, Shamsuddin AM. The effects of leukemic infiltrates in various organs in chronic lymphocytic leukemia. Hum Pathol. 1981;12(5):432–40.
12. Wilputte JY, Martinet JP, Nguyen P, Damoiseaux P, Rahier J, Geubel A. Chronic lymphocytic leukemia with portal hypertension and without liver involvement: a case report underlining the roles of increased spleno-portal blood flow and "protective" sinusoidal vasoconstriction. Acta Gastroenterol Belg. 2003;66(4):303–6.
13. Parikh SA, Rabe KG, Call TG, Zent CS, Habermann TM, Ding W, et al. Diffuse large B-cell lymphoma (Richter syndrome) in patients with chronic lymphocytic leukaemia (CLL): a cohort study of newly diagnosed patients. Br J Haematol. 2013;162(6):774–82. doi:10.1111/bjh.12458.
14. Shehab TM, Kaminski MS, Lok AS. Acute liver failure due to hepatic involvement by hematologic malignancy. Dig Dis Sci. 1997;42(7):1400–5.
15. Punnett A, Tsang RW, Hodgson DC. Hodgkin lymphoma across the age spectrum: epidemiology, therapy, and late effects. Semin Radiat Oncol. 2010;20(1):30–44. doi:10.1016/j.semradonc.2009.09.006.
16. Brinckmeyer LM, Skovsgaard T, Thiede T, Vesterager L, Nissen NI. The liver in Hodgkin's disease – I. Clinico-pathological relations. Eur J Cancer Clin Oncol. 1982;18(5):421–8.
17. Rowbotham D, Wendon J, Williams R. Acute liver failure secondary to hepatic infiltration: a single centre experience of 18 cases. Gut. 1998;42(4):576–80.
18. Nader K, Mok S, Kalra A, Harb A, Schwarting R, Ferber A. Vanishing bile duct syndrome as a manifestation of Hodgkin's lymphoma: a case report and review of the literature. Tumori. 2013;99(4):e164–8. doi:10.1700/1361.15117.
19. Hubscher SG, Lumley MA, Elias E. Vanishing bile duct syndrome: a possible mechanism for intrahepatic cholestasis in Hodgkin's lymphoma. Hepatology. 1993;17(1):70–7.
20. Guliter S, Erdem O, Isik M, Yamac K, Uluoglu O. Cholestatic liver disease with ductopenia (vanishing bile duct syndrome) in Hodgkin's disease: report of a case. Tumori. 2004;90(5):517–20.
21. Leeuwenburgh I, Lugtenburg EP, van Buuren HR, Zondervan PE, de Man RA. Severe jaundice, due to vanishing bile duct syndrome, as presenting symptom of Hodgkin's lymphoma, fully reversible after chemotherapy. Eur J Gastroenterol Hepatol. 2008;20(2):145–7. doi:10.1097/MEG.0b013e3282b9e6c2.
22. Roth A, Kolaric K, Dominis M. Histologic and cytologic liver changes in 120 patients with malignant lymphomas. Tumori. 1978;64(1):45–53.
23. Kolaric K, Roth A, Dominis M, Jakasa V. The diagnostic value of percutaneus liver biopsy in patients with non Hodgkin's lymphoma – a preliminary report. Acta Hepatogastroenterol (Stuttg). 1977;24(6):440–3.
24. Bagley Jr CM, Thomas LB, Johnson RE, Chretien PB, DeVita Jr VT. Diagnosis of liver involvement by lymphoma: results in 96 consecutive peritoneoscopies. Cancer. 1973;31(4):840–7.
25. Scheimberg IB, Pollock DJ, Collins PW, Doran HM, Newland AC, van der Walt JD. Pathology of the liver in leukaemia and lymphoma. A study of 110 autopsies. Histopathology. 1995;26(4):311–21.
26. Salo J, Nomdedeu B, Bruguera M, Ordi J, Gines P, Castells A, et al. Acute liver failure due to non-Hodgkin's lymphoma. Am J Gastroenterol. 1993;88(5):774–6.
27. Ohtani H, Komeno T, Koizumi M, Kimura N, Tanaka S, Nunokawa T, et al. Submassive hepatocellular necrosis associated with infiltration by peripheral T-cell lymphoma of cytotoxic phenotype: report of two cases. Pathol Int. 2008;58(2):133–7. doi:10.1111/j.1440-1827.2007.02201.x.
28. Masood A, Kairouz S, Hudhud KH, Hegazi AZ, Banu A, Gupta NC. Primary non-Hodgkin lymphoma of liver. Curr Oncol. 2009;16(4):74–7.

29. Haider FS, Smith R, Khan S. Primary hepatic lymphoma presenting as fulminant hepatic failure with hyperferritinemia: a case report. J Med Case Rep. 2008;2:279. doi:10.1186/1752-1947-2-279.
30. Baumhoer D, Tzankov A, Dirnhofer S, Tornillo L, Terracciano LM. Patterns of liver infiltration in lymphoproliferative disease. Histopathology. 2008;53(1):81–90. doi:10.1111/j.1365-2559.2008.03069.x.
31. Cameron AM, Truty J, Truell J, Lassman C, Zimmerman MA, Kelly Jr BS, et al. Fulminant hepatic failure from primary hepatic lymphoma: successful treatment with orthotopic liver transplantation and chemotherapy. Transplantation. 2005;80(7):993–6.
32. Thomas FB, Clausen KP, Greenberger NJ. Liver disease in multiple myeloma. Arch Intern Med. 1973;132(2):195–202.
33. Perez-Soler R, Esteban R, Allende E, Tornos Salomo C, Julia A, Guardia J. Liver involvement in multiple myeloma. Am J Hematol. 1985;20(1):25–9.
34. Verdi CJ, Grogan TM, Protell R, Richter L, Rangel C. Liver biopsy immunotyping to characterize lymphoid malignancies. Hepatology. 1986;6(1):6–13.
35. Pastor E, Perella M, Gomez A, Grau E, Perez A, Escandon J. Multiple myeloma of the liver presenting as nonobstructive jaundice. Am J Hematol. 1996;53(3):205–6. doi:10.1002/(SICI)1096-8652(199611)53:3<205::AID-AJH14>3.0.CO;2-C.
36. Solves P, de la Rubia J, Jarque I, Cervera J, Sanz GF, Vera-Sempere FJ, et al. Liver disease as primary manifestation of multiple myeloma in a young man. Leuk Res. 1999;23(4):403–5.
37. Yamamoto T, Maeda N, Kawasaki H. Hepatic failure in a case of multiple myeloma-associated amyloidosis (kappa-AL). J Gastroenterol. 1995;30(3):393–7.
38. Cervantes F, Rozman C. A multivariate analysis of prognostic factors in chronic myeloid leukemia. Blood. 1982;60(6):1298–304.
39. Ondreyco SM, Kjeldsberg CR, Fineman RM, Vaninetti S, Kushner JP. Monoblastic transformation in chronic myelogenous leukemia: presentation with massive hepatic involvement. Cancer. 1981;48(4):957–63.
40. Poreddy V, DeLeve LD. Hepatic circulatory diseases associated with chronic myeloid disorders. Clin Liver Dis. 2002;6(4):909–31.
41. Thurmes PJ, Steensma DP. Elevated serum erythropoietin levels in patients with Budd-Chiari syndrome secondary to polycythemia vera: clinical implications for the role of JAK2 mutation analysis. Eur J Haematol. 2006;77(1):57–60. doi:10.1111/j.1600-0609.2006.00667.x.
42. Briere JB. Essential thrombocythemia. Orphanet J Rare Dis. 2007;2:3. doi:10.1186/1750-1172-2-3.
43. Colaizzo D, Amitrano L, Tiscia GL, Scenna G, Grandone E, Guardascione MA, et al. The JAK2 V617F mutation frequently occurs in patients with portal and mesenteric venous thrombosis. J Thromb Haemost. 2007;5(1):55–61. doi:10.1111/j.1538-7836.2006.02277.x.
44. Brown KE, Tisdale J, Barrett AJ, Dunbar CE, Young NS. Hepatitis-associated aplastic anemia. N Engl J Med. 1997;336(15):1059–64. doi:10.1056/NEJM199704103361504.
45. Lu J, Basu A, Melenhorst JJ, Young NS, Brown KE. Analysis of T-cell repertoire in hepatitis-associated aplastic anemia. Blood. 2004;103(12):4588–93. doi:10.1182/blood-2003-11-3959.
46. Ikawa Y, Nishimura R, Kuroda R, Mase S, Araki R, Maeba H, et al. Expansion of a liver-infiltrating cytotoxic T-lymphocyte clone in concert with the development of hepatitis-associated aplastic anaemia. Br J Haematol. 2013;161(4):599–602. doi:10.1111/bjh.12259.
47. Locasciulli A, Bacigalupo A, Bruno B, Montante B, Marsh J, Tichelli A, et al. Hepatitis-associated aplastic anaemia: epidemiology and treatment results obtained in Europe. A report of The EBMT aplastic anaemia working party. Br J Haematol. 2010;149(6):890–5. doi:10.1111/j.1365-2141.2010.08194.x.
48. Shah A. Acquired hemolytic anemia. Indian J Med Sci. 2004;58(12):533–6.
49. Seve P, Philippe P, Dufour JF, Broussolle C, Michel M. Autoimmune hemolytic anemia: classification and therapeutic approaches. Expert Rev Hematol. 2008;1(2):189–204. doi:10.1586/17474086.1.2.189.

50. Hsu HW, Belfort MA, Vernino S, Moake JL, Moise Jr KJ. Postpartum thrombotic thrombocytopenic purpura complicated by Budd-Chiari syndrome. Obstet Gynecol. 1995;85(5 Pt 2):839–43.
51. Marsella M, Borgna-Pignatti C. Transfusional iron overload and iron chelation therapy in thalassemia major and sickle cell disease. Hematol Oncol Clin North Am. 2014;28(4):703–27, vi. doi:10.1016/j.hoc.2014.04.004.
52. Franchini M, Gandini G, Veneri D, de Matteis G, Federici F, Solero P, et al. Efficacy and safety of phlebotomy to reduce transfusional iron overload in adult, long-term survivors of acute leukemia. Transfusion. 2004;44(6):833–7. doi:10.1111/j.1537-2995.2004.03264.x.
53. Modell B, Khan M, Darlison M. Survival in beta-thalassaemia major in the UK: data from the UK Thalassaemia Register. Lancet. 2000;355(9220):2051–2. doi:10.1016/S0140-6736(00)02357-6.
54. Pattullo V. Hepatitis B, reactivation in the setting of chemotherapy and immunosuppression – prevention is better than cure. World J Hepatol. 2015;7(7):954–67. doi:10.4254/wjh.v7.i7.954.
55. Perrillo RP, Gish R, Falck-Ytter YT. American Gastroenterological Association Institute technical review on prevention and treatment of hepatitis B virus reactivation during immunosuppressive drug therapy. Gastroenterology. 2015;148(1):221–44 e3. doi:10.1053/j.gastro.2014.10.038.
56. Reddy KR, Beavers KL, Hammond SP, Lim JK, Falck-Ytter YT, American Gastroenterological Association I. American Gastroenterological Association Institute guideline on the prevention and treatment of hepatitis B virus reactivation during immunosuppressive drug therapy. Gastroenterology. 2015;148(1):215–9; quiz e16-7. doi:10.1053/j.gastro.2014.10.039.
57. Gooley TA, Rajvanshi P, Schoch HG, McDonald GB. Serum bilirubin levels and mortality after myeloablative allogeneic hematopoietic cell transplantation. Hepatology. 2005;41(2):345–52. doi:10.1002/hep.20529.
58. McDonald GB. Review article: management of hepatic disease following haematopoietic cell transplant. Aliment Pharmacol Ther. 2006;24(3):441–52. doi:10.1111/j.1365-2036.2006.03001.x.

Chapter 15
IgG4-Related Diseases and the Liver

Kenichi Harada

Abstract IgG4-related disease (IgG4-RD) is a systemic illness including autoimmune pancreatitis and IgG4-related sclerosing cholangitis (IgG4-SC). Although hepatic presentation of IgG4-RD has been reported, whether intrahepatic small bile ducts and hepatocytes are direct targets of IgG4-RD is uncertain. IgG4-RD is pathologically characterized by the numerous IgG4^{+} cells found in affected organs, but this IgG4 positivity is also frequently found in extrahepatic cholangiocarcinoma and is prominent, albeit rarely, in other hepatobiliary diseases including primary sclerosing cholangitis and autoimmune hepatitis. Moreover, cholangiocarcinoma arising from precedent IgG4-SC and IgG4-SC accompanying precursor lesions of cholangiocarcinoma (biliary intraepithelial neoplasia) are also reported. Diagnostic criteria for IgG-RD and IgG4-SC were recently proposed, but each individual case should be diagnosed clinicopathologically on the basis of its individual features.

Keywords Cholangiocarcinoma • IgG4-sclerosing cholangitis • IgG4 hepatopathy • IgG4-associated autoimmune hepatitis • Primary biliary cholangitis

15.1 Introduction

IgG4-related disease (IgG4-RD) and its systemic nature were first described in Japan [1–5]. IgG4-RD most profoundly affects the pancreas but involves most organs in the human body, including the pituitary gland, lacrimal glands, salivary glands, lungs, breast, bile duct, aorta, kidney, lymph nodes, retroperitoneum, and prostate. Initial or secondary presentation in the liver, skin, peripheral nerves, and gastrointestinal tract has also been reported. Infiltrates of numerous IgG4^{+} plasma cells in affected organs are important pathological findings of IgG4-RD. Obliterative phlebitis, storiform-type sclerosing fibrosis, and sometimes mass-forming-type sclerosing fibrosis in the lung, pancreas, and liver are also characteristics of this disease. Regardless of the organ in which IgG4-RD develops, elevated serum IgG4

K. Harada (✉)
Department of Human Pathology, Kanazawa University Graduate School of Medical Sciences, Kanazawa 920-8640, Japan
e-mail: kenichih@med.kanazawa-u.ac.jp

H. Ohira (ed.), *The Liver in Systemic Diseases*, DOI 10.1007/978-4-431-55790-6_15

($\geq$135 mg/dL) and marked efficacy of steroid therapy are common characteristics. The prototype IgG4-RD disease is type I autoimmune pancreatitis (AIP). IgG4-related sclerosing cholangitis (IgG4-SC) involves sclerosing cholangitic lesions that arise as complications of AIP or, rarely, are isolated in the biliary tract system. IgG4-SC lesions share the characteristic features of AIP. Hepatic presentation of IgG4-RD has also been described in the literature [6–8]; whether such disease is a primary liver manifestation or simply the extension of IgG4-SC into intrahepatic bile ducts is unclear. In this chapter, we summarize the present knowledge of IgG4-SC and several inflammatory and neoplastic hepatobiliary diseases accompanied by $IgG4^+$ cells.

15.2 IgG4-SC

IgG4 is a minor immunoglobulin subtype composing 3–6 % of the total IgG circulating in adults [1]. Systemic IgG4-RD features elevated serum IgG4 levels and abundant infiltration with $IgG4^+$ plasma cells in affected organs [1, 9, 10]. IgG4-SC can be viewed as a manifestation of IgG4-RD in the bile duct. In the differential diagnosis of IgG4-SC, primary sclerosing cholangitis (PSC, another prototype of sclerosing cholangitis) and cholangiocarcinoma are also clinicopathologically important. Each of these diseases requires an appropriate diagnosis and therapy, but their differentiation is not always easy.

IgG4-SC exhibits severe inflammatory cell infiltrates containing abundant IgG4-bearing plasma cells and biliary sclerosis as a result of progressive fibrosis within the bile duct wall that leads to bile duct stenosis (Fig. 15.1). These diffuse or localized sclerotic and stenotic lesions are found in the large bile ducts of the hepatic hilus, extrahepatic bile ducts, and, in some cases, the gallbladder. These biliary lesions show circumferential wall thickening and are prominent at stenotic sites. Similar inflammatory lesions are also common at non-stenotic biliary sites. IgG4-SC cases not involving other organs are rare; most cases are associated with AIP, particularly those with lesions in the intrapancreatic bile ducts. As with IgG4-RD in other organs, serum IgG4 values of IgG4-SC patients are usually elevated to $\geq$135 mg/dL, and the lesions are reversible and responsive to steroid therapy.

Similar to the pancreatic ducts, the extrahepatic bile duct and gallbladder are covered by a single layer of epithelium and have peribiliary glands [11]. Histologically, bile duct lesions in IgG4-SC resemble the inflammatory and sclerosing lesions found in the pancreatic duct of AIP. Characteristics of IgG4-SC lesions are as follows: (1) inflammation, mainly affecting the bile duct wall (chronic cholangitis) but also particularly prominent around peribiliary glands; the biliary epithelium is relatively preserved; (2) marked lymphoplasmacytic cell infiltration, fibrosis, and luminal stenosis in affected regions of the bile ducts; (3) storiform fibrosis, a characteristic of AIP, is observed in IgG4-SC cases with marked fibrosis; (4) numerous IgG4-bearing plasma cells, as revealed by immunohistochemical staining; and (5) obliterative phlebitis and perineural infiltration of $IgG4^+$ cells

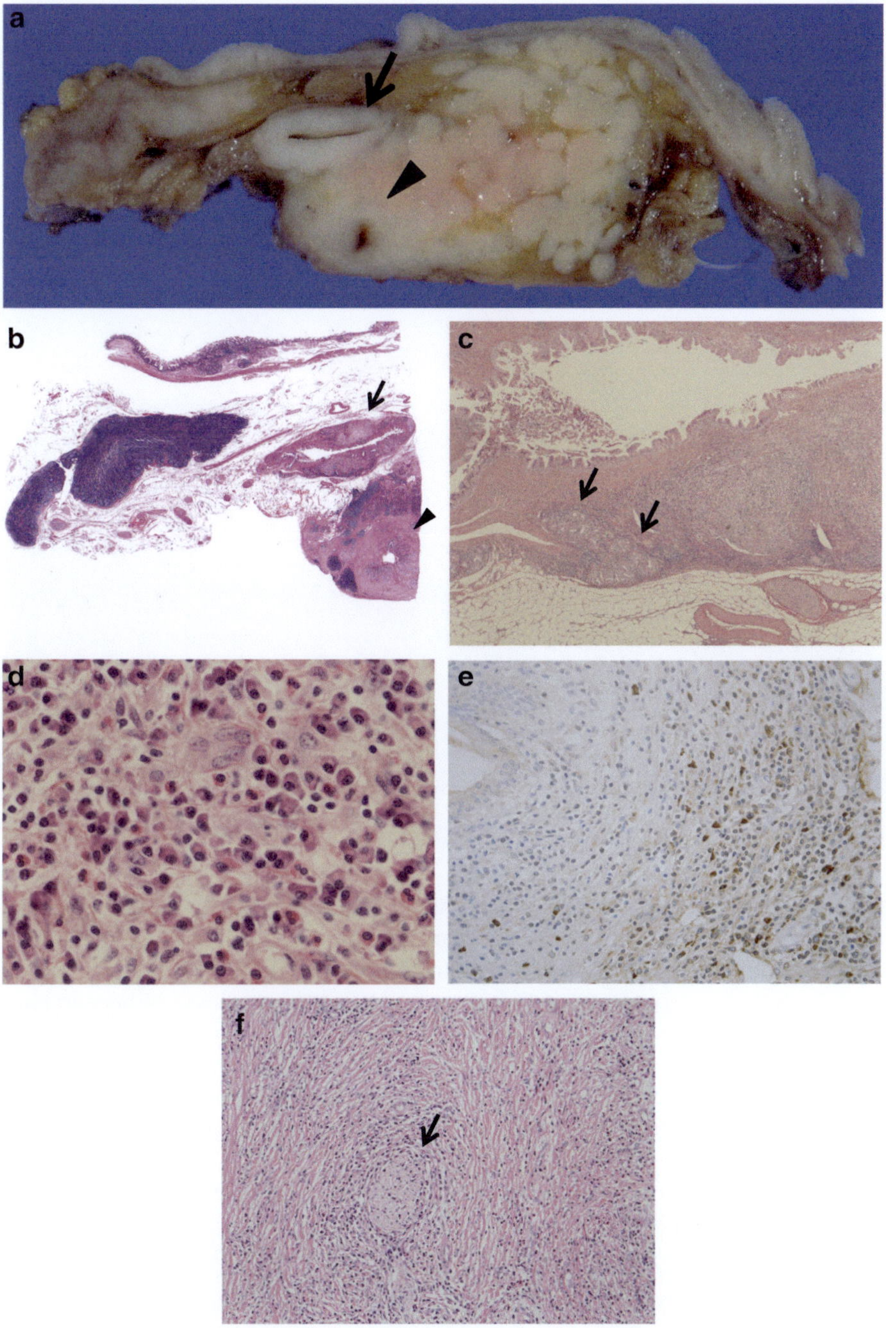

Fig. 15.1 Representative IgG4-related sclerosing cholangitis (IgG4-SC) associated with autoimmune pancreatitis (AIP). (**a**, **b**) Macroscopic and semi-macroscopic findings, respectively. *Arrows* and *arrowheads* denote the stenotic bile duct and pancreatic duct with wall thickening, respectively. (**c**) Inflammation and edema are found in the fibrous-thickened wall and are particularly prominent around the peribiliary gland (*arrows*). The mucosa is relatively preserved, with scant

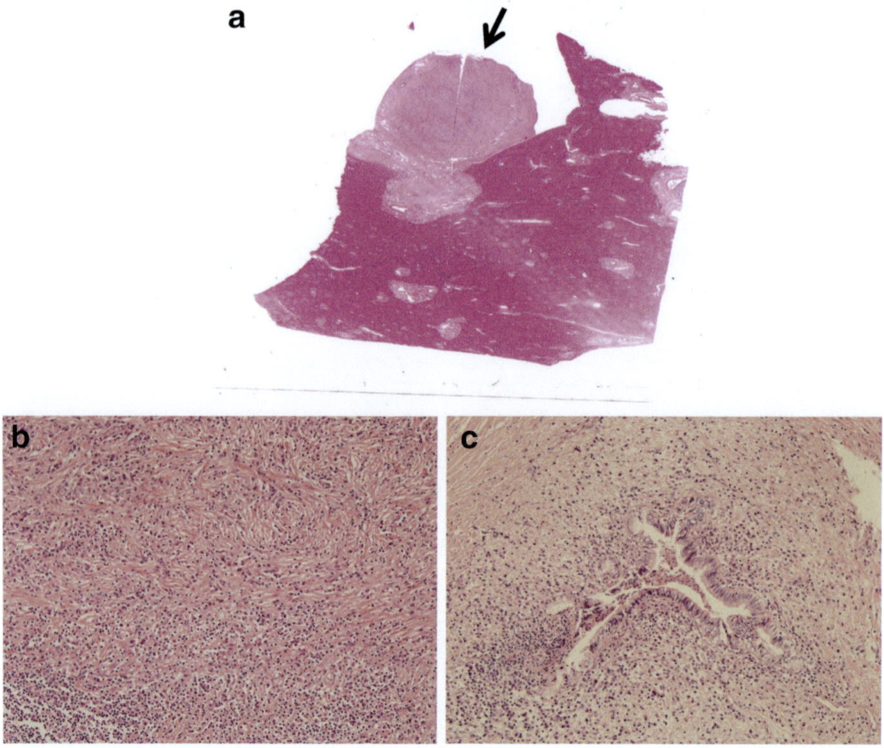

Fig. 15.2 Inflammatory pseudotumor with many IgG4⁺ liver cells. (**a**) Semi-macroscopic findings. Fibrous nodule (*arrow*) is seen. (**b**) Nodule consists of typical storiform fibrosis and inflammation. (**c**) Chronic cholangitis in adjacent portal tract

(Fig. 15.1). As seen in mass-forming pancreatitis, exacerbated inflammation from the hilum to the intrahepatic large bile duct can lead to inflammatory pseudotumors in the liver and hepatic hilus. Before the first report of IgG4-related AIP by Hamano et al. in 2001 [1], Nonomura et al. had reported in 1997 on a case of hepatic hilar inflammatory pseudotumor with cholangitis and phlebitis mimicking cholangiocarcinoma [12]. We later confirmed that the lesions in this case were IgG4-related (Fig. 15.2). At present, two types of inflammatory pseudotumors, fibrohistiocytic and lymphoplasmacytic, have been proposed. The latter is thought to be representative of IgG4-RD [13, 14].

As mentioned above, most IgG4-SC cases accompany IgG4-related AIP, but rare cases without the involvement of other organs are encountered. IgG4-SC cases

Fig. 15.1 (continued) inflammation. (**d**) Higher magnification of inflammatory area. Many scattered plasma cells and eosinophils are seen. (**e**) Immunohistochemistry for IgG4. Abundant positive plasma cells are seen. (**f**) Storiform fibrosis and perineural inflammation (*arrow*) are prominent

without pancreatic lesions are surely present. But whether the presence or absence of pancreatic lesions reflects differences in the pathological features of the IgG4 reaction in IgG4-SC or merely reflects differences in the pathological phenotype of systemic IgG4-RD is unclear. The characteristics of IgG4-SC not associated with pancreatic lesions have been described as follows [15, 16]: (1) it mainly affects middle-aged to elderly men; (2) serum IgG4 is normal or only slightly elevated in most cases; (3) cases with IgE and soluble IL-2 receptor elevation and antinuclear antibody-positive status are frequent; (4) affected bile ducts show relatively long and flat narrowing, but peripheral bile duct stenosis is mild; and (5) affected bile ducts show marked $IgG4^+$ plasmacytic cell infiltration. However, cases of IgG4-SC alone are clinically very hard to differentiate from biliary tumor, particularly cholangiocarcinoma. Although the cases of isolated IgG4-SC mainly display hilar biliary strictures, isolated intrapancreatic IgG4-SC is also reported [16]. Of the five cases included in this report, all patients were male, with a mean age of 74.2 years. Bile duct wall thickening in lesions without luminal stenosis was detected using abdominal computed tomography in all the five cases. Interestingly, in three of the cases, serum IgG4 levels were within normal limits. The mean serum IgG4 level measured before surgery was 202.1 mg/dL (four cases). Isolated intrapancreatic IgG4-SC is difficult to diagnose, particularly if the IgG4 level remains normal [15, 17]. Diagnostic criteria for IgG4-SC have been proposed by two groups in Research on Measures for Intractable Diseases supported by a Health Labour Sciences Research Grant in Japan. Characteristic and diagnostically useful histological findings of bile duct tissue specimens include: (1) $IgG4^+$ plasmacytic cell infiltration ($\geq$10/high-power field (hpf); IgG4/IgG positive cell ratio of $\geq$40 %); (2) marked lymphoplasmacytic cell infiltration and fibrosis, without neutrophil infiltration; (3) obliterative phlebitis or swirling fibrosis; and (4) storiform fibrosis. However, identification of these characteristics in small biopsy specimens obtained from the surface of the bile duct is difficult. Alternatively, the diagnostic criteria for AIP the HISORt Criteria proposed by the Mayo Clinic [18] have been applied to the diagnosis of IgG4-SC [19]. These criteria emphasize $IgG4^+$ plasmacytic cell infiltration, although abundant $IgG4^+$ cell infiltration is important in the histology of IgG4-RD. Because the infiltration of $IgG4^+$ cells is of varying degrees in the cases of cholangiocarcinoma described, care must be taken not to be overly influenced by diagnostic criteria that overemphasize $IgG4^+$ cell infiltration in affected organs. Therefore, no single diagnostic criteria should be strictly followed; rather, each individual case should be clinicopathologically diagnosed on the basis of its own individual features.

In the pathogenesis of IgG4-RD including IgG4-SC, the activation of the Th2 immune response has been confirmed by several studies [20–24]. Two regulatory cytokines, IL-10 and transforming growth factor-beta, are also significantly overexpressed in IgG4-RD [20]. IL-10, a regulatory cytokine mainly produced by $Foxp3^+$ regulatory T cells (Treg cells), Th2 cells, and IL-10-producing regulatory T cells, is thought to induce the differentiation of $IgG4^+$ plasma cells and favor B-cell switching to IgG4 in the presence of IL-4 [25–27]. In the presence of this cytokine milieu, the induction of IgG4$^+$ cells and fibrous sclerosing lesions could occur in other diseases and in coexisting inflammatory lesions in addition to IgG4-RD [28].

15.3 Biliary Distribution of IgG4$^+$ Cells in IgG4-SC

In IgG4-SC, numerous IgG4$^+$ cells are found in the affected regions of bile ducts. These cells accompany other characteristic findings such as a predominance of IgG4$^+$ cells among IgG$^+$ cells and a unique pattern of sclerosing fibrosis. In addition, other regions of the biliary tree are affected. Therefore, biopsies from the papilla of Vater to the peripheral intrahepatic small bile ducts, which are relative easily obtained, are useful for diagnosing IgG4-SC.

Inflammation of the papilla of Vater (papillitis) is commonly found in several inflammatory and neoplastic pancreatobiliary diseases. Although duodenitis, including papillitis, is generally thought to be nonspecific in IgG4-SC and AIP, papillitis accompanying IgG4$^+$ plasmacytic cell infiltration is speculated to be an evidence of IgG4-SC and AIP (Fig. 15.3). Moreover, the IgG4$^+$ cell infiltration found in the papilla of Vater in IgG4-SC and AIP is severe compared with that of PSC, pancreatic cancer, and bile duct cancer, but the swelling and magnitude of IgG4$^+$ cell infiltration do not correlate [29].

Moreover, the site of the biliary tree opposite to the affected bile duct is also involved in IgG4-SC. Therefore, a liver needle biopsy obtained from the periphery of the liver is also useful for diagnosing IgG-SC and AIP [8]. Closed pathological examination of partially hepatectomized or autopsied liver specimens reveals an infiltration of IgG4$^+$ cells that are continuously and broadly distributed among intrahepatic bile ducts; IgG4$^+$ cells are scattered in the small portal tracts containing the interlobular and septal bile ducts found in needle liver biopsies (Fig. 15.4). Although intrahepatic small bile ducts as well as large bile ducts may be the target organs of IgG4-SC, the portal inflammation including IgG4$^+$ cells is thought to result from IgG4$^+$ cells spreading along the biliary tree from IgG4-SC lesions in the hepatic hilus.

15.4 IgG4 Hepatopathy

Varying degrees of liver dysfunction are found in 50–70 % of patients with IgG4-related AIP [8, 30]. Clinicopathological studies reveal an intrahepatic IgG4$^+$ cell infiltration of $\geq$5/hpf in approximately 50 % of AIP patients; the degree of infiltration correlates with serum IgG4 values [8, 30]. A correlation is observed between parenchymal inflammation and AST values and between cholestasis and serum bilirubin levels. The hepatic lesions observed in AIP patients are known as IgG4 hepatopathy [8]. Whether the pathogenesis of IgG4-RD, including IgG4-SC, involves an autoimmune response and whether hepatic parenchymal cells such as

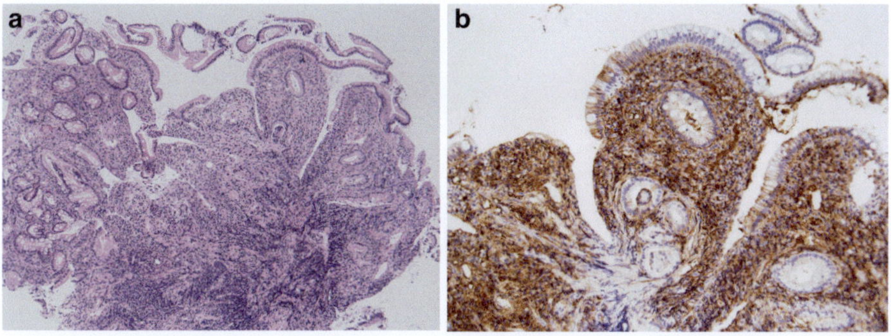

Fig. 15.3 Inflammation of papilla of Vater (papillitis) in IgG4-related sclerosing cholangitis (IgG4-SC) associated with autoimmune pancreatitis (AIP). (**a**) Inflammation is prominent, but differentiating between nonspecific and IgG4-related papillitis is difficult. (**b**) Immunohistochemistry for IgG4 reveals the presence of many IgG4⁺ cells and IgG4 deposition in the stroma and on epithelial cells

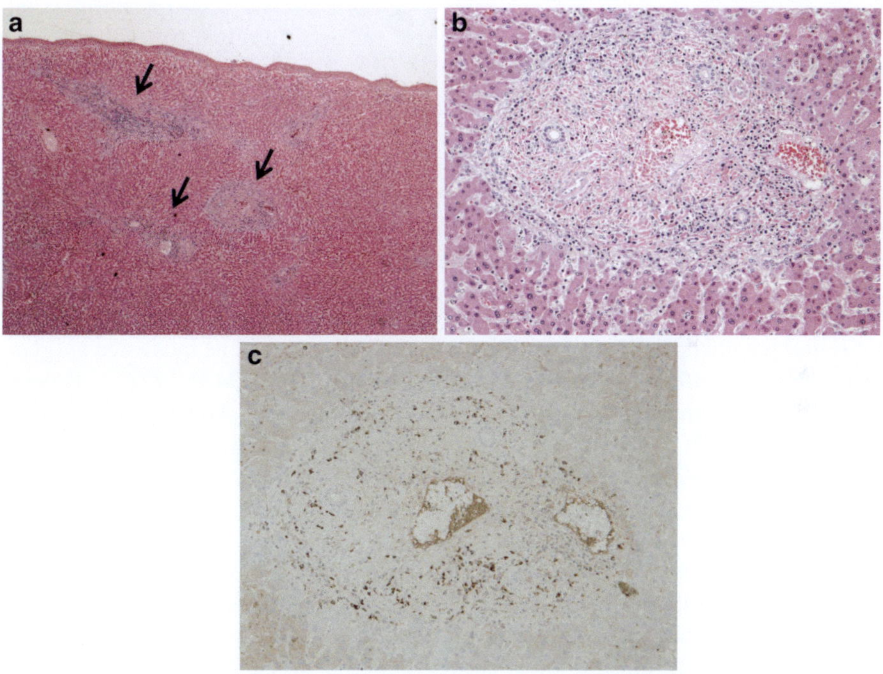

Fig. 15.4 Autopsied live specimens of systemic IgG4-related disease with IgG4-related sclerosing cholangitis. (**a**) In subcapsular area of liver, mild to moderately inflamed portal tracts (*arrows*) are seen. (**b**) Portal tract is mildly sclerotic and a minor scattering of inflammatory cells is seen. (**c**) Immunohistochemistry for IgG4. Many positive cells are found within portal tracts

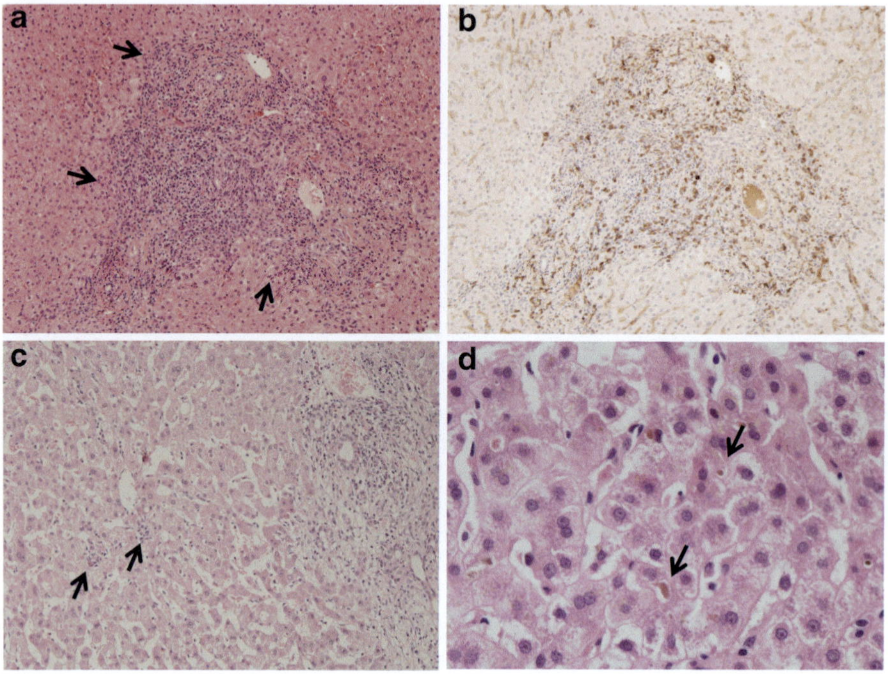

Fig. 15.5 Representative findings of IgG4 hepatopathy. (**a**) Prominent portal inflammation with interface hepatitis (*arrow*). (**b**) Inflamed portal tracts contain many IgG4^{+} cells. Immunohistochemistry for IgG4. (**c**) Lobular hepatitis. Some focal necroses are found (*arrows*). (**d**) Canalicular cholestasis. Bile plugs are found in dilated bile canaliculi (*arrows*)

hepatocytes and cholangiocytes of intrahepatic small bile ducts are target organs of IgG4-RD are unknown. However, the serum IgG4 levels and the incidence of IgG4-bearing cells in affected organs is higher in patients with IgG4-RD than in patients with other autoimmune-mediated liver diseases such as AIH, primary biliary cholangitis (PBC), and PSC [8]. On pathological analysis, liver biopsy specimens from patients with AIP reveal a marked infiltration of inflammatory cells, including IgG4^{+} plasma cells, in small intrahepatic portal tracts [5, 8, 31]. Umemura et al. [8] specifically surveyed the histology of liver biopsies from patients with AIP to clarify the pathogenesis of clinical liver injury, noting five intrahepatic histological patterns: portal inflammation, large bile duct damage, portal sclerosis, lobular hepatitis, and cholestasis (Fig. 15.5). Multiple histological patterns were found to coexist. The portal inflammation pattern consists of an intense infiltration of mononuclear cells containing plasma cells, with or without interface hepatitis. If these intrahepatic findings are isolated in the liver without IgG4-SC, they are presumed to be a liver manifestation of IgG-RD in AIP patients. In contrast, if the histological lesions of IgG4-SC are always present in AIP patients, despite the absence of clinical or radiological findings, all intrahepatic findings identified in AIP patients can be considered secondary to extrahepatic bile duct damage associated with IgG4-SC. Portal inflammation may be involved in IgG4-SC, causing the progression of periductal inflammation along the biliary tracts and the smaller tracts encountered in needle liver biopsies. Moreover, based on our experience of patients with serum IgG4 >1000 mg/dL, interface hepatitis and hepatitis-associated bile duct injury are also found, suggesting a correlation between the severity of inflammation in the affected extrahepatic bile ducts and the degree of inflammatory extension along intrahepatic bile ducts. The pattern of large bile duct damage is characterized by ductular proliferation, neutrophil infiltration, and edematous change in the portal areas. These findings are well known to occur secondarily to stenosis and the obstruction of extrahepatic bile duct, irrespective of any biliary diseases. The portal sclerosis pattern is consistent with dense fibrosis. In general, portal inflammation is scarce in sclerotic portal tracts; however, the sclerotic change may be just a remnant of portal inflammation after the active inflammation subsides, and/or secondary portal tract fibrosis may be associated with sclerosing cholangitis involving the large or extrahepatic bile ducts. The lobular hepatitis pattern may resemble that of viral hepatitis. Pathology reveals a parenchymal inflammation pattern in conjunction with hepatocellular focal necrosis in the parenchyma. Mild parenchymal inflammation is observed in a variety of biliary diseases and is thought to be caused by cholestasis as a nonspecific reactive change. The cholestatic pattern is a canalicular cholestasis found predominantly in the centrilobular area and is consistent with extensive stenosis and obstruction of the affected extrahepatic bile ducts, including intrapancreatic bile ducts. Although the combined findings of parenchymal inflammation (lobular hepatitis) and portal inflammation with an interface hepatitis may indicate a primary liver manifestation [32], all five pathological findings could be explained as secondary to sclerosing cholangitis or obstruction of the extrahepatic biliary tract and may not be specifically related to the histopathogenesis of IgG4-RD.

The liver-related manifestations of IgG4-RD are heterogeneous and not well described within the literature [8, 32, 33]. Whether IgG4 hepatopathy is a primary liver manifestation of systemic IgG4-RD or an excess of $IgG4^{+}$ cells along the biliary tract due to IgG4-SC is unknown. However, IgG4 hepatopathy is an important finding for the diagnosis of IgG4-RD. Diagnosing IgG4-SC in the setting of AIP can be accomplished using the diagnostic criteria for AIP. In cases of IgG4-SC without pancreatic lesions, the presence or absence of IgG4 hepatopathy may be useful to differentiate it from conditions such as PSC and cholangiocarcinoma.

15.5 IgG4-Associated Autoimmune Hepatitis

Elevated serum IgG4 levels have been reported in several patients diagnosed with AIH [6, 7, 34]. IgG4-associated AIH is an identified disease entity characterized by definitive AIH according to the International Autoimmune Hepatitis Group (IAIHG) scoring system [35] and the histopathological features of IgG4-RD. IgG4-associated *de novo* AIH after liver transplantation has also been reported

[36]. In a survey of 60 patients with type 1 AIH, Umemura et al. reported that 2 out of 60 (3.3 %) showed features suggesting IgG4-RD, with elevated serum IgG4 ($\geq$135 mg/dL) and increased IgG4-positive cells in the portal tracts ($\geq$10/hpf); however, liver histology indicated chronic active hepatitis accompanied by liver cell rosette formation, indistinguishable from classic AIH [7]. Bile duct injury and cholestasis found in IgG4 hepatopathy, as mentioned above, were not prominent in these two cases of IgG4-associated AIH [7]. Additionally, Chung et al. [37] reported in a study of 26 AIH patients that AIH can be classified as either IgG4-associated or non-IgG4-associated. IgG4-associated AIH is characterized by higher infiltration of $CD3^+$ T cells, $CD20^+$ B cells, $CD38^+$ plasma cells, and IgG^+ cells as well as $IgG4^+$ cells in the liver. In contrast to classic AIH, these IgG4-associated AIH cases showed a marked response to prednisolone therapy, with improvements in serum IgG4 values, liver function, and liver histology [6, 36, 37]. Some patients developed IgG4-SC during follow-up observation, and others had $IgG4^+$ cell infiltration in both the liver and the gallbladder [6]. The scoring system of the International AIH Group has been widely used to diagnose AIH. Simplified criteria were adopted in 2008 [38], using parameters including autoantibodies, serum IgG values, hepatitis viruses, and pathological hepatic findings of lymphoplasmacytic cell infiltration in the portal tracts, interface hepatitis, hepatocytic rosette formation, and emperipolesis. On the basis of these simplified criteria, most IgG4-associated AIH cases are likely diagnosed as definite AIH. For both AIH diseases, regardless of the presence or absence of prominent $IgG4^+$ cells, immunosuppression with steroids is the mainstay of therapy. Future studies are needed to determine the significance and importance of differentiating between these diseases.

15.6 Overlap Syndrome of IgG4-SC and PBC

PBC mainly affects middle-aged females. Histologically, the interlobular bile ducts are damaged and show characteristic findings of chronic nonsuppurative destructive cholangitis followed by progressive bile duct loss via apoptosis [39–41]. Serologically, the presence of autoantibodies (antimitochondrial antibody (AMA) and anti-M2 antibody) is a specific indicator of PBC. The major proteins recognized by AMA are subunits of the 2-oxo acid dehydrogenase complexes, including the E2 components of the pyruvate dehydrogenase complex (PDC), the 2-oxo-glutarate dehydrogenase complex, the branched-chain 2-oxo acid dehydrogenase complex, and the E3 binding protein (E3BP or Protein X) [42]. The etiopathogenesis of PBC remains speculative, but the cross-reaction of human and bacterial PDC-E2 with AMA and autoreactive T cells in PBC patients suspects the association of molecular mimicry in the pathogenesis of PBC [43–45]. $CD4^+$ helper T cells are essential regulators of immune responses and inflammatory diseases. Immunoreactivity to intra- and extracellular antigens is primarily regulated by two different types of memory $CD4^+$ helper T cells. These Th1 and Th2 cells are principally distinguished by their production of different cytokines as well as their ability to induce either

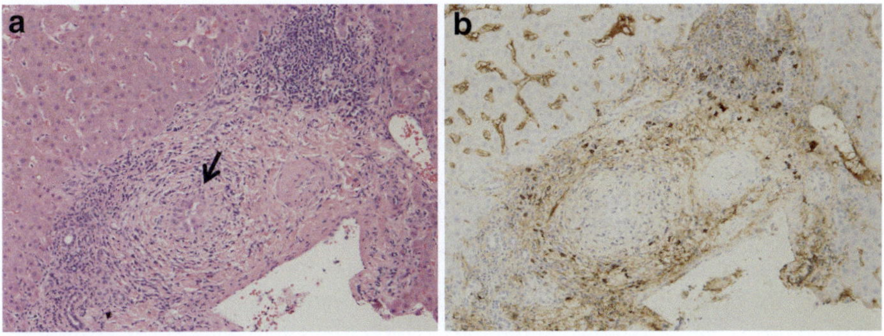

Fig. 15.6 Overlap syndrome of IgG4-related sclerosing cholangitis and primary biliary cholangitis (PBC) in a 61-year-old man. (**a**) In inflamed portal tracts, moderate inflammatory cell infiltrate, and chronic, nonsuppurative destructive cholangitis (CNSDC, *arrow*) are seen. (**b**) Immunohistochemistry for IgG4. Many positive cells are seen. Their distribution is mainly in the peripheral portal tract, but scant cells are located around CNSDC

cellular (Th1) or humoral (Th2) immune reactions. Most studies on the Th1/Th2 balance in liver diseases have been based on the profile of cytokines using peripheral blood lymphocytes or liver tissues; such studies have classified PBC as a Th1-predominant disease [41, 46–48].

Whereas IgG4-SC is associated with systemic IgG4-RD diseases such as AIP, PBC is associated with a variety of autoimmune diseases, irrespective of liver involvement, such as AIH, Sjogren syndrome, rheumatoid arthritis, and Hashimoto's thyroiditis. Although seemingly inconsistent, four cases of concurrent IgG4-RD and PBC have been reported [49–52]. Two of these cases involved PBC and AIP, with elevated serum IgG4 and AMA positivity. One of these cases involved IgG4-SC [49, 50] in a 65-year-old male. In this case, the pathological lesions of PBC and IgG4-SC are speculated to affect the intrahepatic small bile ducts and the large bile ducts of the hepatic hilus, respectively [50]. Moreover, unique overlap cases of isolated IgG4-SC without any other IgG4-RD lesions and of PBC have been reported [51, 52]. Although IgG4-SC and PBC commonly affect older men and middle-aged women, respectively, these overlap cases involved a 61- and a 45-year-old man [51, 52]. Figure 15.6 shows the case of 61-year-old man [52].

With respect to PBC, these patients are not typical, though approximately 15 % of PBC patients are male [53, 54]. Because PBC differs from IgG4-associated AIH as described above, the occurrence of PBC is unlikely to be related to IgG4-RD. In addition, the cytokine milieu differs between PBC (Th1) and IgG4-RD (Th2) [20, 55, 56]. The concomitance of the two diseases associated with opposing cytokine networks is unique. By one interpretation, PBC and IgG4-SC affect bile ducts at different anatomical levels; thus, the peripheral intrahepatic small bile ducts (PBC) and extrahepatic bile ducts (IgG4-SC) are damaged by different mechanisms. However, Li et al. [50] speculate that according to the systemic nature of AIP and PBC, the coexistence of AIP and PBC is not a coincidence. Review of the pathogenesis of both diseases reveals several common features, including genetic susceptibility conferred by HLA-DQB1 [57, 58], dysregulation of cytotoxic T-lymphocyte antigen-4, T-cell-mediated pathogenesis [59, 60], and the involvement of B cells associated with circulating autoantibodies and infiltration of plasma cells [59, 61–63]. The association between the pathogenesis of IgG4-RD and PBC has not been further elucidated. Successful treatment of concomitant disease requires combination therapy with prednisolone for the IgG4-SC and ursodeoxycholic acid for the PBC [51].

Elevated serum IgG subclasses are associated with numerous autoimmune diseases, including primary Sjögren syndrome, systemic sclerosis, systemic lupus erythematosus, and PBC [64]. Serum IgG1 (IgG1/IgG) and/or IgG3 (IgG3/IgG) are significantly increased in these autoimmune diseases, with serum IgG subclass levels presenting distinct patterns in different autoimmune diseases. For IgG4-RD, 6.34 % of patients have serum IgG4 >135 mg/dL, but there are no significant differences in the frequency of elevated serum IgG4 levels between patients and healthy controls. We should reconsider the pathological significance of increased serum IgG4 levels. Further studies of serum IgG subclass distribution will help to elucidate the immunopathogenesis of autoimmune diseases, including IgG4-RD [64].

15.7 Cholangiocarcinoma with Histological IgG4 Positivity

Differentiating between IgG4-SC and cholangiocarcinoma is clinically important but very difficult, even with the use of recent modalities. The infiltration of IgG4$^+$ cells is very characteristic and useful in the diagnosis of IgG4-RD, but histological IgG4 positivity is found in several other inflammatory and neoplastic lesions, including PSC [24, 65]. Moreover, patients with pancreatic adenocarcinoma accompanied by histological IgG4 positivity and/or elevated serum IgG4 levels [66–69] and those with pancreatic and biliary cancers arising from IgG4-RD [68, 70, 71] have been reported. However, a cause-and-effect relationship between histological IgG4 positivity and these cancers has not been demonstrated. Our retrospective survey [72] of 68 surgical specimens from patients with extrahepatic biliary cancers including common bile duct cancers, gallbladder cancer, and cancers of the papilla of Vater reports that ten or more IgG4$^+$ cells/hpf were observed in 37 % of cases. Cases resembling IgG4-RD and having marked infiltration ($\geq$50 IgG4$^+$ cells/hpf) made up 9 % of the total (Fig. 15.7). In contrast, intrahepatic bile ducts and hepatocellular carcinoma mostly lack the prominent IgG4$^+$ cells (unpublished data), although the reason is unknown. IgG4$^+$ cells are found within and around the tumor area, predominantly in the invasive front of the carcinoma tissue. Therefore, the presence of IgG4$^+$ cells is not a histological hallmark of IgG4-RD, and histological IgG4 positivity is speculated to occur nonspecifically in carcinoma tissues [72]. Several cancers involving remarkable infiltration of IgG4$^+$ cells ($\geq$50 cells/hpf) are speculated to originate from precedent IgG4-SC, but data

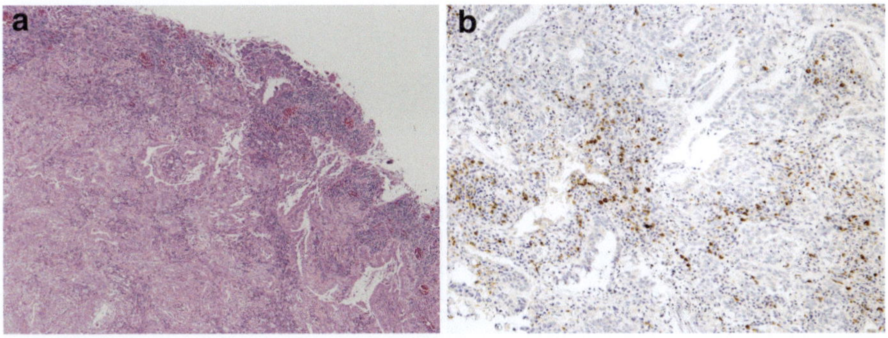

Fig. 15.7 Extrahepatic cholangiocarcinoma. (**a**) Primary carcinoma nest consists of adenocarcinoma with abundant inflammatory cells. (**b**) Immunohistochemistry for IgG4 reveals the presence of many IgG4$^+$ cells within cancer nests

collected before the diagnosis of each cancer is needed to demonstrate the presence of IgG4-SC.

Patients with IgG4-SC are generally older men (85 %) [19], but this male preponderance is not found in histological IgG4 positivity concomitant with cholangiocarcinoma according to our survey [72]. As a histological characteristic of cholangiocarcinoma, irrespective of intra- vs. extrahepatic location, desmoplastic change consisting of fibrosis occurs. However, storiform fibrosis and obliterative phlebitis, other characteristics of IgG4-RD, are not prominent in cholangiocarcinoma. These observations indicate that IgG4-SC and cholangiocarcinoma share features, including increased fibrosis and histological IgG4 positivity, but the pathogenetic mechanisms underlying these features are speculated to differ.

The expression of the Th2-type cytokine milieu and IL-10 produced by Treg cells is assumed to involve IgG4 class switching and/or the progressive proliferation/differentiation of IgG4$^+$ plasma cells [20, 24, 26, 73, 74]. The induction of IgG4$^+$ cells is directly regulated by IL-10 [25]. This known regulatory/inhibitory cytokine plays the main role in the inhibition of the general immune reaction and possibly in IgG4-RD. The clinicopathological significance of histological IgG4 positivity in biliary tract cancers is still unknown, but our studies suggest that IgG4 positivity in cancer reflects the immune escape from cancer immunity [28, 72]. In fact, the degree of IgG4$^+$ infiltration in biliary tract cancers correlates with the degree of CD8$^+$ cytotoxic T-cell invasion into cancer cell layers [72]. Moreover, patients with IgG4-rich tissues in biliary tract cancers have a poor prognosis compared with those having IgG4-poor tissues [72]. Because the cancer cells as well as Treg cells produce IL-10, the cancer cells themselves take part in the IL10-induced milieu [28].

In biliary cancers, IgG4$^+$ cells are not only found in cancer nests but are also scattered in the nonneoplastic biliary mucosa adjacent to the cancerous mucosa [75, 76]. As shown in Fig. 15.8, many IgG4$^+$ cells are found within and peripheral to the invasive regions of submucosal layers. A similar IgG4 positivity is prominent in

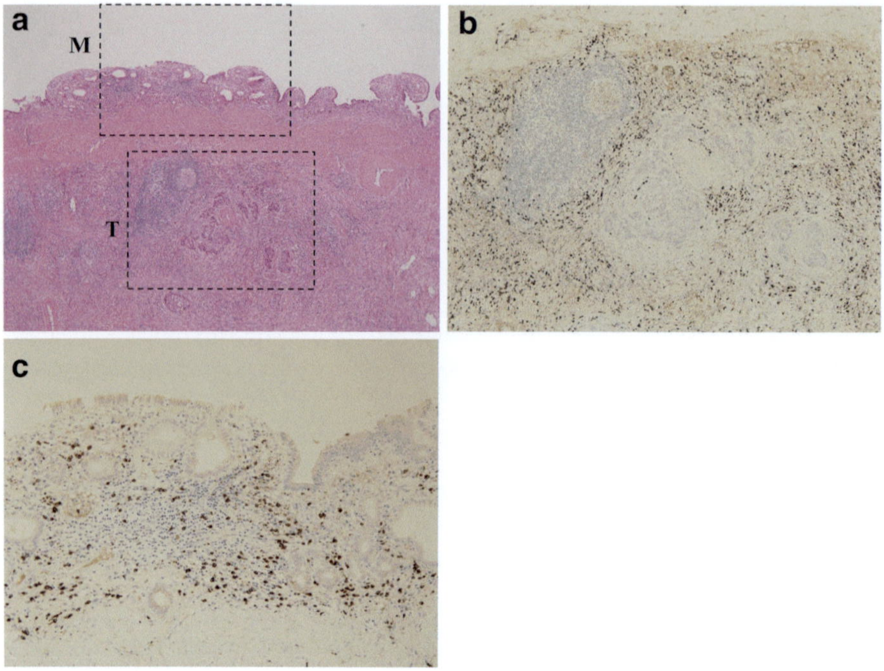

Fig. 15.8 Gallbladder cancer. (**a**) Section adjacent to the primary cancer area, but a cancer nest (*T*) invades the subserosal layer with marked inflammatory cells. Nonneoplastic surface mucosa (*M*) also accompanies inflammation. (**b**, **c**) Immunohistochemistry for IgG4. In the cancerous region (*B*) and the nonneoplastic superficial mucosa (*C*), many IgG4$^+$ cells are intermixed with inflammatory infiltrate

the nonneoplastic mucosa around the primary cancer lesion. Although a biopsy of the bile duct is the best modality for diagnosing cholangiocarcinoma, such examination is unfortunately limited in the superficial biliary mucosa using biopsy specimens. Therefore, if a biopsy specimen is obtained from this IgG4-rich, nonneoplastic biliary mucosa in patients with increased serum IgG4 levels, the condition could be diagnosed as "cholangitis with IgG4$^+$ cells, consistent with IgG4-SC." Another informative case involves that of a 70-year-old male with serum IgG4 of 113 mg/dL, the borderline zone for IgG4-RD. Radiologically, IgG4-SC, PSC, and cholangiocarcinoma of the hepatic hilus were included in the differential diagnosis. Cytologically, no atypical cells were detected in bile specimens. Biopsies of the ampulla of Vater and liver revealed infiltration of numerous IgG4$^+$ cells (Fig. 15.9), consistent with IgG4-SC. However, the biopsy of the stenotic biliary region indicated the presence of adenocarcinoma (cholangiocarcinoma) (Fig. 15.9). The bile duct biopsy from the stenotic region is the cornerstone of differential diagnosis; the pathological diagnosis of cancer is very easy in appropriate specimens. This case emphasizes the importance of using appropriate specimens for pathological diagnosis and understanding the

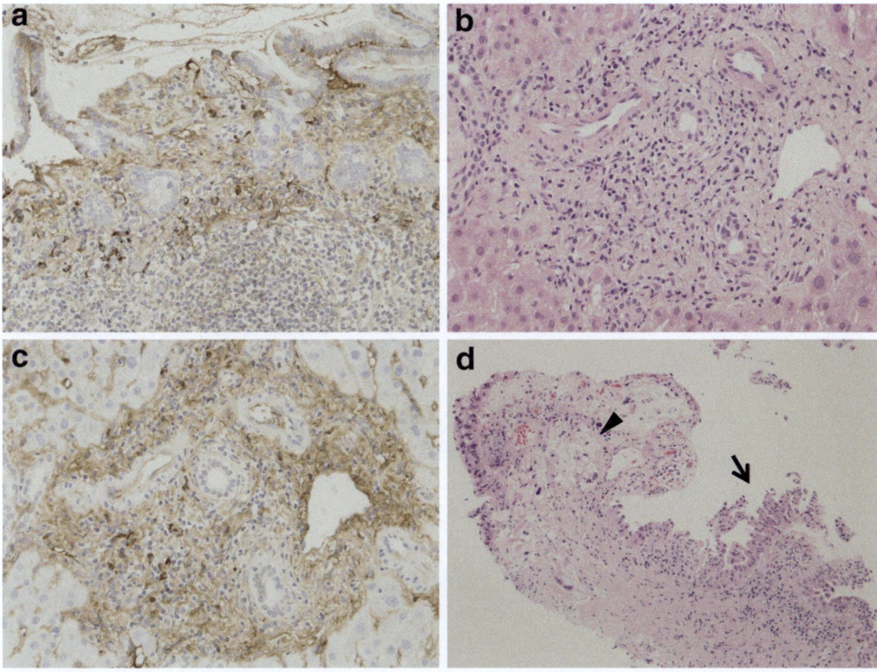

Fig. 15.9 Cholangiocarcinoma of the hepatic hilus accompanying IgG4 positivity in the ampulla of Vater and peripheral liver. (**a**) Biopsy of the ampulla of Vater. Immunohistochemistry for IgG4 demonstrates the presence of several positive cells within papillitis. (**b, c**) Liver needle biopsy. Mild portal inflammation (*b*) and several IgG4$^+$ cells (*c*) are found in peripheral small portal tracts. (**d**) Biopsy from the stenotic large bile duct in the hepatic hilus. Well- (*arrow*) and poorly (*arrowhead*) differentiated adenocarcinomas (cholangiocarcinoma) are present

distribution of IgG4$^+$ cells in cholangiocarcinoma. That is, histological IgG4 positivity is not only localized in and around the primary cancer but also broadly distributed into the distal and proximal regions of the biliary tree. Although few in number, cholangiocarcinoma cases arising from preceding IgG4-SC have been reported [68, 70, 71]; in addition, the precursor lesions of cholangiocarcinoma (BilIN lesions) are often encountered in IgG4-SC (Fig. 15.10) [77]. Therefore, in practice, it is impossible to completely exclude the possibility of cholangiocarcinoma in the diagnosis of IgG4-SC. Elevated serum IgG4 values are an important finding when diagnosing AIP and IgG4-SC but are not sufficient to definitively diagnose IgG4-RD. Rather, a danger lurks that IgG4-RD may be diagnosed or excluded too readily, and serum IgG4 values should not be regarded as more than an adjuvant diagnostic clue.

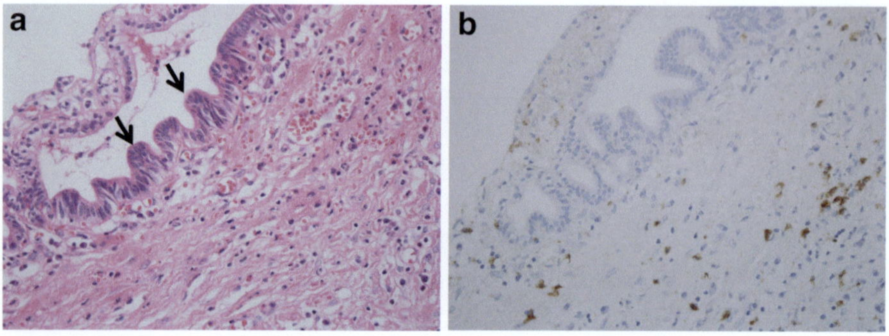

Fig. 15.10 IgG4-related sclerosing cholangitis affecting the common bile duct. (**a**) Biliary intraepithelial neoplasia (BilIN) is found in the preserved biliary epithelium (*arrows*). (**b**) Immunohistochemistry for IgG4. Several positive cells are scattered

15.8 Concluding Remarks

IgG4-RD is a systemic disease that affects most organs. Most patients synchronously or metachronously suffer from multiple organ involvement. AIP is the prototype of IgG4-RD, and extrahepatic biliary tracts, including the gallbladder, are also surely a manifestation of IgG4-RD. However, whether intrahepatic small bile ducts and hepatocytes are direct targets in IgG4-RD is unknown. Moreover, an increase in $IgG4^+$ cells is highly sensitive but not highly specific for IgG4-DR. In contrast, several cases of IgG4-RD with low serum IgG4 levels and/or scant $IgG4^+$ cell infiltration in target organs have also been reported. Although IgG4-related lesions present numerous oddities, further studies will surely resolve these challenges by accumulating more cases and experience.

References

1. Hamano H, Kawa S, Horiuchi A, Unno H, Furuya N, Akamatsu T, Fukushima M, et al. High serum IgG4 concentrations in patients with sclerosing pancreatitis. N Engl J Med. 2001;344:732–8.
2. Umehara H, Okazaki K, Masaki Y, Kawano M, Yamamoto M, Saeki T, Matsui S, et al. Comprehensive diagnostic criteria for IgG4-related disease (IgG4-RD), 2011. Mod Rheumatol. 2012;22:21–30.
3. Stone JH, Zen Y, Deshpande V. IgG4-related disease. N Engl J Med. 2012;366:539–51.
4. Kamisawa T, Zen Y, Pillai S, Stone JH. IgG4-related disease. Lancet. 2015;385:1460–71.
5. Kamisawa T, Funata N, Hayashi Y, Eishi Y, Koike M, Tsuruta K, Okamoto A, et al. A new clinicopathological entity of IgG4-related autoimmune disease. J Gastroenterol. 2003;38:982–4.
6. Umemura T, Zen Y, Hamano H, Ichijo T, Kawa S, Nakanuma Y, Kiyosawa K. IgG4 associated autoimmune hepatitis: a differential diagnosis for classical autoimmune hepatitis. Gut. 2007;56:1471–2.

7. Umemura T, Zen Y, Hamano H, Joshita S, Ichijo T, Yoshizawa K, Kiyosawa K, et al. Clinical significance of immunoglobulin G4-associated autoimmune hepatitis. J Gastroenterol. 2011;46 Suppl 1:48–55.
8. Umemura T, Zen Y, Hamano H, Kawa S, Nakanuma Y, Kiyosawa K. Immunoglobin G4-hepatopathy: association of immunoglobin G4-bearing plasma cells in liver with autoimmune pancreatitis. Hepatology. 2007;46:463–71.
9. Hamano H, Kawa S, Ochi Y, Unno H, Shiba N, Wajiki M, Nakazawa K, et al. Hydronephrosis associated with retroperitoneal fibrosis and sclerosing pancreatitis. Lancet. 2002;359:1403–4.
10. Zen Y, Nakanuma Y. IgG4-related disease: a cross-sectional study of 114 cases. Am J Surg Pathol. 2010;34:1812–9.
11. Nakanuma Y. A novel approach to biliary tract pathology based on similarities to pancreatic counterparts: is the biliary tract an incomplete pancreas? Pathol Int. 2010;60:419–29.
12. Nonomura A, Minato H, Shimizu K, Kadoya M, Matsui O. Hepatic hilar inflammatory pseudotumor mimicking cholangiocarcinoma with cholangitis and phlebitis – a variant of primary sclerosing cholangitis? Pathol Res Pract. 1997;193:519–25; discussion 526.
13. Zen Y, Fujii T, Sato Y, Masuda S, Nakanuma Y. Pathological classification of hepatic inflammatory pseudotumor with respect to IgG4-related disease. Mod Pathol. 2007;20:884–94.
14. Ahn KS, Kang KJ, Kim YH, Lim TJ, Jung HR, Kang YN, Kwon JH. Inflammatory pseudotumors mimicking intrahepatic cholangiocarcinoma of the liver; IgG4-positivity and its clinical significance. J Hepatobiliary Pancreat Sci. 2012;19:405–12.
15. Hamano H, Kawa S, Uehara T, Ochi Y, Takayama M, Komatsu K, Muraki T, et al. Immunoglobulin G4-related lymphoplasmacytic sclerosing cholangitis that mimics infiltrating hilar cholangiocarcinoma: part of a spectrum of autoimmune pancreatitis? Gastrointest Endosc. 2005;62:152–7.
16. Nakazawa T, Ikeda Y, Kawaguchi Y, Kitagawa H, Takada H, Takeda Y, Makino I, et al. Isolated intrapancreatic IgG4-related sclerosing cholangitis. World J Gastroenterol. 2015;21:1334–43.
17. Hayashi K, Nakazawa T, Ohara H, Ando T, Takada H, Tanaka H, Sasaki M, et al. Autoimmune sclerosing cholangiopancreatitis with little pancreatic involvements by imaging findings. Hepatogastroenterology. 2007;54:2146–51.
18. Chari ST, Smyrk TC, Levy MJ, Topazian MD, Takahashi N, Zhang L, Clain JE, et al. Diagnosis of autoimmune pancreatitis: the Mayo Clinic experience. Clin Gastroenterol Hepatol. 2006;4:1010–6; quiz 1934.
19. Ghazale A, Chari ST, Zhang L, Smyrk TC, Takahashi N, Levy MJ, Topazian MD, et al. Immunoglobulin G4-associated cholangitis: clinical profile and response to therapy. Gastroenterology. 2008;134:706–15.
20. Zen Y, Fujii T, Harada K, Kawano M, Yamada K, Takahira M, Nakanuma Y. Th2 and regulatory immune reactions are increased in immunoglobin G4-related sclerosing pancreatitis and cholangitis. Hepatology. 2007;45:1538–46.
21. Akitake R, Watanabe T, Zaima C, Uza N, Ida H, Tada S, Nishida N, et al. Possible involvement of T helper type 2 responses to Toll-like receptor ligands in IgG4-related sclerosing disease. Gut. 2010;59:542–5.
22. Suzuki K, Tamaru J, Okuyama A, Kameda H, Amano K, Nagasawa H, Nishi E, et al. IgG4-positive multi-organ lymphoproliferative syndrome manifesting as chronic symmetrical sclerosing dacryo-sialadenitis with subsequent secondary portal hypertension and remarkable IgG4-linked IL-4 elevation. Rheumatology (Oxford). 2010;49:1789–91.
23. Miyake K, Moriyama M, Aizawa K, Nagano S, Inoue Y, Sadanaga A, Nakashima H, et al. Peripheral CD4+ T cells showing a Th2 phenotype in a patient with Mikulicz's disease associated with lymphadenopathy and pleural effusion. Mod Rheumatol. 2008;18:86–90.
24. Koyabu M, Uchida K, Miyoshi H, Sakaguchi Y, Fukui T, Ikeda H, Takaoka M, et al. Analysis of regulatory T cells and IgG4-positive plasma cells among patients of IgG4-related sclerosing cholangitis and autoimmune liver diseases. J Gastroenterol. 2010;45:732–41.

25. Robinson DS, Larche M, Durham SR. Tregs and allergic disease. J Clin Invest. 2004;114:1389–97.
26. Jeannin P, Lecoanet S, Delneste Y, Gauchat JF, Bonnefoy JY. IgE versus IgG4 production can be differentially regulated by IL-10. J Immunol. 1998;160:3555–61.
27. Koyabu M, Uchida K, Fukata N, Kusuda T, Ikeura T, Sakaguchi Y, Yoshida K, et al. Primary sclerosing cholangitis with elevated serum IgG4 levels and/or infiltration of abundant IgG4-positive plasma cells. J Gastroenterol. 2010;45:122–9.
28. Harada K, Shimoda S, Kimura Y, Sato Y, Ikeda H, Igarashi S, Ren XS, et al. Significance of immunoglobulin G4 (IgG4)-positive cells in extrahepatic cholangiocarcinoma: molecular mechanism of IgG4 reaction in cancer tissue. Hepatology. 2012;56:157–64.
29. Kawakami H, Zen Y, Kuwatani M, Eto K, Haba S, Yamato H, Shinada K, et al. IgG4-related sclerosing cholangitis and autoimmune pancreatitis: histological assessment of biopsies from Vater's ampulla and the bile duct. J Gastroenterol Hepatol. 2010;25:1648–55.
30. Kawa S, Hamano H, Kiyosawa K. Pancreatitis. St. Louis: Elsevier; 2006.
31. Hirano K, Shiratori Y, Komatsu Y, Yamamoto N, Sasahira N, Toda N, Isayama H, et al. Involvement of the biliary system in autoimmune pancreatitis: a follow-up study. Clin Gastroenterol Hepatol. 2003;1:453–64.
32. Joshi D, Webster GJ. Letter: IgG4-hepatopathy and IgG4-associated autoimmune hepatitis--authors' reply. Aliment Pharmacol Ther. 2015;41:327.
33. Perricone G. Hepatic involvement in IgG4-related disease: IgG4-hepatopathy and IgG4-autoimmune hepatitis. Autoimmun Rev. 2015;14:268.
34. Umemura T, Zen Y, Nakanuma Y, Kiyosawa K. Another case of autoimmune hepatitis. Hepatology. 2010;52:389–90.
35. Alvarez F, Berg PA, Bianchi FB, Bianchi L, Burroughs AK, Cancado EL, Chapman RW, et al. International Autoimmune Hepatitis Group Report: review of criteria for diagnosis of autoimmune hepatitis. J Hepatol. 1999;31:929–38.
36. Zhao XY, Rakhda MI, Wang TI, Jia JD. Immunoglobulin G4-associated de novo autoimmune hepatitis after liver transplantation for chronic hepatitis B- and C-related cirrhosis and hepatocellular carcinoma: a case report with literature review. Transplant Proc. 2013;45:824–7.
37. Chung H, Watanabe T, Kudo M, Maenishi O, Wakatsuki Y, Chiba T. Identification and characterization of IgG4-associated autoimmune hepatitis. Liver Int. 2010;30:222–31.
38. Hennes EM, Zeniya M, Czaja AJ, Pares A, Dalekos GN, Krawitt EL, Bittencourt PL, et al. Simplified criteria for the diagnosis of autoimmune hepatitis. Hepatology. 2008;48:169–76.
39. Nakanuma Y, Ohta G. Histometric and serial section observations of the intrahepatic bile ducts in primary biliary cirrhosis. Gastroenterology. 1979;76:1326–32.
40. Kaplan MM, Gershwin ME. Primary biliary cirrhosis. N Engl J Med. 2005;353:1261–73.
41. Harada K, Ozaki S, Gershwin ME, Nakanuma Y. Enhanced apoptosis relates to bile duct loss in primary biliary cirrhosis. Hepatology. 1997;26:1399–405.
42. Gershwin ME, Mackay IR, Sturgess A, Coppel RL. Identification and specificity of a cDNA encoding the 70 kd mitochondrial antigen recognized in primary biliary cirrhosis. J Immunol. 1987;138:3525–31.
43. Shimoda S, Nakamura M, Ishibashi H, Hayashida K, Niho Y. HLA DRB4 0101-restricted immunodominant T cell autoepitope of pyruvate dehydrogenase complex in primary biliary cirrhosis: evidence of molecular mimicry in human autoimmune diseases. J Exp Med. 1995;181:1835–45.
44. Kita H, Lian ZX, Van de Water J, He XS, Matsumura S, Kaplan M, Luketic V, et al. Identification of HLA-A2-restricted CD8(+) cytotoxic T cell responses in primary biliary cirrhosis: T cell activation is augmented by immune complexes cross-presented by dendritic cells. J Exp Med. 2002;195:113–23.
45. Shimoda S, Ishikawa F, Kamihira T, Komori A, Niiro H, Baba E, Harada K, et al. Autoreactive T-cell responses in primary biliary cirrhosis are proinflammatory whereas those of controls are regulatory. Gastroenterology. 2006;131:606–18.

46. Dienes HP, Lohse AW, Gerken G, Schirmacher P, Gallati H, Lohr HF, Buschenfelde KH M z. Bile duct epithelia as target cells in primary biliary cirrhosis and primary sclerosing cholangitis. Virchows Arch. 1997;431:119–24.
47. Harada K, Isse K, Kamihira T, Shimoda S, Nakanuma Y. Th1 cytokine-induced downregulation of PPARgamma in human biliary cells relates to cholangitis in primary biliary cirrhosis. Hepatology. 2005;41:1329–38.
48. Bertoletti A, D'Elios MM, Boni C, De Carli M, Zignego AL, Durazzo M, Missale G, et al. Different cytokine profiles of intraphepatic T cells in chronic hepatitis B and hepatitis C virus infections. Gastroenterology. 1997;112:193–9.
49. Wiegand J, Neid M, Kaiser T, Wittekind C, Mossner J, Tillmann HL, Schiefke I. Coexistence of autoimmune pancreatitis and primary biliary cirrhosis in a Caucasian patient - a rare cause of cholestasis. Z Gastroenterol. 2006;44:1227–9.
50. Li A, Wang Y, Deng Z. Concurrent autoimmune pancreatitis and primary biliary cirrhosis: a rare case report and literature review. BMC Gastroenterol. 2014;14:10.
51. Naitoh I, Nakazawa T, Hayashi K, Miyabe K, Shimizu S, Kondo H, Yoshida M, et al. A case of IgG4-related sclerosing cholangitis overlapped with primary biliary cirrhosis. Intern Med. 2012;51:1695–9.
52. Takemoto R, Miyake Y, Harada K, Nakanuma Y, Moriya A, Ando M, Hirohata M, et al. Overlap of IgG4-related sclerosing cholangitis and primary biliary cirrhosis. Intern Med. 2014;53:1429–33.
53. Harada K, Hirohara J, Ueno Y, Nakano T, Kakuda Y, Tsubouchi H, Ichida T, et al. Incidence of and risk factors for hepatocellular carcinoma in primary biliary cirrhosis: national data from Japan. Hepatology. 2013;57:1942–9.
54. Harada K, Nakanuma Y. Prevalence and risk factors of hepatocellular carcinoma in Japanese patients with primary biliary cirrhosis. Hepatol Res. 2014;44:133–40.
55. Harada K, Van de Water J, Leung PS, Coppel RL, Nakanuma Y, Gershwin ME. In situ nucleic acid hybridization of pyruvate dehydrogenase complex-E2 in primary biliary cirrhosis: pyruvate dehydrogenase complex-E2 messenger RNA is expressed in hepatocytes but not in biliary epithelium. Hepatology. 1997;25:27–32.
56. Harada K, Tsuneyama K, Yasoshima M, Kanemori Y, Ohta H, Masuda S, Onai N, et al. Type1 and type2 memory T cells imbalance shown by expression of intrahepatic chemokine receptors relates to pathogenesis of primary biliary cirrhosis. Hepatol Res. 2002;24:290–9.
57. Hirschfield GM, Liu X, Xu C, Lu Y, Xie G, Lu Y, Gu X, et al. Primary biliary cirrhosis associated with HLA, IL12A, and IL12RB2 variants. N Engl J Med. 2009;360:2544–55.
58. Kawa S, Ota M, Yoshizawa K, Horiuchi A, Hamano H, Ochi Y, Nakayama K, et al. HLA DRB10405-DQB10401 haplotype is associated with autoimmune pancreatitis in the Japanese population. Gastroenterology. 2002;122:1264–9.
59. Hart PA, Zen Y, Chari ST. Recent advances in autoimmune pancreatitis. Gastroenterology. 2015;149:39–51.
60. Poupon R. Primary biliary cirrhosis: a 2010 update. J Hepatol. 2010;52:745–58.
61. Myers RP, Swain MG, Lee SS, Shaheen AA, Burak KW. B-cell depletion with rituximab in patients with primary biliary cirrhosis refractory to ursodeoxycholic acid. Am J Gastroenterol. 2013;108:933–41.
62. Imam MH, Talwalkar JA, Lindor KD. Clinical management of autoimmune biliary diseases. J Autoimmun. 2013;46:88–96.
63. Takahashi T, Miura T, Nakamura J, Yamada S, Miura T, Yanagi M, Matsuda Y, et al. Plasma cells and the chronic nonsuppurative destructive cholangitis of primary biliary cirrhosis. Hepatology. 2012;55:846–55.
64. Zhang L, Lewis JT, Abraham SC, Smyrk TC, Leung S, Chari ST, Poterucha JJ, et al. IgG4+ plasma cell infiltrates in liver explants with primary sclerosing cholangitis. Am J Surg Pathol. 2010;34:88–94.

65. Deshpande V, Sainani NI, Chung RT, Pratt DS, Mentha G, Rubbia-Brandt L, Lauwers GY. IgG4-associated cholangitis: a comparative histological and immunophenotypic study with primary sclerosing cholangitis on liver biopsy material. Mod Pathol. 2009;22:1287–95.
66. Raina A, Krasinskas AM, Greer JB, Lamb J, Fink E, Moser AJ, Zeh 3rd HJ, et al. Serum immunoglobulin G fraction 4 levels in pancreatic cancer: elevations not associated with autoimmune pancreatitis. Arch Pathol Lab Med. 2008;132:48–53.
67. Ghazale A, Chari ST, Smyrk TC, Levy MJ, Topazian MD, Takahashi N, Clain JE, et al. Value of serum IgG4 in the diagnosis of autoimmune pancreatitis and in distinguishing it from pancreatic cancer. Am J Gastroenterol. 2007;102:1646–53.
68. Kamisawa T, Chen PY, Tu Y, Nakajima H, Egawa N, Tsuruta K, Okamoto A, et al. Pancreatic cancer with a high serum IgG4 concentration. World J Gastroenterol. 2006;12:6225–8.
69. Dhall D, Suriawinata AA, Tang LH, Shia J, Klimstra DS. Use of immunohistochemistry for IgG4 in the distinction of autoimmune pancreatitis from peritumoral pancreatitis. Hum Pathol. 2010;41:643–52.
70. Motosugi U, Ichikawa T, Yamaguchi H, Nakazawa T, Katoh R, Itakura J, Fujii H, et al. Small invasive ductal adenocarcinoma of the pancreas associated with lymphoplasmacytic sclerosing pancreatitis. Pathol Int. 2009;59:744–7.
71. Oh HC, Kim JG, Kim JW, Lee KS, Kim MK, Chi KC, Kim YS, et al. Early bile duct cancer in a background of sclerosing cholangitis and autoimmune pancreatitis. Intern Med. 2008;47:2025–8.
72. Kimura Y, Harada K, Nakanuma Y. Pathologic significance of immunoglobulin G4-positive plasma cells in extrahepatic cholangiocarcinoma. Hum Pathol. 2012;43:2149–56.
73. Nouri-Aria KT, Wachholz PA, Francis JN, Jacobson MR, Walker SM, Wilcock LK, Staple SQ, et al. Grass pollen immunotherapy induces mucosal and peripheral IL-10 responses and blocking IgG activity. J Immunol. 2004;172:3252–9.
74. Okazaki K, Uchida K, Fukui T. Recent advances in autoimmune pancreatitis: concept, diagnosis, and pathogenesis. J Gastroenterol. 2008;43:409–18.
75. Harada K, Nakanuma Y. Cholangiocarcinoma with respect to IgG4 Reaction. Int J Hepatol. 2014;2014:803876.
76. Resheq YJ, Quaas A, von Renteln D, Schramm C, Lohse AW, Luth S. Infiltration of peritumoural but tumour-free parenchyma with IgG4-positive plasma cells in hilar cholangiocarcinoma and pancreatic adenocarcinoma. Dig Liver Dis. 2013;45:859–65.
77. Ohtani H, Ishida H, Ito Y, Yamaguchi T, Koizumi M. Autoimmune pancreatitis and biliary intraepithelial neoplasia of the common bile duct: a case with diagnostically challenging but pathogenetically significant association. Pathol Int. 2011;61:481–5.

Chapter 16
Infectious Diseases (Non-hepatitis Virus Infection) and the Liver

Hiroshi Yotsuyanagi

Abstract Many microorganisms are related to liver injury. Several representative viral diseases are shown and discussed in this chapter. Epstein Barr virus, human cytomegalovirus, herpes simplex virus, herpes zoster virus and human herpesvirus 6 belong to the *genus herpesviridae*. Most of them may cause severe hepatitis in immunocompromised hosts with symptoms. Liver injury is milder in immunocompetent patients. Diagnosis of hepatitis caused by these viruses are based on nucleic acid and serological tests. However, the diagnosis remains unestablished in most viruses. The treatment and prevention are just symptomatic in most occasion. Parvovirus B19 infection causes liver injury with typical eruption and red cell aplasia. Dengue, which belongs to the *genus flaviviridae* and is transmitted by mosquito are also discussed.

Keywords *Genus herpesviridae* • Atypical lymphocytes • Mononucleosis

16.1 Hepatitis by Viruses Belonging to the Genus *Herpesviridae*

There are various kinds of human herpes viruses, most of which infect latently after initial infection. Herpesviruses are characterized as follows: [1] reactivation may occur spontaneously or after immunosuppressive treatment and [2] although infection in infancy and school age is usualy subclinical, infection in adolescence is often symptomatic.

Viruses belonging to the genus *Herpesviridae* have double-stranded DNA that encodes proteins required for viral morphogenesis, replication, and latent infection.

Among human herpesviruses, HHV-4 (human herpesvirus 4, Epstein-Barr virus) and HHV-5 (human herpesvirus 5, human cytomegalovirus) may cause infectious mononucleosis, which is characterized by atypical lymphocytes, lymphadenopathy, and systemic symptoms, on primary infection. Liver dysfunction is noted in most symptomatic patients.

H. Yotsuyanagi (✉)
Department of Infectious Diseases, Internal Medicine, Graduate School of Medicine, University of Tokyo, 7-3-1, Hongo, Bunkyo, Tokyo 113-8655, Japan
e-mail: hyotsu-tky@umin.ac.jp

H. Ohira (ed.), *The Liver in Systemic Diseases*, DOI 10.1007/978-4-431-55790-6_16

16.1.1 Epstein-Barr Virus (EBV) Infection

EBV can attach and enter CD21, which is expressed mainly on B cells but on many kinds of cells including T cells, NK cells, and pharyngeal mucosal epithelial cells. Therefore, primary infection of EBV may occur readily by contact with the family members and close friends [1].

Acute infection with primary infection of the viruses belonging to the genus *Herpesviridae* is called "infectious mononucleosis (IM)," characterized by fever, lymphadenopathy, and atypical lymphocytes in the peripheral blood. As described above, infection occurs mainly in B cells.

In contrast, infection of EBV in T cells and NK cells, which may lead to lymphoproliferative disorder, is called chronic active EB virus infection (CAEBV).

Primary infection of EBV in adolescence occurs in pharyngeal epithelial cells through the kiss, expanding to B cells.

The precise mechanism of liver injury in EBV-associated IM is not clear. However, liver cell injury is presumably induced by a bystander reaction from activated lymphocytes in the sinusoids [2].

Various tumors including Burkitt's lymphoma, nasopharyngeal carcinoma, Hodgkin's disease, and peripheral T-cell lymphoma may be related to chronic EBV infection. Recently, EBV is proposed as a possible regulator of autoimmune diseases including multiple sclerosis and lupus.

16.1.1.1 Route of Infection and Clinical Course

Approximately 90 % of adults have been already infected with EBV and may excrete viruses intermittently from the pharynx. About 15–25 % of healthy adults with past EBV infection excrete EBV. Accordingly, infection occurs from infancy and nearly half of the children are infected by 2 years of age. Infection rate increases with age, until adolescence more than 80 % is infected [3]. Infection from infancy to school age is usually asymptomatic. In contrast, about half of the adolescent cases develop infectious mononucleosis.

Infectious mononucleosis associated with EBV develops fever and pharyngitis/tonsillitis after 4–6 weeks of incubation period. Fever, which often exceeds 38 °C, lasts 1–2 weeks in many cases. Pharyngitis/tonsillitis often accompanies pseudomembrane.

Clinical features of infectious mononucleosis caused by EBV include lymphadenopathy in the cervix and skin eruption. Rash, which appears mainly in trunk and upper limbs, is macular and resembles that observed in measles or rubella. Hepatomegaly and splenomegaly are noted in 80 % and 60 %, respectively. Eyelid edema, which is observed in about 30 % of cases, is specific to EBV-associated IM. Common symptoms and their frequencies are listed in Table 16.1.

Central nervous system diseases (aseptic meningitis, encephalitis, acute hemiplegia, Guillain-Barre syndrome, optic neuritis, cranial nerve palsy, peripheral neuritis, transverse myelitis, acute cerebellar ataxia, lymphoma of the central

Table 16.1 Common symptoms in EBV-associated infectious mononucleosis

Signs and symptoms	Note
General malaise	
Headache	
Fever	Moderate to high grade after appearance of mononucleosis
Tonsillitis	Accompanies white or dirty exudate
Cervical lymph node swelling	Painful and prominent in posterior region
Palatal petechiae	
Periorbital and palpebral edema	Specific to EBV-associated IM
Nausea/vomiting/anorexia	
Hepatosplenomegaly	
Rash	Typically maculopapular or morbilliform

Up-to-date "clinical manifestations and treatment of Epstein-Barr virus infection"

nervous system), myocarditis, and hematological abnormalities (hemolytic anemia, thrombocytopenia, aplastic anemia, B-cell lymphoma) are commonly observed concurrent diseases in EBV-associated infectious mononucleosis.

Liver involvement is characterized by mild elevation of aminotransferases accompanied by elevated lactic dehydrogenase. The liver injury tends to be more severe in older patients. Fulminant hepatitis, which is rarely observed, is also reported [4]. Granulomatous hepatitis is also noted [5]. Chronic hepatitis presumably caused by EBV is also reported [6].

EBV primary infection in the posttransplant setting lacks clinical symptoms in most cases. Posttransplant lymphoproliferative disease is a main problem [7].

16.1.1.2 Laboratory Data and Diagnosis

Peripheral blood test shows an increase of lymphocyte with atypical lymphocytes. Atypical lymphocytes are not infected B lymphocytes but are CD8-positive T cells activated by cytokines produced by CD4 + T cells and NK cells.

For the diagnosis of EB-associated IM, at least 50 % lymphocytosis and 10 % atypical lymphocytosis are necessary.

Liver dysfunction is noted in 80–90 % of EBV-associated IM [8].

Liver dysfunction is most remarkable 1–2 weeks after the onset. ALT sometimes rises over 500 IU/L. Compared with other types of acute hepatitis, EBV-associated hepatitis shows higher levels of LDH. Five to seven percent of patients showed jaundice.

EBV-associated-specific antibody comprises antivirus capsid antigen (VCA), anti-early antigen (EA), and anti-EBV nuclear antigen (EBNA).

Three classes (IgM, IgA, and IgG) of anti-VCA are measurable. IgM anti-VCA is used for the diagnosis of IM. However, IgM anti-VCA may remain negative at the disease onset. IgG anti-VCA is often already seroconverted of even in such a case. IgG anti-VCA is detectable for a long time since disease onset. IgA anti-VCA is detected in specific conditions, such as nasopharyngeal cancer and chronic active

EBV infection. IgG anti-EA is detected earlier than anti-EBNA from the end of the acute phase of IM and turned negative within few months.

Anti-EBNA, which is detected 3–6 weeks after infection, is negative at the onset of IM. Some patients with IM show negative IgM anti-VCA, negative anti-EBNA, and positive IgG anti-VCA. The results should be carefully interpreted because elevation of IgG anti-VCA may be nonspecific.

Heterophile agglutinin antibodies to sheep and horse red cell antibody (monospot) test are used for the definite diagnosis in many countries. The test remains positive for 1 year in about 70 % of the cases.

Polyclonal gammopathy, rheumatoid factors, cold agglutinin, or antinuclear antibody are sometimes detected. Nonspecific elevation of antibodies against several viruses (e.g., cytomegalovirus) is noted, which should be carefully interpreted at diagnosis of EBV-associated IM.

16.1.1.3 Treatment

The efficacy of antiviral treatment (acyclovir or valacyclovir) for the treatment of EBV-associated infectious mononucleosis has not been established yet. Therefore, the treatment of EBV-associated infectious mononucleosis is just symptomatic.

Inadvertent use of ampicillin or amoxicillin may cause drug eruption in more than 90 % of the cases, which warrants careful management of IM.

The symptoms of EBV-associated IM may disappear within a month in 80 % of the adult cases. The symptoms last longer in the rest 20 % but disappear within a few months unless chronic active EBV infection occurs. However, EBV, like other herpesviruses, is not cleared from the body and leads to latent infection. The latent virus may be reactivated under immunosuppressive state, and shedding of EBV into saliva may happen.

As written above, splenomegaly is noted in 60 % of IM. Patients with marked splenomegaly, which is observed occasionally, should refrain from hard exercise for the prevention of splenic rupture.

16.1.2 Human Cytomegalovirus (HCMV) Infection

Human cytomegalovirus (HHV-5) is a double-stranded DNA virus belonging to the *Betaherpesvirinae* subfamily. HCMV can be transmitted only to human.

Epidermal growth factor receptor (EGF-R), platelet-derived growth factor receptor (PDGFR)-α, DC-SIGN, and integrins mediate HCMV attachment, and entry and are regarded as co-receptors. HCMV can infect many kinds of cells including endothelial cells, epithelial cells, smooth muscle cells, fibroblasts, neuronal cells, hepatocytes, trophoblasts, monocytes/macrophages (Mφs), and dendritic cells (DCs) [9].

Also HCMV, mainly viral envelope glycoprotein gB, activates innate immunity via toll-like receptor (TLR)-2 [10].

16.1.2.1 Route of Infection and Clinical Course

HCMV is excreted into various body fluids (saliva, semen, and mucus), urine, and breast milk. Transmission to infants may happen at any time. Most of the infected infants are asymptomatic but excrete large amounts of HCMV into urine and saliva. Therefore, transmission to infants may happen in the nursery.

Women who catch HCMV during pregnancy can transmit HCMV to fetus via the placenta. Congenital CMV infection may cause hearing disturbance and mental retardation. Mothers who are negative for anti-CMV in early stage of pregnancy should be careful not to have CMV during pregnancy.

Improved hygiene and health education decreased the prevalence of anti-CMV among general people to less than 60 %, which shows that more than 40 % of the general public is susceptible to HCMV. Transmission of CMV happens on exposure to body fluid during close contact.

Infectious mononucleosis occurs in 10 % of the exposed people after 20–60 days of incubation period. The symptoms resemble those observed in EBV-associated IM. The frequency of lymphadenopathy and tonsillitis is lower in HCMV-associated IM. On the contrary, the frequency of systemic symptoms such as high fever, headache, and muscle pain is higher in HCMV-associated IM.

Neurological and hematological complications are not common in HCMV-associated IM. Interstitial pneumonitis may be complicated in severe cases.

Lymphocytosis with atypical lymphocytes and elevation of liver enzymes are observed in HCMV-associated IM as well as EBV-associated IM.

After primary HCMV infection, latent infection is maintained in circulating lymphocytes, monocytes, and polymorphonuclear leukocytes. Reactivation usually happens in immunocompromised cases mainly caused by decreased cellular immunity. Extensive and severe infection involving the lung, gastrointestinal tract, retina, nervous system, and liver may happen and be fatal without adequate treatment. Additionally, immunocompetent patients may experience reactivation under severe comorbidities [11].

Liver injury in immunocompetent adults is usually mild. Hepatosplenomegaly and mild to moderate liver dysfunction are noted. Cholestatic syndrome caused by sclerosing cholangitis is observed in patients with HIV.

De novo cytomegalovirus hepatitis after liver transplantation occurs in about two-thirds of the cases, the donor of whom were positive for anti-CMV. CMV hepatitis was mild. Treatment by ganciclovir may eradicate CMV in this setting [12].

16.1.2.2 Laboratory Data and Diagnosis

Diagnosis of HCMV-associated IM is based on serological tests. IgM anti-HCMV is used for the diagnosis of HCMV-associated IM. The results should be carefully interpreted because low-tittered antibody may be nonspecific.

For further assessment, HCMV DNA can be measured by PCR. Moreover, HCMV mRNA in PBMC can be measured by NASBA (nucleic acid sequence-based amplification) test. HCMV antigenemia test, which counts the number of white blood cells positive for HCMV antigen, shows positive results only in immune-compromised patients.

For the diagnosis of HCMV-related hepatitis, histological findings of the liver give useful information. Giant multinucleated cell reaction is often observed with lymphocyte infiltration and hepatocyte necrosis. Hepatocytes and bile duct epithelial cells typically contain large inclusion body in the nucleus which look like "owl's eye."

16.1.2.3 Treatment

HCMV-associated IM is self-limited in immune-competent patients. Treatment of HCMV-associated IM is indicated only in immune-compromised (posttransplantation and HIV-coinfected) patients. For severe cases, mainly immunocompromised ones, antiviral treatment is indicated. Ganciclovir is considered first against CMV [13]. The duration of therapy should be determined by repeated measurements of CMV in the blood. Valganciclovir is expected to have stronger effect.

16.1.3 Herpes Simplex Infection

Herpes simplex viruses, HSV-1 and HSV-2, infect humans via mucosal surfaces or abraded skin and replicate in cells of the epidermis and dermis. Then viral replication continues in the neuronal cells. Latent infection develops in the ganglia, which often reactivate with reappearance of the virus on the surface of the mucosa.

Viremia may be complicated on the spread of the virus. Visceral involvement of HSV is seen in the esophagus, lung, and liver. HSV hepatitis is rare in the immunocompetent adults. HSV hepatitis is mainly reported in immunocompromised hosts [14], pregnant women [15], neonates [16].

More than 80 % of neonatal HSV infection is caused by mother-to-infant transmission on delivery. Eighty percent of neonatal HSV cases are attributed to HSV-2 infection. Nearly 25 % of the neonatal HSV infection is classified as disseminated form. Hepatitis occurs with multiorgan involvement and usually carries a high mortality rate for lack of immunity [17] Therefore, starting antivirals early in the disease is essential [18].

HSV hepatitis in pregnant women is seen in the third trimester of pregnancy. Preeclampsia/HELLP syndrome, acute fatty liver of pregnancy (AFLP), and cholestasis of pregnancy are to be ruled out because prompt delivery is indicated for the treatment of these diseases. Because of impaired immunity, the primary infection of HSV may be disseminated and may present as fulminant hepatitis [15]. Abdominal tenderness may also be noted. Lack of specific signs and symptoms may make early diagnosis difficult but important because initiation of antiviral therapy may save the life of patient and fetus [19].

HSV hepatitis in the posttransplant setting might cause fulminant hepatitis but needs further evidence [20].

Liver biopsy in the immunocompromised cases discloses extensive hemorrhagic necrosis with mild inflammatory cells. Intranuclear inclusion body called "Cowdry type A" is often observed [19].

HSV can cause hepatitis even in immunocompetent patients. Slight elevation of aminotransferase levels may be present in 14 % of healthy adults with acute genital infection [21]. Fulminant hepatitis was reported and associated with a favorable outcome after antiviral therapy [22].

16.1.4 Varicella-Zoster Infection

Varicella-Zoster virus (VZV) enters and replicates in epithelial cells in the upper respiratory tract on primary infection. The infected virus spreads to the local lymphoid tissues. The infected lymphocytes transport VZV to the skin, which causes viremic state [23] occurring 4–6 days after infection. Dissemination of VZV to other organs, such as the liver, spleen, and sensory ganglia, may be complicated. Virions simultaneously reached sensory nerve cells in ganglia and cause latent infection [24].

When viral replication is reactivated, VZV reaches the skin via anterograde axonal transport to cause the symptoms of zoster, which is characterized by a vesicular rash in the dermatome that is innervated by the affected ganglion. In immunocompromised persons, zoster may disseminate, causing generalized skin lesions and central nervous system, pulmonary, and hepatic involvement.

Primary varicella in posttransplant patients and patients with malignant disease may be disseminated leading to fulminant hepatitis [25–28].

Reactivation of VSV after liver transplantation was reported. Antiviral treatment was effective [29].

Mild and transient liver enzyme abnormalities can occur in up to 25 % of children with varicella [30].

Reactivation of VZV in immunocompetent adults usually runs a mild course. However, severe case involving liver was reported [31, 32].

16.1.5 Human Herpesvirus 6 (HHV-6) Infection

Human herpesvirus 6 (HHV-6) is a lymphotropic virus that mainly infects CD4+ lymphocytes. More than 90 % of humans catch HHV-6 by the age of 2 [33]. HHV-6 persists lifelong like other herpesviruses and sheds from saliva, which is a main transmission route. Children who catch HHV-6 before age 2 may suffer exanthema subitum, and those who catch after age of 2 may suffer mononucleosis syndromes. Although liver involvement is considered rare in infants and immunocompetent adults, severe hepatitis cases have been reported [34–37].

HHV-6 hepatitis is often complicated in immunocompromised patients. Liver transplantation recipients may have mild to severe hepatitis. They may have pneumonitis, syncytial giant-cell hepatitis, and disseminated disease. The presence of confluent periportal necrosis on liver graft biopsy suggests HHV-6-induced graft hepatitis and should be considered for antiviral treatment [38, 39].

Reactivation of virus after transplantation occurs in one-third of organ and one-half of bone marrow recipients within 4 weeks of transplantation. High intrahepatic HHV-6 virus loads may be associated with decreased graft survival [40].

16.2 Hepatitis Caused by Other Viruses

16.2.1 Human Parvovirus B19 Infection

Human parvovirus B19 (HPV-B19) is a single-stranded DNA virus that can induce erythema infectiosum. However, many adult patients show subclinical course and result in long memory. Cryptogenic hepatitis caused by HPV-B19 was reported more than 10 years ago [41], which suggests liver enzymes might be rarely complicated.

Infection of HPV-B19 was most often reported as acute hepatitis [42]. Many adult cases have been reported. Some cases, many of which were immunocompetent, showed mild liver injury. On the contrary, fulminant hepatitis was reported in children or immunocompromised adults [43, 44].

16.2.2 Dengue

Dengue virus (DENV) is the most common arbovirus infection. Dengue virus is a single-stranded, enveloped RNA flavivirus, containing antigens that cross-react with yellow fever virus, West Nile virus, and Japanese encephalitis virus. The genome structure of dengue virus is similar to hepatitis C virus.

Dengue fever (DF) accompanies ocular pain, muscle or joint pains, headache, and cutaneous rash. Dengue hemorrhagic fever (DHF) is a severe form of DF, which is characterized by thrombocytopenia, bleeding tendency, and plasma leakage. DHF with systemic circulatory failure is called as dengue shock syndrome (DSS).

Hepatocytes and Kupffer cells may be prime targets for dengue virus infection [45, 46]. Although the precise mechanisms of the DENV are not clarified, high levels of viremia facilitate DENV to attach and infect hepatocytes via heparin sulfates and dendritic cell-specific intercellular adhesion molecule-3-grabbing non-integrin [47]. DENV causes liver injury by direct viral toxicity or dysregulated immunologic injury in response to the virus.

Elevation of liver enzyme is observed in 80–90 % of the cases [48]. Abnormal liver tests are generally present in the first days of clinical infection and peak during the second week of illness [49]. In some cases, elevation of AST is more prominent than that of ALT, which suggests that damaged muscle is the origin of elevated enzymes.

The degree of liver enzyme elevation is variable, from mild, asymptomatic liver enzyme elevation to liver failure. The majority of liver failure cases are children [50]. Acute liver failure is seen more frequently among DF than DHF patients. Higher levels of viremia are associated with more severe liver damage [51].

References

1. Cohen JI. Epstein-Barr virus infection. N Engl J Med. 2000;343:481–92.
2. Dienes HP, Drebber U. Pathology of immune-mediated liver injury. Dig Dis. 2010; 28:57–62. Drebber U et al. The role of Epstein-Barr virus in acute and chronic hepatitis. J Hepatol. 2006; 44: 879–885.
3. Takeuchi K, Tanaka-Taya K, Kazuyama Y, Ito YM, Hashimoto S, Fukayama M, Mori S. Prevalence of Epstein-Barr virus in Japan: trends and future prediction. Pathol Int. 2006;56:112–6.
4. Papatheodoridis GV, Delladetsima JK, Kavallierou L, Kapranos N, Tassopoulos NC. Fulminant hepatitis due to Epstein-Barr virus infection. J Hepatol. 1995;23:348–50.
5. Harrington P, Gutiérrez J, Ramírez-Ronda C, Quinones-Soto R, Bermúdez R, Chaffey J. Granulomatous hepatitis. Rev Infect Dis. 1982;4:638–55.
6. Petrova M, Muhtarova M, Nikolova M, Magaev S, Taskov H, Nikolovska D, Krastev Z. Chronic Epstein-Barr virus-related hepatitis in immunocompetent patients. World J Gastroenterol. 2006;12:5711–6.
7. Smets F, Bodeus M, Goubau P, Reding R, Otte JB, Buts JP, Sokal EM. Characteristics of Epstein-Barr virus primary infection in pediatric liver transplant recipients. J Hepatol. 2000;32:100–4.
8. Kofteridis DP, Koulentaki M, Valachis A, et al. Epstein Barr virus hepatitis. Eur J Intern Med. 2011;22:73–6.
9. Sinzger C, Digel M, Jahn G. Cytomegalovirus cell tropism. Curr Top Microbiol Immunol. 2008;325:63–83.
10. Boehme KW, Guerrero M, Compton T. Human cytomegalovirus envelope glycoproteins B and H are necessary for TLR2 activation in permissive cells. J Immunol. 2006;177 (10):7094–102.
11. von Muller L, Klemm A, Durmus N, Weiss M, Suger-Wiedeck H, Schneider M, Hampl W, Mertens T. Cellular immunity and active human cytomegalovirus infection in patients with septic shock. J Infect Dis. 2007;196:1288–95.
12. Paya CV, Hermans PE, Wiesner RH, Ludwig J, Smith TF, Rakela J, Krom RA. Cytomegalovirus hepatitis in liver transplantation: prospective analysis of 93 consecutive orthotopic liver transplantations. J Infect Dis. 1989;160:752–8.

13. Balfour HJ. Antiviral drugs. N Engl J Med. 1999;340:1255–68.
14. Montalbano M, Slapak-Green GI, Neff GW. Fulminant hepatic failure from herpes simplex virus: post liver transplantation acyclovir therapy and literature review. Transplant Proc. 2005;37:4393–6.
15. Kang AH, Graves CR. Herpes simplex hepatitis in pregnancy: a case report and review of the literature. Obst Gynecol Survey. 1999;54:463–8.
16. Benador N, Mannhardt W, Schranz D, Braegger C, Fan- coni S, Hassam S, et al. Three cases of neonatal herpes simplex virus infection presenting as fulminant hepatitis. Eur J Pediatr. 1990;149:555–9.
17. Whitley RJ. Neonatal herpes simplex virus infections. Presentation and management. J Reprod Med. 1986;31(5 Suppl):426–32.
18. Kimberlin DW, Lin CY, Jacobs RF, Powell DA, Frenkel LM, Gruber WC, Rathore M, Bradley JS, Diaz PS, Kumar M, Arvin AM, Gutierrez K, Shelton M, Weiner LB, Sleasman JW, de Sierra TM, Soong SJ, Kiell J, Lakeman FD, Whitley RJ, National Institute of Allergy and Infectious Diseases Collaborative Antiviral Study Group. Natural history of neonatal herpes simplex virus infections in the acyclovir era. Pediatrics. 2001;108:223–9.
19. Klein NA, Mabie WC, Shaver DC, Latham PS, Adamec TA, Pinstein ML, Riely CA. Herpes simplex virus hepatitis in pregnancy. Two patients successfully treated with acyclovir. Gastroenterology. 1991;100:239–44.
20. Yuasa M, Ishiwata K, Sugio T, Kaji D, Ota H, Tsuji M, Yamamoto H, Yamamoto G, Asano-Mori Y, Uchida N, Izutsu K, Taniguchi S. Herpes simplex virus type 2 fulminant hepatitis after umbilical cord blood transplantation for acute myeloid leukemia. Rinsho Ketsueki. 2014;55:682–6 [Article in Japanese].
21. Minuk G, Nicolle L. Genital herpes and hepatitis in healthy young adults. J Med Virol. 1986;19:269–75.
22. Velasco M, Llamas E, Guijarro-Rojas M, Ruiz-Yague M. Fulminant herpes hepatitis in a healthy adult: a treatable disorder? J Clin Gastroenterol. 1999;28:386–9.
23. Ku CC, et al. Varicella-zoster virus transfer to skin by T cells and modulation of viral replication by epidermal cell interferon-α. J Exp Med. 2004;200:917–25.
24. Gilden DH, et al. Varicella-zoster virus DNA in human sensory ganglia. Nature. 1983;306:478–48.
25. Morishita K, Kodo H, Asano S, Fujii H, Miwa S. Fulminant varicella hepatitis following bone marrow transplantation. JAMA. 1985;253:511.
26. Plisek S, Pliskova L, Bostik V, Prasil P, Laco J, Chlibek R, Vyroubal P, Kosina P, Bostik P. Fulminant hepatitis and death associated with disseminated varicella in an immunocompromised adult from the Czech Republic caused by a wild-type clade 4 varicella-zoster virus strain. J Clin Virol. 2011;50:72–5.
27. Okamoto A, Abe A, Okamoto M, Kobayashi T, Terazawa T, Inaguma Y, Tokuda M, Yanada M, Morishima S, Kanie T, Yamamoto Y, Tsuzuki M, Akatsuka Y, Mizuta S, Yoshikawa T, Emi N. Severe hepatitis associated with varicella zoster virus infection in a patient with diffuse large B cell lymphoma treated with rituximab-CHOP chemotherapy. Int J Hematol. 2012;96:516–20.
28. Alonso EM, Fox AS, Franklin WA, Whitington PF. Post- necrotic cirrhosis following varicella hepatitis in a liver transplant patient. Transplantation. 1990;49:650–3.
29. Yamada N, Sanada Y, Okada N, Wakiya T, Ihara Y, Urahashi T, Mizuta K. Successful rescue of disseminated varicella infection with multiple organ failure in a pediatric living donor liver transplant recipient: a case report and literature review. Virol J. 2015;12:91.
30. Plotkin SA. Clinical and pathogenetic aspects of varicella-zoster. Postgrad Med J. 1985;61 Suppl 4:7–14.
31. Beby-Defaux A, Brabant S, Chatellier D, Bourgoin A, Robert R, Ruckes T, Agius G. Disseminated varicella with multiorgan failure in an immunocompetent adult. J Med Virol. 2009;81:747–9.
32. Petrun B, Williams V, Brice S. Disseminated varicella-zoster virus in an immunocompetent adult. Dermatol Online J. 2015; 21: pii: 13030/qt3cz2x99b.

33. Huang LM, Lee CY, Chen JY, Yang CS, Wang JD, Chang MH, Hsu CY, Kuo PF. Primary human herpesvirus 6 infections in children: a prospective serologic study. J Infect Dis. 1992;165:1163–4.
34. Aita K, Jin Y, Irie H, Takahashi I, Kobori K, Nakasato Y, Kodama H, Yanagawa Y, Yoshikawa T, Shiga J. Are there histopathologic characteristics particular to fulminant hepatic failure caused by human herpesvirus-6 infection? A case report and discussion. Hum Pathol. 2001;32:887–9.
35. Ohashi M, Yoshikawa T, Asonuma K, Iwasaki T, Nishiyama Y, Asano Y, Kimoto Y, Yagi T, Urushihara N, Tanaka N, Baba K. Human herpesvirus 6 fulminant hepatic failure treated by living donor liver transplantation. Pediatr Int. 2004;46:730–2.
36. Härmä M, Höckerstedt K, Lautenschlager I. Human herpesvirus-6 and acute liver failure. Transplantation. 2003;76:536–9.
37. Buyse S, Roque-Afonso AM, Vaghefi P, Gigou M, Dussaix E, Duclos-Vallée JC, Samuel D, Guettier C. Acute hepatitis with periportal confluent necrosis associated with human herpesvirus 6 infection in liver transplant patients. Am J Clin Pathol. 2013;140:403–9.
38. Kuntzen T, Friedrichs N, Fischer HP, Eis-Hübinger AM, Sauerbruch T, Spengler U. Postinfantile giant cell hepatitis with autoimmune features following a human herpesvirus 6-induced adverse drug reaction. Eur J Gastroenterol Hepatol. 2005;17:1131–4.
39. Potenza L, Luppi M, Barozzi P, Rossi G, Cocchi S, Codeluppi M, Pecorari M, Masetti M, Di Benedetto F, Gennari W, Portolani M, Gerunda GE, Lazzarotto T, Landini MP, Schulz TF, Torelli G, Guaraldi G. HHV-6A in syncytial giant-cell hepatitis. N Engl J Med. 2008;359:593–602.
40. Pischke S, Gösling J, Engelmann I, Schlue J, Wölk B, Jäckel E, Meyer-Heithuis C, Lehmann U, Strassburg CP, Barg-Hock H, Becker T, Manns MP, Schulz T, Wedemeyer H, Heim A. High intrahepatic HHV-6 virus loads but neither CMV nor EBV are associated with decreased graft survival after diagnosis of graft hepatitis. J Hepatol. 2012;56:1063–9.
41. Arista S, DeGrazia S, DiMarco V, DiStefano R, Craxı A. Arvovirus B19 and "cryptogenic" chronic hepatitis. J Hepatol. 2003;38:375–6.
42. Bihari C, Rastogi A, Saxena P, Rangegowda D, Chowdhury A, Gupta N, Sarin SK. Parvovirus B19 associated hepatitis. Hepat Res Treat. 2013. http://dx.doi.org/10.1155/2013/472027
43. Langnas AN, Markin RS, Cattral MS, Naides SJ. Parvovirus B19 as a possible causative agent of fulminant liver failure and associated aplastic anemia. Hepatology. 1995;22:1661–5.
44. Sokal EM, Melchior M, Cornu C, et al. Cute parvovirus B19 infection associated with fulminant hepatitis of favourable prognosis in young children. Lancet. 1998;352:1739–41.
45. Marianneau P, Steffan AM, Royer C, Drouet MT, Jaeck D, Kirn A, Deubel V. Infection of primary cultures of human Kupffer cells by Dengue virus: no viral progeny synthesis, but cytokine production is evident. J Virol. 1999;73:5201–6.
46. Thongtan T, Panyim S, Smith DR. Apoptosis in dengue virus infected liver cell lines HepG2 and Hep3B. J Med Virol. 2004;72:436–44.
47. Miller JL, de Wet BJ, Martinez-Pomares L, Radcliffe CM, Dwek RA, Rudd PM, Gordon S. The mannose receptor mediates dengue virus infection of macrophages. PLoS Pathog. 2008;4, e17.
48. Parkash O, Almas A, Jafri SW, Hamid S, Akhtar J, Alishah H. Severity of acute hepatitis and its outcome in patients with dengue fever in a tertiary care hospital Karachi, Pakistan (South Asia). BMC Gastroenterol. 2010;10:43–50.
49. Trung DT, le Thao TT, Hien TT, et al. Liver involvement associated with dengue infection in adults in Vietnam. Am J Trop Med Hyg. 2010;83:774–80.
50. Samanta J, Sharma V. Dengue and its effects on liver. World J Clin Cases. 2015;3:125–31.
51. Thomas L, Verlaeten O, Cabié A, Kaidomar S, Moravie V, Martial J, Najioullah F, Plumelle Y, Fonteau C, Dussart P, Césaire R. Influence of the dengue serotype, previous dengue infection, and plasma viral load on clinical presentation and outcome during a dengue-2 and dengue-4 co-epidemic. Am J Trop Med Hyg. 2008;78:990–8.

Index

H. Ohira (ed.), *The Liver in Systemic Diseases*, DOI 10.1007/978-4-431-55790-6

MIX
Papier aus verantwortungsvollen Quellen
Paper from responsible sources
FSC® C105338

FSC
www.fsc.org

If you have any concerns about our products,
you can contact us on
ProductSafety@springernature.com

In case Publisher is established outside the EU,
the EU authorized representative is:
Springer Nature Customer Service Center GmbH
Europaplatz 3, 69115 Heidelberg, Germany

Printed by Libri Plureos GmbH
in Hamburg, Germany